# ALPHA 1–ANTITRYPSIN DEFICIENCY

# LUNG BIOLOGY IN HEALTH AND DISEASE

*Executive Editor*

**Claude Lenfant**
*Director, National Heart, Lung and Blood Institute*
*National Institutes of Health*
*Bethesda, Maryland*

1. Immunologic and Infectious Reactions in the Lung, *edited by Charles H. Kirkpatrick and Herbert Y. Reynolds*
2. The Biochemical Basis of Pulmonary Function, *edited by Ronald G. Crystal*
3. Bioengineering Aspects of the Lung, *edited by John B. West*
4. Metabolic Functions of the Lung, *edited by Y. S. Bakhle and John R. Vane*
5. Respiratory Defense Mechanisms (in two parts), *edited by Joseph D. Brain, Donald F. Proctor, and Lynne M. Reid*
6. Development of the Lung, *edited by W. Alan Hodson*
7. Lung Water and Solute Exchange, *edited by Norman C. Staub*
8. Extrapulmonary Manifestations of Respiratory Disease, *edited by Eugene Debs Robin*
9. Chronic Obstructive Pulmonary Disease, *edited by Thomas L. Petty*
10. Pathogenesis and Therapy of Lung Cancer, *edited by Curtis C. Harris*
11. Genetic Determinants of Pulmonary Disease, *edited by Stephen D. Litwin*
12. The Lung in the Transition Between Health and Disease, *edited by Peter T. Macklem and Solbert Permutt*
13. Evolution of Respiratory Processes: A Comparative Approach, *edited by Stephen C. Wood and Claude Lenfant*
14. Pulmonary Vascular Diseases, *edited by Kenneth M. Moser*
15. Physiology and Pharmacology of the Airways, *edited by Jay A. Nadel*
16. Diagnostic Techniques in Pulmonary Disease (in two parts), *edited by Marvin A. Sackner*
17. Regulation of Breathing (in two parts), *edited by Thomas F. Hornbein*
18. Occupational Lung Diseases: Research Approaches and Methods, *edited by Hans Weill and Margaret Turner-Warwick*
19. Immunopharmacology of the Lung, *edited by Harold H. Newball*
20. Sarcoidosis and Other Granulomatous Diseases of the Lung, *edited by Barry L. Fanburg*
21. Sleep and Breathing, *edited by Nicholas A. Saunders and Colin E. Sullivan*
22. *Pneumocystis carinii* Pneumonia: Pathogenesis, Diagnosis, and Treatment, *edited by Lowell S. Young*

23. Pulmonary Nuclear Medicine: Techniques in Diagnosis of Lung Disease, *edited by Harold L. Atkins*
24. Acute Respiratory Failure, *edited by Warren M. Zapol and Konrad J. Falke*
25. Gas Mixing and Distribution in the Lung, *edited by Ludwig A. Engel and Manuel Paiva*
26. High-Frequency Ventilation in Intensive Care and During Surgery, *edited by Graziano Carlon and William S. Howland*
27. Pulmonary Development: Transition from Intrauterine to Extrauterine Life, *edited by George H. Nelson*
28. Chronic Obstructive Pulmonary Disease: Second Edition, Revised and Expanded, *edited by Thomas L. Petty*
29. The Thorax (in two parts), *edited by Charis Roussos and Peter T. Macklem*
30. The Pleura in Health and Disease, *edited by Jacques Chrétien, Jean Bignon, and Albert Hirsch*
31. Drug Therapy for Asthma: Research and Clinical Practice, *edited by John W. Jenne and Shirley Murphy*
32. Pulmonary Endothelium in Health and Disease, *edited by Una S. Ryan*
33. The Airways: Neural Control in Health and Disease, *edited by Michael A. Kaliner and Peter J. Barnes*
34. Pathophysiology and Treatment of Inhalation Injuries, *edited by Jacob Loke*
35. Respiratory Function of the Upper Airway, *edited by Oommen P. Mathew and Giuseppe Sant'Ambrogio*
36. Chronic Obstructive Pulmonary Disease: A Behavioral Perspective, *edited by A. John McSweeny and Igor Grant*
37. Biology of Lung Cancer: Diagnosis and Treatment, *edited by Steven T. Rosen, James L. Mulshine, Frank Cuttitta, and Paul G. Abrams*
38. Pulmonary Vascular Physiology and Pathophysiology, *edited by E. Kenneth Weir and John T. Reeves*
39. Comparative Pulmonary Physiology: Current Concepts, *edited by Stephen C. Wood*
40. Respiratory Physiology: An Analytical Approach, *edited by H. K. Chang and Manuel Paiva*
41. Lung Cell Biology, *edited by Donald Massaro*
42. Heart–Lung Interactions in Health and Disease, *edited by Steven M. Scharf and Sharon S. Cassidy*
43. Clinical Epidemiology of Chronic Obstructive Pulmonary Disease, *edited by Michael J. Hensley and Nicholas A. Saunders*
44. Surgical Pathology of Lung Neoplasms, *edited by Alberto M. Marchevsky*
45. The Lung in Rheumatic Diseases, *edited by Grant W. Cannon and Guy A. Zimmerman*
46. Diagnostic Imaging of the Lung, *edited by Charles E. Putman*
47. Models of Lung Disease: Microscopy and Structural Methods, *edited by Joan Gil*

48. Electron Microscopy of the Lung, *edited by Dean E. Schraufnagel*
49. Asthma: Its Pathology and Treatment, *edited by Michael A. Kaliner, Peter J. Barnes, and Carl G. A. Persson*
50. Acute Respiratory Failure: Second Edition, *edited by Warren M. Zapol and Francois Lemaire*
51. Lung Disease in the Tropics, *edited by Om P. Sharma*
52. Exercise: Pulmonary Physiology and Pathophysiology, *edited by Brian J. Whipp and Karlman Wasserman*
53. Developmental Neurobiology of Breathing, *edited by Gabriel G. Haddad and Jay P. Farber*
54. Mediators of Pulmonary Inflammation, *edited by Michael A. Bray and Wayne H. Anderson*
55. The Airway Epithelium, *edited by Stephen G. Farmer and Douglas Hay*
56. Physiological Adaptations in Vertebrates: Respiration, Circulation, and Metabolism, *edited by Stephen C. Wood, Roy E. Weber, Alan R. Hargens, and Ronald W. Millard*
57. The Bronchial Circulation, *edited by John Butler*
58. Lung Cancer Differentiation: Implications for Diagnosis and Treatment, *edited by Samuel D. Bernal and Paul J. Hesketh*
59. Pulmonary Complications of Systemic Disease, *edited by John F. Murray*
60. Lung Vascular Injury: Molecular and Cellular Response, *edited by Arnold Johnson and Thomas J. Ferro*
61. Cytokines of the Lung, *edited by Jason Kelley*
62. The Mast Cell in Health and Disease, *edited by Michael A. Kaliner and Dean D. Metcalfe*
63. Pulmonary Disease in the Elderly Patient, *edited by Donald A. Mahler*
64. Cystic Fibrosis, *edited by Pamela B. Davis*
65. Signal Transduction in Lung Cells, *edited by Jerome S. Brody, David M. Center, and Vsevolod A. Tkachuk*
66. Tuberculosis: A Comprehensive International Approach, *edited by Lee B. Reichman and Earl S. Hershfield*
67. Pharmacology of the Respiratory Tract: Experimental and Clinical Research, *edited by K. Fan Chung and Peter J. Barnes*
68. Prevention of Respiratory Diseases, *edited by Albert Hirsch, Marcel Goldberg, Jean-Pierre Martin, and Roland Masse*
69. *Pneumocystis carinii* Pneumonia: Second Edition, Revised and Expanded, *edited by Peter D. Walzer*
70. Fluid and Solute Transport in the Airspaces of the Lungs, *edited by Richard M. Effros and H. K. Chang*
71. Sleep and Breathing: Second Edition, Revised and Expanded, *edited by Nicholas A. Saunders and Colin E. Sullivan*
72. Airway Secretion: Physiological Bases for the Control of Mucous Hypersecretion, *edited by Tamotsu Takishima and Sanae Shimura*
73. Sarcoidosis and Other Granulomatous Disorders, *edited by D. Geraint James*
74. Epidemiology of Lung Cancer, *edited by Jonathan M. Samet*
75. Pulmonary Embolism, *edited by Mario Morpurgo*

76. Sports and Exercise Medicine, *edited by Stephen C. Wood and Robert C. Roach*
77. Endotoxin and the Lungs, *edited by Kenneth L. Brigham*
78. The Mesothelial Cell and Mesothelioma, *edited by Marie-Claude Jaurand and Jean Bignon*
79. Regulation of Breathing: Second Edition, Revised and Expanded, *edited by Jerome A. Dempsey and Allan I. Pack*
80. Pulmonary Fibrosis, *edited by Sem Hin Phan and Roger S. Thrall*
81. Long-Term Oxygen Therapy: Scientific Basis and Clinical Application, *edited by Walter J. O'Donohue, Jr.*
82. Ventral Brainstem Mechanisms and Control of Respiration and Blood Pressure, *edited by C. Ovid Trouth, Richard M. Millis, Heidrun F. Kiwull-Schöne, and Marianne E. Schläfke*
83. A History of Breathing Physiology, *edited by Donald F. Proctor*
84. Surfactant Therapy for Lung Disease, *edited by Bengt Robertson and H. William Taeusch*
85. The Thorax: Second Edition, Revised and Expanded (in three parts), *edited by Charis Roussos*
86. Severe Asthma: Pathogenesis and Clinical Management, *edited by Stanley J. Szefler and Donald Y. M. Leung*
87. *Mycobacterium avium*–Complex Infection: Progress in Research and Treatment, *edited by Joyce A. Korvick and Constance A. Benson*
88. Alpha 1–Antitrypsin Deficiency: Biology • Pathogenesis • Clinical Manifestations • Therapy, *edited by Ronald G. Crystal*

## ADDITIONAL VOLUMES IN PREPARATION

Respiratory Sensation, *edited by Lewis Adams and Abraham Guz*

Adhesion Molecules and the Lung, *edited by Peter A. Ward and Joseph C. Fantone*

Pulmonary Rehabilitation, *edited by Alfred P. Fishman*

Acute Respiratory Failure in Chronic Obstructive Pulmonary Disease, *edited by Jean-Philippe Derenne, W. A. Whitelaw, and Thomas Similowski*

Environmental Impact on the Airways: From Injury to Repair, *edited by Jacques Chrétien and Daniel Dusser*

Primary Pulmonary Hypertension, *edited by Lewis J. Rubin and Stuart Rich*

Tissue Oxygen Deprivation: From Molecular to Integrated Function, *edited by Gabriel G. Haddad and George Lister*

Inhalation Aerosols: Physical and Biological Basis for Therapy, *edited by Anthony J. Hickey*

# ALPHA 1–ANTITRYPSIN DEFICIENCY

## BIOLOGY • PATHOGENESIS • CLINICAL MANIFESTATIONS • THERAPY


*Edited by*

Ronald G. Crystal

*The New York Hospital–*
*Cornell Medical Center*
*New York, New York*



**Marcel Dekker, Inc.** **New York • Basel • Hong Kong**

ISBN: 0-8247-8848-6

The publisher offers discounts on this book when ordered in bulk quantities. For more information, write to Special Sales/Professional Marketing at the address below.

This book is printed on acid-free paper.



Marcel Dekker, Inc.
270 Madison Avenue, New York, New York 10016

Current printing (last digit):
10 9 8 7 6 5 4 3 2 1

PRINTED IN THE UNITED STATES OF AMERICA

To Janet and Zachary,
whose support over many years has allowed me to focus on
the basic and clinical investigation of lung disease

# INTRODUCTION

> Our ideas are only intellectual instruments which we are to break into phenomena; we must change them when they have served their purpose, as we change a blunt lancet that we have used long enough.
>
> —Claude Bernard

In his book *The Morbid Anatomy of Some of the Most Important Parts of the Human Body*, Matthew Baillie (1793) pointed out that in emphysematous lungs "the air-cells are seen much enlarged beyond their natural size, so as to resemble the air cells of the lung in amphibious animals." A few years later, in *A Treatise on the Diseases of the Chest and on Mediate Auscultation*, Rene Laënnec (1819) also described emphysema as "an anatomical state of hypertrophy of the lungs which go out of the thoracic cavity of the aperture of the mediastinum instead of collapsing."

That the enlargement of the alveoli is, in fact, the result of partial tissue destruction was described later, but it was really the discovery of alpha 1–antitrypsin deficiency by Laurell and Eriksson (1963) and the demonstration of the association between antitrypsin deficiency and emphysema by Eriksson (1965) that revolutionized our thinking about emphysema and brought into focus the concept of proteolysis in the lungs. Since then, an enormous amount of work has been done on alpha 1–antitrypsin, on its deficiency, and on other proteolytic enzymes and their relation to lung and other diseases.

Alpha 1–antitrypsin deficiency is not a very common disease, particularly compared with the garden variety of emphysema. However, it underscores the contribution that genetics makes to chronic obstructive pulmonary disease and the promise that identification of genetic determinants may eventually allow us to pinpoint the individuals who may be adversely affected by environmental influences.

This book provides a retrospective assessment of the observations that have accumulated since the pioneering discovery of Lowell and Eriksson, but it also paves the way for new research. Its editor, Ronald Crystal, has assembled a group of investigators who have devoted years of work to uncovering the structure and function of alpha 1–antitrypsin and the clinical consequences of its deficiency. Although this knowledge has not yet led to a cure for this disease, the ideas put forth will, undoubtedly, be the "intellectual instrument" of tomorrow, as well as the vehicles that will bring us ultimately to a cure.

Twenty years ago, Dr. Crystal's book *The Biochemical Basis of Pulmonary Function* was published as part of this series of monographs. It was a prelude to the concepts of lung biology that have emerged since. This volume will likewise be a stimulus for years to come. I am grateful to Dr. Crystal and to his colleagues for the opportunity to add it to the series Lung Biology in Health and Disease.

**Claude Lenfant, M.D.**
Bethesda, Maryland

# PREFACE

Alpha 1–antitrypsin ($\alpha$1AT) deficiency is a "new" disease, having been discovered only 32 years ago by Laurell and Eriksson in 1963. The tale of $\alpha$1AT deficiency, described in detail in the 25 chapters in this book, is a remarkable story of the power of modern biomedical research to define a clinical entity, unravel the complex pathobiological processes underlying its pathogenesis, and conceive and put into practice a therapy that should prevent the major clinical manifestations of the disorder. As will be apparent to the reader of *Alpha 1–Antitrypsin Deficiency*, this is a disorder that is remarkably well understood in all aspects, from the gene to the patient.

The book is divided into four sections. Part I provides a broad overview of basic and clinical aspects of the disorder, including a review of the 32 years of successful research by many groups of investigators throughout the world. Part II, "Biology and Pathobiology," contains chapters describing the $\alpha$1AT gene and its promoter, the evolution of the $\alpha$1AT gene, its genotypes and phenotypes, the neutrophil elastase (NE) gene and its promoter, the three-dimensional protein structures of $\alpha$1AT and NE, the kinetics of the interactions of $\alpha$1AT and NE, $\alpha$1AT gene expression, and the chemistry and biology of secretory leukoprotease inhibitor, the other major lung antiprotease. Part III, "Clinical Manifestations," comprises chapters summarizing all clinical aspects of $\alpha$1AT deficiency, including laboratory diagnosis, the overall clinical manifestations of the disease, lung function, the associated reactive airway disease, natural history, prevalence, and the National Heart and Lung Institute's national registry for patients with this disorder. Finally, Part IV, "Treatment," details the available therapeutic strategies for treating the lung and liver disease, including intravenous and aerosol augmentation therapy with human antiproteases, attempts at augmenting liver production of α1AT, low-molecular-weight inhibitors of NE, lung and liver transplantation, and demonstration of the feasibility of gene therapy.

α1AT deficiency has been an important focus of the research of my laboratory for more than 17 years. Our interest in this disorder started in 1978 when James Gadek, then a fellow in the National Institute of Allergy and Infectious Diseases at the National Institutes of Health, suggested that Danazol, and impeded androgen that enhances C1-esterase inhibitor levels in hereditary angioedema, might function to enhance serum levels of α1AT. This led to clinical studies on defining the protease-antiprotease imbalance in the lower respiratory tract of normal persons and individuals with α1AT deficiency. Eventually, this led to development of the strategy to use weekly infusions of α1AT purified from human plasma as the therapy for this disorder. Along the way, we carried out a variety of studies of normal and abnormal α1AT genes, α1AT gene expression, cloning and characterization of the NE gene, understanding of the biology of protease and antiprotease function in the human lung, the demonstration of aerosol strategies to deliver protein antiproteases to humans, and finally, the development of strategies for gene therapy of a α1AT deficiency. To all the scientists who joined me on that quest over many years, I am very grateful.

The successful story of the understanding of α1AT deficiency and the development of widely used augmentation therapy to prevent the pulmonary manifestations of this disorder could not have been done without the support of Claude Lenfant, the Director of the National Heart, Lung, and Blood Institute and the Executive Editor of the Marcel Dekker, Inc., series relating to lung disease. He saw the importance of understanding α1AT deficiency as a model for many lung disorders and helped to develop support at the national level for basic and applied studies of this disorder, including establishment of the National Registry for Alpha 1-Antitrypsin Deficiency. On a personal note, his support, over more than 20 years, when I was Chief of the Pulmonary Branch of the Division of Intramural Research of the National Heart, Lung, and Blood Institute, and more recently since my move to The New York Hospital–Cornell Medical Center, has been instrumental to our efforts to understand α1AT deficiency and to develop a treatment for it. I am grateful for the encouragement he has given me over these many years, and for his friendship.

**Ronald G. Crystal**

# CONTRIBUTORS

**Dalila Ali-Hadji, M.Sc.** Department of Molecular and Cellular Biology, Transgene, Strasbourg, France

**Alan F. Barker, M.D.** Associate Professor of Medicine, Department of Pulmonary and Critical Care, Oregon Health Sciences University, Portland, Oregon

**Joseph G. Bieth, Ph.D.** INSERM Research Director, Laboratory of Enzymology, Louis Pasteur University, INSERM U 392, Strasbourg, France

**Wolfram Bode, Ph.D.** Max-Planck-Institut für Biochemie, Martinsried, Germany

**Mark Brantly** Senior Investigator, Pulmonary–Critical Care Medicine Branch, National Heart, Lung, and Blood Institute, National Institutes of Health, Bethesda, Maryland

**A. Sonia Buist, M.D.** Professor of Medicine and Physiology and Head of Pulmonary, and Critical Care Division, Department of Medicine, Oregon Health Sciences University, Portland, Oregon

**David F. Carmichael, Ph.D.** Aerie Consulting Group, Boulder, Colorado

**Joel D. Cooper, M.D.** Joseph C. Bancroft Professor of Surgery and Head, Section of General Thoracic Surgery, Department of Cardiothoracic Surgery, Washington University School of Medicine, and Co-director, Lung Transplantation Program, Barnes Hospital, St. Louis, Missouri

**Ronald G. Crystal, M.D.** Professor of Medicine and Chief, Division of Pulmonary and Critical Care Medicine, The New York Hospital–Cornell Medical Center, New York, New York

**Wilfried Dalemans, Ph.D.** Department of Molecular and Cellular Biology, Transgene, Strasbourg, France

**Ray G. D'Silva, B.S., RPFT** Research Associate, Department of Pulmonary and Critical Care, Oregon Health Sciences University, Portland, Oregon

**Roland M. du Bois, M.D.** Head, Interstitial Lung Disease Unit, Department of Occupational and Environmental Medicine, Royal Brompton Hospital, and National Heart and Lung Institute, London, England

**Richard A. Engh, Ph.D.** Max-Planck-Institut für Biochemie, Martinsried, Germany

**Robert J. Fallat, M.D.** Director of Pulmonary Physiology and Research, Department of Medicine, California Pacific Medical Center, San Francisco, California

**John G. Hay, M.D.** Instructor, Division of Pulmonary and Critical Care Medicine, The New York Hospital–Cornell Medical Center, New York, New York

**Sophie Jallat, Ph.D.** Department of Molecular and Cellular Biology, Transgene, Strasbourg, France

**Gregg Joslin, M.D., Ph.D.** Department of Obstetrics and Gynecology, Washington University School of Medicine, St. Louis, Missouri

**Chih-Min Kam, Ph.D.** Senior Research Scientist, School of Chemistry and Biochemistry, Georgia Institute of Technology, Atlanta, Georgia

**Shiro Kira, M.D., Ph.D.** Professor, Department of Respiratory Medicine, Juntendo University School of Medicine, Tokyo, Japan

**Andrea Mastrangeli, M.D.** Assistant Professor in Medicine, Department of Medicine-Division of Pulmonary and Critical Care, The New York Hospital–Cornell Medical Center, New York, New York

**Noel G. McElvaney, M.D.** Senior Staff Fellow, Pulmonary and Critical Care Medicine Branch, National Heart, Lung, and Blood Institute, Bethesda, Maryland

**Paolo Monaci, M.D.** Group Leader, Department of Biotechnology, Istituto di Richerche di Biologica Molecolare P. Angeletti, Pomezia, Rome, Italy

**Alfredo Nicosia, M.D.** Project Leader, Department of Biotechnology, Istituto di Richerche di Biologica Molecolare P. Angeletti, Pomezia, Rome, Italy

**Toshihiro Nukiwa, M.D., Ph.D.** Professor, Department of Respiratory Oncology and Molecular Medicine, Institute of Development, Aging and Cancer, Tohoku University, Sendai, Japan

**Fumitaka Ogushi, M.D., Ph.D.** Assistant Professor, Third Department of Internal Medicine, Tokushima University School of Medicine, Tokushima, Japan

**Kjell Ohlsson, Ph.D., M.D.** Professor, Department of Surgical Pathophysiology, University of Lund, Lund, and Malmö General Hospital, Malmö, Sweden

**Andrea Pavirani, Ph.D.** Assistant Scientific Director and Department Head, Department of Molecular and Cellular Biology, Transgene, Strasbourg, France

**David H. Perlmutter, M.D.** Professor of Pediatrics, Cell Biology and Physiology, Washington University School of Medicine, St. Louis, Missouri

**Frédéric Perraud, Ph.D.** Department of Molecular and Cellular Biology, Transgene, Strasbourg, France

**R. Richard Plaskon, Ph.D.** Research Scientist, School of Chemistry and Biochemistry, Georgia Institute of Technology, Atlanta, Georgia

**James C. Powers, Ph.D.** Regents' Professor, School of Chemistry and Biochemistry, Georgia Institute of Technology, Atlanta, Georgia

**Kuniaki Seyama, M.D., Ph.D.** Assistant Professor, Department of Respiratory Medicine, Juntendo University School of Medicine, Tokyo, Japan

**Thomas E. Starzl, M.D., Ph.D.** Director of the Pittsburgh Transplantation, Department of Transplantation, University of Pittsburgh Medical Center, Pittsburgh, Pennsylvania

**James K. Stoller, M.D.** Head, Section of Respiratory Therapy, Director, I. H. Page Center for Medical Effectiveness Research, Department of Pulmonary and Critical Care Medicine, Cleveland Clinic Foundation, Cleveland, Ohio

**Motoyoshi Suzuki, M.D.** Visiting Fellow, Division of Pulmonary and Critical Care Medicine, Department of Medicine, The New York Hospital–Cornell Medical Center, New York, New York

**Elbert P. Trulock, M.D.** Associate Professor of Medicine, Washington University School of Medicine, and Medical Director, Lung Transplantation Program, Barnes Hospital, St. Louis, Missouri

**David H. Van Thiel, M.D.** Medical Director of Transplantation, Department of Transplantation, Baptist Medical Center of Oklahoma, Oklahoma City, Oklahoma

**Mark D. Wewers, M.D.** Associate Professor of Medicine, Department of Pulmonary and Critical Care Division, The Ohio State University Hospital, Columbus, Ohio

**Janet Wittes, Ph.D.** President, Statistics Collaborative, Inc., Washington, D.C.

**Margaret C. Wu, Ph.D.** Statistician, Office of Biostatistics Research, National Heart, Lung, and Blood Institute, National Institutes of Health, Bethesda, Maryland

**Kunihiko Yoshimura, M.D., Ph.D.** Assistant Professor, Department of Internal Medicine II, Daisan Hospital, The Jikei University School of Medicine, Tokyo, Japan

# CONTENTS

## Part II: BIOLOGY AND PATHOBIOLOGY

# ALPHA 1–ANTITRYPSIN DEFICIENCY

# Part One

## INTRODUCTION

# 1

# Alpha 1–Antitrypsin Deficiency: An Introduction

**ANDREA MASTRANGELI and RONALD G. CRYSTAL**

The New York Hospital–Cornell Medical Center
New York, New York

## I. Introduction

Alpha 1–antitrypsin (α1AT) deficiency is a common hereditary disorder characterized by a reduction of serum levels of α1AT, emphysema, and liver disease (1–8). The description of α1AT deficiency is an account of the power of modern biomedical research to link human disease to a pathobiological problem, define the pathogenesis of the disease state, and develop therapies to suppress the pathobiological processes and thus treat the disease. It is the purpose of this chapter to provide an overview of the biological and pathological underpinnings of α1AT deficiency and to summarize the clinical manifestations of the disease and its treatment. Details of each of the topics discussed in this chapter can be found in the relevant specific chapters that follow.

α1AT is a 52 kDa molecule synthesized primarily by liver hepatocytes (9–11). The α1AT molecule is abundant in human plasma, with concentrations normally in the 20 to 53 μM range (12,13). Although α1AT diffuses through all organs of the body, its primary function is in the lung parenchyma, where it serves to protect the fragile alveolar tissues from destruction by neutrophil elastase (NE), an omnivorous protease capable of destroying the major structural proteins of the alveolar wall (9,14–16). Mutations of the α1AT gene result in an inability of the gene to direct the synthesis and secretion of normal amounts of α1AT (10,17–19). When the abnormal α1AT gene is inherited from both parents, and the α1AT serum levels are below 11 μM, the amounts of α1AT available to diffuse through the lung are insufficient to protect the alveoli from NE, resulting in progressive lung destruction and emphysema by ages 35 to 50 years (5,18,20). In a small fraction of those affected, the abnormal α1AT accumulates in the hepatocytes and causes neonatal jaundice and/or hepatitis and cirrhosis in children and adults (21–27). Very rarely, α1AT deficiency is associated with relapsing panniculitis (28).

## II. History

The hereditary disorder α1AT deficiency was discovered in 1963 by C.-B. Laurell and S. Eriksson in Malmo, Sweden. The seminal observation was the link of a decrease in the α1-globulin band of protein electrophoretic analysis of human serum and the presence of chronic lung disease in the affected individuals (6–8). It was known that about 90% of the α1-globulin band was a single protein capable of inhibiting the proteolytic enzyme trypsin; hence, the term *alpha 1–antitrypsin deficiency* was used to define the disease state (29,30). Over the next several years, more cases were observed, but it was not until the studies of Gross et al. (31,32) and Janoff et al. (33) that the function of α1AT in the lung was understood. In the mid-1960s, Gross et al. (31,32) showed that emphysema could be induced in experimental animals by introducing papain (a proteolytic enzyme) into the lungs of experimental animals, establishing the concept that an excess proteolysis in the lung leads to lung destruction. Later in the decade, Janoff et al. (33–35) discovered that neutrophils carry and release the potent proteolytic enzyme neutrophil elastase. It was soon recognized that neutrophil elastase was the natural target of α1AT, and thus was likely the proteolytic enzyme that was responsible for the lung destruction in α1AT deficiency.

Through the late 1960s and early 1970s, methods were developed to carefully separate the hereditary α1AT variants in serum on the basis of their electric charge, such that the disease could easily be diagnosed on the basis of measuring serum α1AT levels together with α1AT molecules migrating in abnormal positions on electrophoretic analyses (36). Although partial sequence data of tryptic peptides of abnormal α1AT variants strongly suggested the genetic basis of the disease, it was not until the human α1AT gene was cloned and sequenced by Long et al. (37) and the common Z variant was cloned and sequenced by Nukiwa et al. (38) that the true genetic basis of α1AT deficiency was clearly defined. The pathogenesis of emphysema associated with α1AT deficiency was definitively demonstrated through the work of Gadek et al. (39) showing that the levels of α1AT were decreased in the fluid lining of the lungs of affected individuals, as was the ability of the lung fluid to inhibit neutrophil elastase, the proteolytic enzyme responsible for destruction of the lung parenchyma in α1AT deficiency. Finally, Gadek et al. (40) and Wewers et al. (41) showed that it was possible to administer purified human α1AT into the circulation of α1AT-deficient individuals and raise lung levels of α1AT and augment lung anti-NE defenses. As a result of these studies, a purified preparation of α1AT (Prolastin) is available to treat this disease in the United States and in several European countries.

## III. Nomenclature

Based on an understanding of the pathobiology of α1AT deficiency, it is apparent that *alpha 1–antitrypsin* is a misnomer; i.e., while it is correct that "α1AT" inhibits trypsin, its true target is neutrophil elastase. This fact, together with the realization that α1AT inhibits a number of serine proteases (proteolytic enzymes with serine at the active site), has led some investigators to use the term *alpha 1–antiprotease* or *alpha 1–antiproteinase* in place of *alpha 1– antitrypsin* to reflect the broad inhibitory nature of the α1AT molecule (8,9,29). While these new terms are correct in the biological sense, their use leads to some confusion, because the clinical disorder is broadly referred to as *alpha 1–antitrypsin deficiency*. In this context, most clinical investigators continue to use the term *alpha 1–antitrypsin* to refer to the molecule, with full understanding that it really refers to a broad-spectrum inhibitor of serine proteases.

## IV. Biology

The α1AT gene occupies a 12.2 segment of chromosome 14 at q32.1, and is composed of four coding exons and three untranslated exons in the 5′ region (11, 18,19,37,42). The mRNA for α1AT is 1.6 kb in length in hepatocytes, but in the minor extrahepatocyte sites where the α1AT gene is expressed (such as mononuclear phagocytes), the mRNA transcripts are 1.8 and 2.0 kb (11,43). The sequences 5′ to the α1AT coding exons contain a number of putative transcription regulatory sites, including NFIL-6, HNF-1, HNF-2, C/EBP, SPI, EGRI, NFkB, and AP-1. Consistent with these observations, acute-phase stimuli that up-regulate a variety of serum proteins produced by the liver also up-regulate α1AT serum levels (44,49).

The α1AT molecule is a 394-residue, 52kDa glycoprotein with three asparagine-linked carbohydrate side chains (42,50,51). The carbohydrate side chains are either biantennary or triantennary complex carbohydrates. Approximately 34 mg/kg body weight of α1AT is secreted into the serum daily, and the glycosylated molecule has a serum half-life of 4 to 5 days (52,53). The α1AT molecule is globular, with the active inhibitory site positioned on a protrusion from the surface of the molecule (54). α1AT inhibits NE and other serine proteases by combining the α1AT inhibitory site with the active proteolytic site of the protease (Fig. 1). The attraction of the α1AT and NE molecules is great, with an association constant of $10^7$ $M^{-1}$ $sec^{-1}$ (55). In this regard, should the two molecules come into contact, the attraction is sufficiently great that the NE will be inhibited (9,54,56,57). Once that interaction occurs, the inhibition is "pseudo-irreversible"—the α1AT molecule is clipped (and thus can no longer function) and the NE stays attached to the active site of the clipped α1AT molecule (the complex can come apart, but does so rarely) (14,58,59).

The center of the active site of the α1AT molecule is $Met^{358}$ (54). When the $Met^{358}$ is oxidized to a methione sulfoxide or sulfone, the association rate constant of the inhibition of NE by the α1AT is markedly reduced (60–62). This biological phenomenon has major implications for α1AT deficiency, because neutrophils and alveolar macrophages in the lower respiratory tract can release oxidants that can oxidize the α1AT active site $Met^{358}$ and the lung is constantly exposed to inhaled oxidants (14,63–66). Importantly, cigarette smoke can easily oxidize the $Met^{358}$ in α1AT and render it impotent as an inhibitor of NE (62). This fact is likely

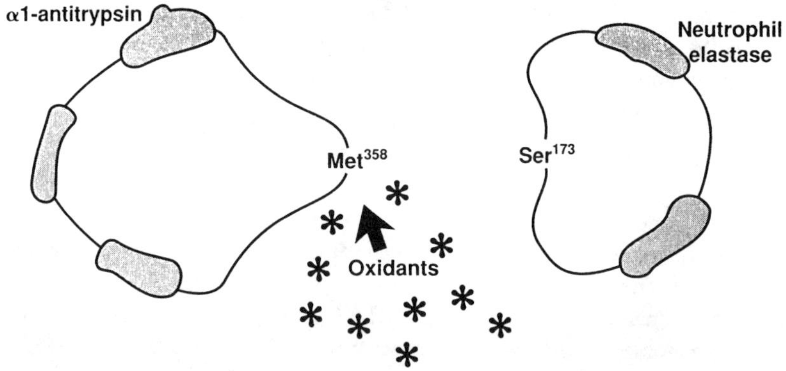


**Figure 1** Inhibition of the neutrophil elastase (NE) molecule by alpha 1–antitrypsin. The α1AT molecule is globular, with its active inhibitory site ($Met^{358}$–$Ser^{359}$) protruding from the opposite end of the molecule from the carbohydrate side chains at asparaginyl residues 46, 83, and 247. The NE enzyme is also globular and is glycosylated at $Asn^{95}$ and $Asn^{144}$. The active site of NE is centered in a pocket that contains the catalytic triad $Ser^{173}$–$His^{41}$–$Asp^{88}$. When NE attacks a protein substrate such as elastin, a portion of this protein is locked into this pocket, triggering the transfer of an electron within the catalytic triad and converting the $Ser^{173}$ into a reactive nucleophile that attacks and cleaves a peptide bond of the target. The cleaved protein is released, allowing NE to attack again. In contrast, when NE interacts with α1AT, the $Met^{358}$–$Ser^{359}$ of α1AT fits into the active-site pocket of NE and the catalytic triad is activated, but the interaction is such that the α1AT-NE complex remains intact, resulting in inhibition of the NE.

responsible for the clinical observation that the large majority of individuals with α1AT who develop clinically apparent emphysema have a history of cigarette smoking; i.e., while α1AT deficiency is a hereditary disorder, the clinical phenotype of emphysema usually results from the combination of inheritance of two abnormal α1AT genes (resulting in reduced amounts of α1AT) plus acquired factors (such as cigarette smoking) interfering with NE inhibitory function of the mutant α1AT molecule.

α1AT will inhibit a broad variety of serine proteases, but only a few of these proteases are relevant to the lung (9,51,67). The most important, by far, is neutrophil elastase, a 29 kDa protease released by activated or effete neutrophils (68,69). NE is synthesized in the promyelocytic stage of neutrophil development in bone marrow and stored in the azurophilic (primary) granules of neutrophils (68). When the neutrophil is activated—for example, when it is attracted to lung tissues by chemoattractants, or when the cell dies—the preformed NE is released into the lung tissue (69). In this context, a very relevant question is: why is it that the lung is destroyed in α1AT deficiency and not other tissues? The most likely explanations relate to three facts: 1) the alveolar structures are among the most fragile tissues of the body and are thus vulnerable to proteolytic attack; 2) there are large numbers of neutrophils that marginate in the pulmonary capillaries, and thus there is a high potential burden of NE in the lung; and 3) the α1AT in the lung is rendered impotent by oxidants, particularly oxidants in cigarette smoke (62).

## V. Pathobiology

The pathobiology of α1AT deficiency is directly related to mutations of the α1AT gene (10,17–19). α1AT deficiency is an autosomal recessive disorder, and thus an abnormal α1AT gene must be inherited from both parents for the clinical disorder to be manifest.

There are at least 20 known α1AT alleles associated with α1AT deficiency, and several different mechanisms by which these mutant alleles cause the deficiency state (Fig. 2). Most of these produce some α1AT protein, but there are a few α1AT mutant alleles for which no α1AT protein can be detected. Normal α1AT serum levels are 20 to 53 μM, and specific α1AT genes are associated with specific ranges of α1AT levels in the serum (12,13). The several normal variants of α1AT genes are all associated with normal serum levels of α1AT; these genes are referred to mostly as M variants because of the middle position of migration of the α1AT variant on isoelectric focusing gels commonly used to identify α1AT phenotypes (70–72). The most common α1AT deficiency variant, referred to as the Z variant because of its electrophoretic mobility, differs from the common normal M1($Val^{213}$) variant by a single base substitution ($Glu^{342} \rightarrow Lys$) (Fig. 2). The Z mutation is responsible for >95% of all α1AT-deficiency alleles (12).

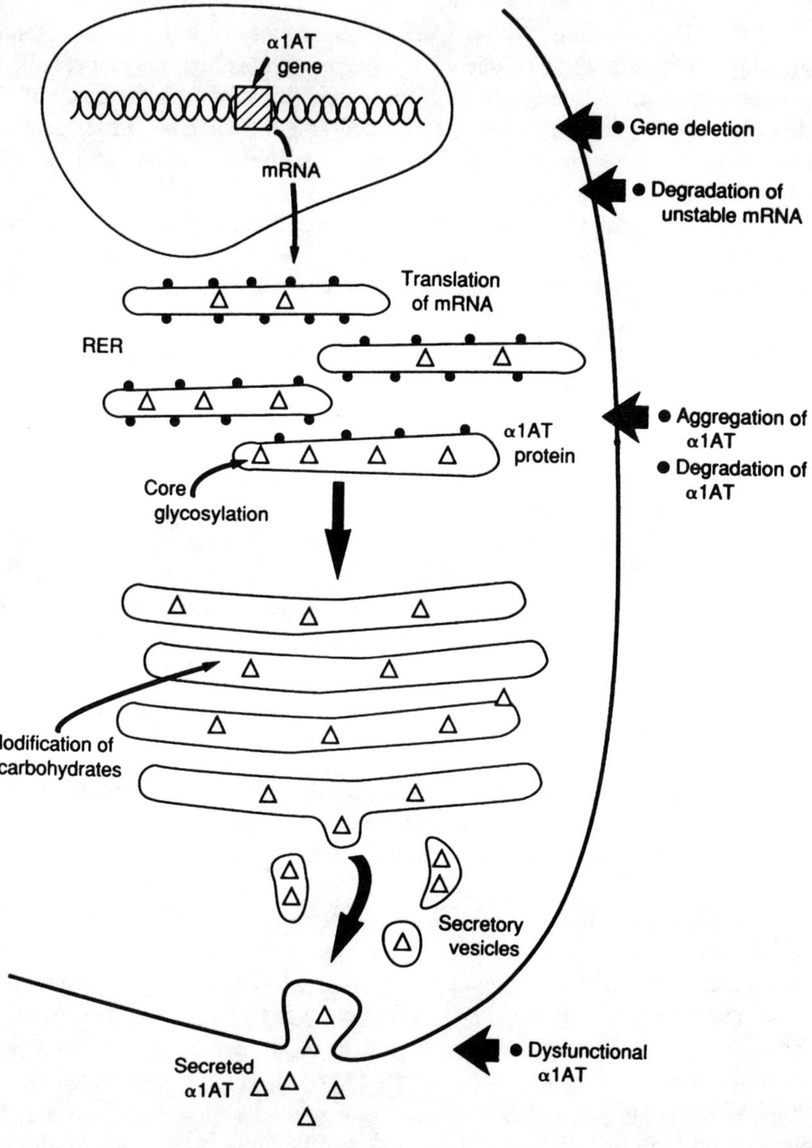


**Figure 2** Pathway of α1-antitrypsin synthesis and secretion showing sites at which mutations of the α1AT gene result in α1AT deficiency. These mutations have consequences at several levels, including gene deletion, degradation of unstable mRNA transcripts, aggregation of α1AT in the rough endoplasmic reticulum (RER), degradation of the α1AT protein prior to translocation to the Golgi complex, and release of dysfunctional α1AT. See Refs. 18 and 19 for details. (From Crystal RG. α1-antitrypsin deficiency. In: Fishman AP, ed. Update: Pulmonary Disease and Disorders. New York: McGraw-Hill, 1992.)

Homozygous inheritance of the Z allele is associated with an average α1AT serum level of 5.8 μM, and a range of 2 to 10.2 μM (73). The Z protein can function as an inhibitor of NE, albeit with a lower association rate constant than the normal M variants (74). However, because of the low concentrations of the Z protein in the serum, and hence in the lung, the alveolar structures are vulnerable to attack by NE.

The pathogenesis of the liver disease associated with α1AT deficiency is not as well understood as the pathogenesis of the lung disease (19). The liver disease occurs in only a small fraction of individuals with α1AT deficiency, and the lung disease and liver disease rarely coexist in the same individual (17,75). Whereas the lung disease can occur in any α1AT-deficiency individual with an α1AT serum level of <11 μM, the liver disease occurs only in association with the Z allele and a few other rare alleles such as $M_{malton}$ (10,17). Histological evaluation of the liver parenchyma in α1AT deficiency of Z homozygotes shows an accumulation of α1AT in the rough endoplasmic reticulum of the hepatocytes, leading to the hypothesis that the liver abnormalities result from the local accumulation of the α1AT molecule (19) (Fig. 3). The mechanism by which the Z molecule accumulates is likely through interaction of hydrophobic residues of the mutant α1AT molecule that are exposed due to changes in the three-dimensional structure secondary to the $Glu^{342}$→Lys substitution (54).

## VI. Clinical Manifestations

The two major clinical manifestations of α1AT deficiency are emphysema and liver disease. The following is an overview of the clinical presentations of these manifestations; for more details regarding each, and the rare manifestation of relapsing panniculitis, detailed reviews are available in this text elsewhere (5,12, 18,75–78).

### A. Lung Disease

The lung disease associated with α1AT deficiency rarely starts before the age of 30 years. It is always characterized by lung destruction, but in 10 to 20% of affected individuals, there is also reactive airways disease (12). There is evidence that only a fraction of individuals with α1AT deficiency develop symptomatic lung disease. There are probably many reasons for this, including the possibility that many of these individuals are not identified as such. However, as discussed above, it is clear that cigarette smoking plays a major role in the pathogenesis of the lung disease associated with α1AT deficiency, with the large majority of identified individuals with α1AT deficiency and clinically symptomatic lung disease having a history of cigarette smoking (18,19,75).

Typically, the symptoms associated with the lung destruction start with dyspnea, usually with exercise (12). This is progressive, evolving into respiratory

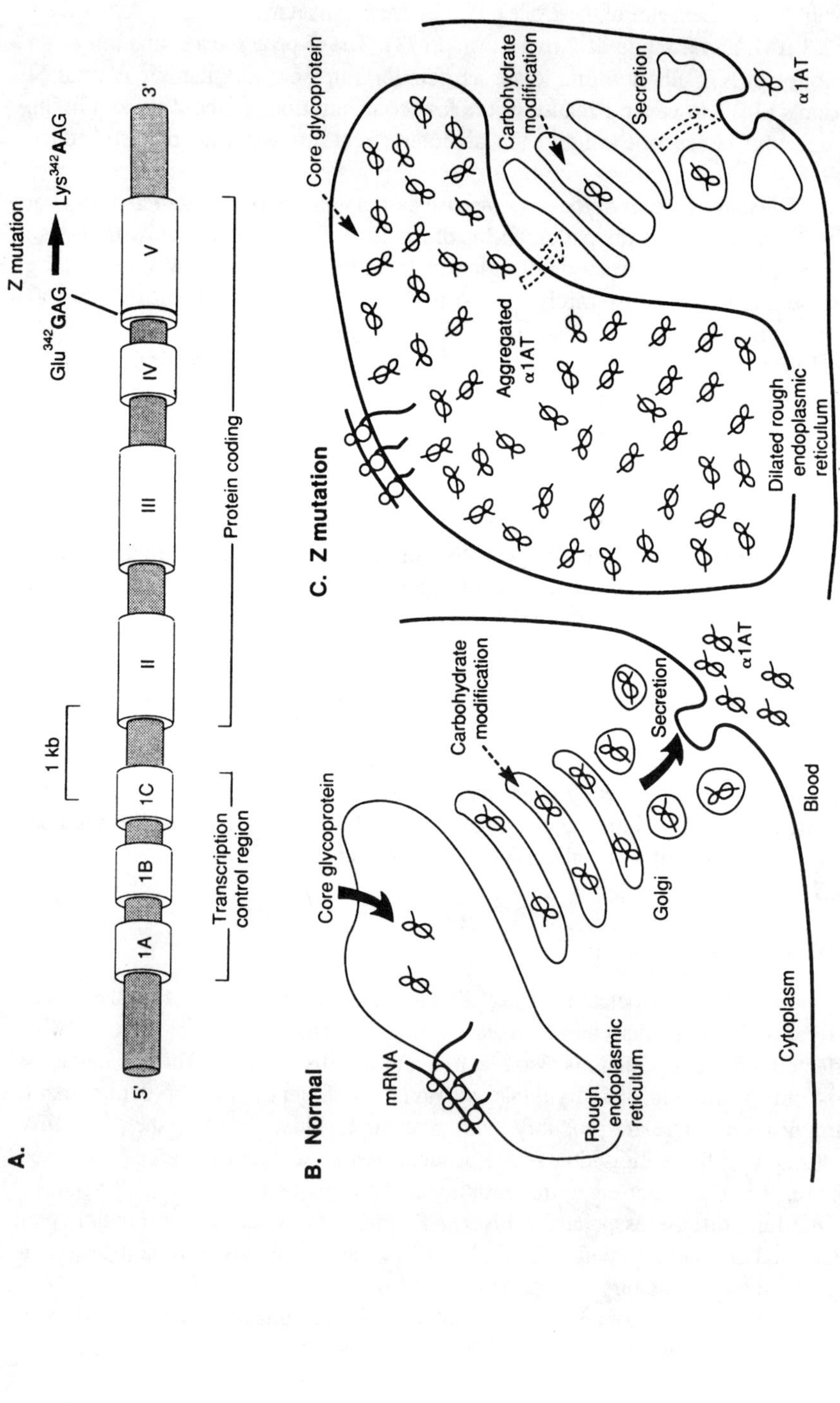
A.
Z mutation
Glu$^{342}$GAG → Lys$^{342}$AAG
5'
3'
1A
1B
1C
II
III
IV
V
1 kb
Transcription control region
Protein coding
B. Normal
mRNA
Core glycoprotein
Rough endoplasmic reticulum
Carbohydrate modification
Golgi
Secretion
α1AT
Cytoplasm
Blood
C. Z mutation
Core glycoprotein
Aggregated α1AT
Dilated rough endoplasmic reticulum
Carbohydrate modification
Secretion
α1AT

Figure 3

insufficiency. The chest roentgenogram shows a loss of vascularity at the bases, increased vascularity in the upper lung zones, flattened diaphragms, and a widened retrosternal air space (12,76). The computerized axial tomography scan is much more sensitive to the emphysema than the conventional chest film, with evidence of lower-lobe lung destruction evident on thin sections even when there is normal lung function (76). A scintigraphic ventilation-perfusion scan shows evidence of destruction of the lower lung zones, with retention of gas in lower lung zones in the washout phase and a loss of capillary bed in the lower zones, and a shift in the perfusion to the upper zones (76,79). Finally, lung-function tests are typical for individuals with emphysema, with a loss in vital capacity, a normal or mildly increased total lung capacity, an increase in the residual volume with an increased residual volume to total lung capacity, a reduced forced expiratory volume in 1 second, a markedly coved flow-volume loop with decease in the flows at all volumes, and a decreased diffusing capacity (12). Typically, the $Po_2$ is mildly reduced at rest, as is the $Pco_2$, with a normal pH. With exercise, the $Po_2$ drops markedly (12).

The subgroup of individuals with α1AT deficiency and reactive airways disease have clinical findings similar to those described above, but have superimposed findings typical of an asthmatic. The pathogenesis of the reactive airways disease is not understood, but the airway obstruction is partially reversible with bronchodilators.

### B. Liver Disease

The liver disease associated with α1AT deficiency occurs in the neonatal period (as obstructive jaundice), later in childhood (as hepatitis and cirrhosis), and in

---

**Figure 3** Mechanisms of the deficiency of alpha 1–antitrypsin in the serum secondary to the common Z mutation of the alpha 1–antitrypsin gene. (A) Schematic of the α1–antitrypsin gene. Shown (5′ to 3′) are exons $I_A$–$I_C$ (part of transcription control region) and exons II–V (the protein coding exons). The common mutation is in exon V. (B) Shown is a hepatocye with the normal pathway of a α1AT transcription, translation, posttranslational modification with core glycosylation in the rough endoplasmic reticulum, carbohydrate modification in the Golgi and secretion of α1AT. (C) The hepatocyte in individuals homozygous for the Z mutation. The Z α1AT molecule is modified with core glycosylation, but then aggregates prior to being translocated to the Golgi. The rough endoplasmic reticulum becomes dilated with the accumulated α1AT. The result is decreased secretion of α1AT, and hence a deficiency of α1AT in the circulation, placing the lung at high risk for destruction by neutrophil elastase. In some individuals, the accumulation of α1AT in the hepatocyte causes liver disease. (From Jennings CA, Crystal RG. In: Gallin JI, Goldstein IM, Snyderman R, eds. Inflammation: Basic Principles and Clinical Correlates. New York: Raven Press, 1992.)

adults (as hepatitis and cirrhosis) (77). The neonatal disease is reversible in about 90% of affected infants, and neonatal jaundice associated with α1AT deficiency is not a necessary precedent of the late-childhood or adult disease. There are also reports of an increased incidence of primary hepatocellular cellular carcinoma in association with the cirrhosis of α1AT deficiency in adults (27,80,81).

### C. Relapsing Panniculitis

A rare form of skin disease, relapsing panniculitis, is clearly associated with α1AT deficiency. The pathogenesis of the disease, and why it occurs so rarely in individuals with the same α1AT genotype, is not known (28,82).

## VII. Therapy

The major focus in treating α1AT deficiency has been on correcting the deficiency state and preventing the lung destruction. There is no specific therapy for the liver disease, and the hepatitis and cirrhosis are treated as if they were idiopathic.

Therapy for the lung disease is focused on augmenting serum α1AT levels or providing an alternative anti-NE inhibitory defense for the alveolar structures. Based on the knowledge that α1AT is an acute-phase reactant, and that serum α1AT levels increased in normal individuals during stress and in females during pregnancy or while on birth-control pills, strategies were developed to assess the possibility of raising serum α1AT levels in Z homozygotes with endotoxin or estrogens. Unfortunately, none of these strategies worked (18,19), nor did attempts to raise serum levels with the testosterone analogs danazol (based on the knowledge that these drugs are useful in treating hereditary angioedema, another hereditary disorder associated with mutations of another serine protease inhibitor gene—C1 esterase inhibitor—expressed in hepatocytes) or tamoxifen (based on the concept that it interacts with estrogen receptors) (49,83). It is not completely understood why strategies to raise the liver production and/or secretion of α1AT do not work, but it likely is related to the mechanisms of accumulation of the Z form of α1AT aggregating in the liver.

The triumph of understanding the biology and pathobiology of α1AT deficiency culminated in the development of a therapy for α1AT deficiency based on augmenting serum levels of α1AT with partially purified human α1AT prepared from the serum of donors (41,84). The studies of Gadek et al. (39) showed that this was feasible, and that lung levels and function of α1AT could be restored with the intravenous administration of 60 mg/kg of human α1AT administered once weekly. This observation was verified in a larger series by Wewers et al. (41) and Hubbard et al. (85), demonstrating that this therapy was safe and the lung anti-NE activity on the epithelial surface of the lower respiratory tract could be restored with intravenous doses of 60 mg/kg once weekly or 240 mg/kg once monthly (85).

The once-weekly form of therapy is approved by the Food and Drug Administration in the United States and by the regulatory agencies in several other countries, and more than 2500 individuals receive this therapy worldwide.

Several alternative approaches have been investigated to augment lung anti-NE levels in α1AT deficiency, including the aerosol administration of purified human α1AT, recombinant α1AT, recombinant secretory leukoprotease inhibitor, and several small molecules with anti-NE activity (62,86,87). Although several of these strategies are rational in the context of the pathobiology of the disease, none is currently available for administration to patients with α1AT deficiency other than in the clinical investigational setting.

The newest strategy to augment the anti-NE protection of the alveoli in α1AT deficiency is gene therapy, in which the human α1AT cDNA is administered in a vector (a viral vector, such as a retrovirus or adenovirus, or nonviral vector, such as a liposome). Studies in experimental animals have shown that this is feasible in experimental animals, particularly with replication-deficient recombinant adenovirus vectors administered to the liver or peritoneum, or directly to the lung (88–90).

## References

1. Morse JO. Alpha$_1$-antitrypsin deficiency. N Engl J Med 1978; 299:1045–1048, 1099–1105.
2. Sharp HL, Bridges RA, Krivit W, Freir EF. Cirrhosis associated with alpha-1 antitrypsin deficiency: a previously unrecognized inherited disorder. J Lab Clin Med 1969; 73:934–939.
3. Kueppers F, Black LF. α1-Antitrypsin and its deficiency. Am Rev Respir Dis 1974; 110:176–194.
4. Carrell RW, Owen MC. α1-Antitrypsin: structure, variation and disease. Essays Med Biochem 1979; 4:83–119.
5. Gadek JE, Crystal RG. α1-antitrypsin deficiency. In: Stanbury JB, Wyngaarden JB, Fredrickson DS, Goldstein JL, Brown MS, eds. The Metabolic Basis of Inherited Disease. New York: McGraw-Hill 1982:1450–1467.
6. Laurell C-B, Eriksson S. The electrophoretic α1-globulin pattern of serum in α1-antitrypsin deficiency. Scand J Clin Lab Invest 1963; 15:132–140.
7. Eriksson S. Pulmonary emphysema and alpha-1 antitrypsin deficiency. Acta Med Scand 1964; 175:197–205.
8. Eriksson S. Studies in α1-antitrypsin deficiency. Acta Med Scand 1965; 177: 421–428.
9. Travis J, Salvesen GS. Human plasma proteinase inhibitors. Annu Rev Biochem 1983; 52:655–709.
10. Crystal RG. The α1-antitrypsin gene and its deficiency states. Trends Genet 1989; 5:411–417.
11. Perlino E, Cortese R, Ciliberto G. The human alpha 1-antitrypsin gene is transcribed

from two different promoters in macrophages and hepatocytes. EMBO J 1987; 6: 2767–2771.
12. Brantly ML, Paul LD, Miller BH, Falk RT, Wu M, Crystal RG. Clinical features and natural history of the destructive lung disease associated with alpha 1-antitrypsin deficiency of adults with pulmonary symptoms. Am Rev Respir Dis 1988; 138: 327–336.
13. Brantly ML, Wittes JT, Vogelmeier CF, Hubbard RC, Fells GA, Crystal RG. Use of a highly purified α1-antitrypsin standard to establish ranges for the common normal and deficient α1-antitrypsin phenotypes. Chest 1991; 100:703–708.
14. Beatty K, Bieth J, Travis J. Kinetics of association of serine proteinases with native and oxidized α-1-proteinase inhibitor and α-1-antichymotrypsin. J Biol Chem 1980; 55:3931–3934.
15. Bieth JG, Elastases: catalytic and biologic properties. In: Medcham R, ed. Regulation of Matrix Accumulation. New York: Academic Press, 1986:217–320.
16. Heidtmann H, Travis J. Human α1-proteinase inhibitor. In: Barrett AJ, Salvesen G, eds. Proteinase Inhibitors. Amsterdam: Elsevier, 1986:441–445.
17. Crystal RG. α1-antitrypsin deficiency, emphysema, and liver disease: Genetic basis and strategies for therapy. J Clin Invest 1990; 85:1343–1352.
18. Crystal RG, Brantly ML, Hubbard RC, Curiel DT, States DJ, Holmes MD. The α1-antitrypsin gene and its mutations: Clinical consequences and strategies for therapy. Chest 1989; 95:196–208.
19. Brantly M, Nukiwa T, Crystal RG. Molecular basis of α1-antitrypsin deficiency. Am J Med 1988; 84:13–31.
20. Hubbard RC, Crystal RG. Alpha 1-antitrypsin augmentation therapy for alpha 1-antitrypsin deficiency. Am J Med 1988; 84:52–62.
21. Sharp HL, Bridges RA, Krivit W, Freier EF. Cirrhosis associated with alpha$_1$-antitrypsin deficiency: a previously unrecognized inherited disorder. J Lab Clin Med 1969; 73:934–939.
22. Sharp HL. Alpha$_1$-antitrypsin deficiency. Hosp Pract 1971; 6:83–86.
23. Lieberman J. Mittman C, Gordon HW. Alpha$_1$-antitrypsin in livers of patient with emphysema. Science 1972; 175:63–65.
24. Eriksson S. Liver disease in alpha$_1$-antitrypsin deficiency. Scand J Gastroenterol 1985; 20:907–911.
25. Berg NO, Eriksson S. Liver disease in adults with alpha$_1$-antitrypsin deficiency. N Engl J Med 1972; 287:1264–1267.
26. Cox DW, Smyth S. Risk for liver disease in adults with alpha$_1$-antitrypsin deficiency. Am J 1983; 74:221–227.
27. Eriksson S, Carlson J, Velez R. Risk of cirrhosis and primary liver cancer in alpha$_1$-antitrypsin deficiency. N Engl J Med 1986; 314:736–739.
28. Pittelkow MR, Smith KC, Daniel WP. Alpha-1-antitrypsin deficiency and panniculitis: Perspectives on disease relationship and replacement therapy. Am J Med 1988; 84:80–86.
29. Jacobsson K. Studies on the trypsin and plasmin inhibitors in human blood serum. Scand J Clin Lab Invest 1955; 7:55–102.

30. Schultze HE, Heide K, Haupt H. Alpha$_1$-antitrypsin aus human-serum. Klin Wochenschr 1962; 40:427–429.
31. Gross P, Pfitzer EA, Tolker E, et al. Experimental emphysema: Its production with papain in normal and silicotic rats. Arch Environ Health 1965; 11:50–58.
32. Gross P, Babyak MA, Tolker E, Kaschak M. Enzymatically produced pulmonary emphysema, a preliminary report. J Occup Med. 1964; 6:481–484.
33. Janoff A, White R, Carp H, et al. Lung injury induced by leukocytic proteases. Am J Pathol 1979; 97:111–136.
34. Janoff A, Schaefer S. Mediators of acute inflammation in leucocyte lysosomes. Nature 1967; 213:144–147.
35. Janoff A, Zeligs JD. Vascular injury and lysis of basement membrane in vitro by neutral protease of human leukocytes. Science 1968; 161:702–704.
36. Seal LA, Carp DA, George RB. Comparison of commercially available radial immunodiffusion kits for the determination of serum α1-antitrypsin concentrations. Am Rev Respir Dis 1975; 111:97–100.
37. Long GL, Chandra I, Woo SLC, Davie EW, Kurachi K. Complete sequence of the cDNA for human α1-antitrypsin and the gene for the S variant. Biochemistry 1984; 23:4828–4837.
38. Nukiwa T, Satoh K, Brantly ML, Ogushi F, Fells GA, Courtney M, Crystal RG. Identification of a second mutation in the protein coding sequence of the Z-type alpha 1-antitrypsin gene. J Biol Chem 1986; 261:15989–15994.
39. Gadek JE, Zimmerman RL, Fells GA, Rennard SI, Crystal RG. Antielastases of the human alveolar structures: implications for the protease-antiprotease theory of emphysema. J Clin Invest 1981; 68:889–898.
40. Gadek JE, Klein H. Holland PV, Crystal RG. Replacement therapy of alpha 1-antitrypsin deficiency: reversal of protease-antiprotease imbalance within the alveolar structures of PiZZ subjects. J Clin Invest 1981; 68:1158–1165.
41. Wewers MD, Casolaro MA, Sellers SE, Swayze SC, McPaul KM, Crystal RG. Replacement therapy for alpha$_1$-antitrypsin deficiency associated with emphysema. N Engl J Med 1987; 316:1055–1062.
42. Carrell RW, Jeppsson J-O, Laurell C-B, et al. Structure and variation of human α1-antitrypsin. Nature 1982; 298:329–334.
43. Rogers J, Kalsheker N, Wallis S, et al. The isolation of a clone of α1-antitrypsin and the detection of a α1-antitrypsin in mRNA from liver and leukocytes. Biochem Biophys Res Commun 1983; 116:375–382.
44. Kueppers F. Genetically determined differences in the response of alpha-1-antitrypsin levels in human serum to typhoid vaccine. Huma Genetik 1968; 6:207–214.
45. Laurell C-B, Kullander S, Thorell J. Effect of administration of a combined estrogen-progestin contraceptive on the level of individual plasma proteins. Scand J Clin Lab Invest 1967; 21:337–343.
46. Aronsen K-F, Ekelund G, Kindmark C-O, Laurell C-B. Sequential changes of plasma proteins after surgical trauma. Scand J Clin Lab Invest 1972; 29:127–136.
47. Eriksson S. The effect of tamoxifen in intermediate alpha-1-antitrypsin deficiency associated with the phenotype PiSZ. Ann Clin Res 1983; 15:95–98.

48. Gadek JE, Fulmer JD, Gelfand JA, Frank MM, Petty TL, Crystal RG. Danazol-induced augmentation of serum α1-antitrypsin levels in individuals with marked deficiency this antiprotease. J Clin Invest 1980; 66:82–87.
49. Wewers MD, Brantly ML, Casolaro MA, Crystal RG. Evaluation of tamoxifen as a therapy to augment alpha 1-antitrypsin levels in Z homozygous alpha-1-antitrypsin deficient individuals. Am Rev Respir Dis 1987; 135:401–402.
50. Jeppsson J-O, Lilja H, Johansson M. Isolation and characterization of minor fractions of α1-antitrypsin by high-performance liquid chromatographic chromato-focusing. J Chromatogr 1985; 327:173–177.
51. Mega T, Lujan E, Yoshida A. Studies on the oligosaccharide chains of human α1-protease inhibitor: I. Isolation of glycopeptides. J Biol Chem 1980; 255:4053–4056.
52. Jones EA, Vergalla J, Steer CJ, Bradley-Moore PR, Vierling JM. Metabolism of intact and desialylated α1-antitrypsin. Clin Sci Mol Med 1978; 55:139–148.
53. Jeppsson J-O, Laurell C-B, Nosslin B, Cox DW. Catabolic rate of α1-antitrypsin of Pi types S, and $M_{malton}$ and of asialylated M-protein in man. Clin Sci Mol Med 1978; 55:103–107.
54. Loebermann H, Tokuoka R, Deisenhofer J, Huber R. Human α1-proteinase inhibitor: crystal structure analysis of two crystal modifications, molecular model and preliminary analysis of the implications for function. J Mol Biol 1984; 177:531–556.
55. Smith CE, Johnson DA. Human bronchial leucocyte proteinase inhibitor. Biochem J 1985; 225:463–472.
56. McRae B, Nakajima K, Travis J, Powers JC. Studies on reactivity of human leukocyte elastase, cathepsin G, and porcine pancreatic elastase toward peptides including sequences related to the reactive site of α1-protease inhibitor (α1-antitrypsin). Biochemistry 1980; 19:3973–3978.
57. Bode W, Wei A, Huber R, Meyer E, Travis J, Neumann S. X-ray crystal structure of human leukocyte elastase (PMN elastase) and the third domain of the turkey ovomucoid inhibitor. EMBO J 1986; 5:2453–2458.
58. Johnson DA, Travis J. Human alpha-1-protease inhibitor mechanism of action: evidence for activation by limited proteolysis. Biochem Biophys Res Commun 1976; 72: 33–39.
59. Ogushi F, Fells GA, Hubbard RC, Straus SD, Crystal RG. Z-type α1-antitrypsin is less competent then M1-type α1-antitrypsin as an inhibitor of neutrophil elastase. J Clin Invest 1987; 80:1366–1374.
60. Johnson D, Travis J. The oxidative inactivation of human α1-proteinase inhibitor—further evidence for methionine at the reactive center. J Biol Chem 1979; 254:4022–4026.
61. Carp H, Jannoff A. Potential mediator of inflammation—phagocyte-derived oxidants suppress the elastase-inhibitory capacity of $alpha_1$-proteinase inhibitor *in vitro*. J Clin Invest 1980; 66:987–995.
62. Hubbard RC, Ogushi F, Fells GA, Cantin AM, Jallat S, Courtney M, Crystal RG. Oxidants spontaneously released by alveolar macrophages of cigarette smokers can inactivate the active site of α1-antitrypsin, rendering it ineffective as an inhibitor of neutrophil elastase. J Clin Invest 1987; 80:1289–1295.

63. Gadek JE, Fells GA, Crystal RG. Cigarette smoking induces functional antiprotease deficiency in the lower respiratory tract of humans. Science 1979; 206:1315–1316.
64. Johnson D, Travis J. The oxidative inactivation of human alpha-1-proteinase inhibitor: further evidence of methionine at the reactive center. J Biol Chem 1979; 254: 4022–4026.
65. Johnson D, Travis J. Structural evidence for methionine at the reactive site of human alpha-1-proteinase inhibitor. J Biol Chem 1978; 253:7142–7144.
66. Beatty K, Matheson N, Travis J. Kinetic and chemical evidence for the inability of oxidized alpha-1-proteinase inhibitor to protect lung elastin from elastolytic degradation. Hoppe-Seylers Z Physiol Chem 1984; 365:731–736.
67. Heidmann H, Travis J. Human α1-proteinase inhibitor. In: Barrett AJ, Salvesen G, eds. Proteinase Inhibitors. Amsterdam: Elsevier, 1986:441–445.
68. Wright DG. Human neutrophil degranulation. Methods Enzymol 1988; 162:538–551.
69. Travis J. Structure, function, and control of neutrophil proteinases. Am J Med 1988; 84:37–43.
70. Allen RC, Harley RA, Talamo RC. A new method for determination of alpha-1-antitrypsin phenotypes using isoelectric focusing on polyacrylamide gel slabs. Am J Clin Pathol 1974; 62:732–739.
71. Frants RR, Eriksson AW. α1-Antitrypsin: common subtypes of piM. Hum Hered 1976; 26:435–440.
72. Kueppers F. α1-Antitrypsin M1: a new common genetically determined variant. Am J Hum Genet 1976; 28:370–377.
73. Registry of the National Heart, Lung, and Blood Institute for Patients with α1-Antitrypsin Deficiency. Bethesda, MD, 1994.
74. Ogushi F, Hubbard R, Fells G, et al. Evaluation of the S-type of α1-antitrypsin as an in vivo and in vitro inhibitor of neutrophil elastase. Am Rev Respir Dis 1988; 137: 364–370.
75. Cox DW. α1-antitrypsin deficiency. In: Scriver CR, Beaudet AL, Sly WS, Valle D, eds. The Metabolic Basis of Inherited Diseases. 6th ed. New York: McGraw-Hill, 1989: 2409–2437.
76. McElvaney NG, Birrer P, Chang-Stroman LM, Crystal RG. In: Grassi C, Travis J, Casali L. Luisetti M, eds. Current Concepts in the Biochemistry of Pulmonary Emphysema. London: Springer Verlag, and Verona, Italy: B1 & G1 Publishers, 1992; 89:1478–1484.
77. Birrer P, McElvaney NG, Chang-Stroman LM, Crystal RG. α1-antitrypsin deficiency and liver disease. J Inher Metab Dis 1991; 14:512–525.
78. Hutchison CS. Natural history of alpha-1-protease inhibitor deficiency. Am J Med 1988; 89:3–12.
79. McElvaney NG, Feuerstein I, Simon TR, Hubbard RC, Crystal RG. Comparison of the relative sensitivity of routine pulmonary function tests, scintigraphy, and computed axial tomography in detecting "early" lung abnormalities associated with α1-antitrypsin deficiency. Am Rev Respir Dis 1989; 139:A122.
80. Carlson J, Eriksson S. Chronic "cryptogenic" liver disease and malignant hepatoma in intermediate $alpha_1$-antitrypsin deficiency identified by a $P_iZ$-specific monoclonal antibody. Scand J Gastroenterol 1985; 20:835–842.

81. Chan CH, Steer CJ, Vergalla J, Jones EA. Alpha$_1$-antitrypsin deficiency with cirrhosis associated with the protease inhibitor phenotype SZ. Am J Med 1978; 65:978–986.
82. Fagerhol MK, Cox DW. The P$_i$polymorphism: genetic, biochemical and clinical aspects of human alpha$_1$-antitrypsin. Adv Hum Genet 1981; 11:1–62.
83. Wewers MD, Gadek JE, Keogh BA, Fells GA, Crystal RG. Evaluation of danazol therapy for patients with PiZZ alpha-1-antitrypsin deficiency. Am Rev Respir Dis 1986; 134:476–480.
84. Gadek JE, Fells GA, Zimmerman RL, Rennard SI, Crystal RG. Anti-elastases of the human alveolar structures: implications for the protease-antiprotease theory of emphysema. J Clin Invest 1981; 68:889–898.
85. Hubbard RC, Sellers S, Czerski D, Stephens L, Crystal RG. Biochemical efficacy and safety of monthly augmentation therapy for α1-antitrypsin deficiency. JAMA 1988; 260:1259–1264.
86. Hubbard RC, Brantly ML, Sellers SE, Mitchell ME, Crystal RG. Delivery of proteins for therapeutic purposes by aerosolization: direct augmentation of anti-neutrophil elastase defenses of the lower respiratory tract in deficiency with an aerosol of α1-antitrypsin. Ann Intern Med 1989; 111:206–212.
87. Birrer P, McElvaney NG, Gillissen A, Hoyt RF, Bloedow DC, Hubbard RC, Crystal RG. Intravenous administration of recombinant secretory leukoprotease inhibitor as strategy to augment antineutrophil elastase protective screen of the lung. J Appl Physiol 1992; 317–323.
88. Jaffe HA, Danel C, Longenecker G, Metzger M, Setoguchi Y, Rosenfeld MA, Gant TW, Thorgeirsson SS, Stratford-Perricaudet LD, Perricaudet M, Pavirani A, Lecocq J-P, Crystal RG. Adenovirus-mediated *in vivo* gene transfer and expression in normal rat liver. Nature Genet 1992; 1:372–378.
89. Setoguchi Y, Jaffe HA, Chu C-S, Crytsal RG. Intraperitoneal *in vivo* gene therapy to deliver α1-antitrypsin to the systemic circulation. Am J Respir Cel Mol Biol 1994; 10:369–377.
90. Rosenfeld M, Siegfried W, Yoshimura K, Yoneyama K, Fukayama M, Stier LE, Paakko PK, Gilardi P, Stratford-Perricaudet LD, Perricaudet M, Jallat S, Pavirani A, Lecocq J-P, Crystal RG. Adenovirus-mediated transfer of a recombinant α1-antitrypsin gene to the lung epithelium *in vivo*. Science 1991; 252:431–434.

# Part Two

## BIOLOGY AND PATHOBIOLOGY

# 2

# Alpha 1–Antitrypsin Gene and Promoter

**JOHN G. HAY, MOTOYOSHI SUZUKI, and RONALD G. CRYSTAL**

The New York Hospital–Cornell Medical Center
New York, New York

## I. Introduction

The alpha 1–antitrypsin (α1AT) gene is located on the q arm of human chromosome 14 (1). The gene is 12.2 kb in length and consists of seven exons designated IA, IB, IC, II, III, IV, and V. The protein coding region is contained within exons II–V (2,3).

## II. Chromosomal Location

The α1AT gene product is a protease inhibitor, a member of a family of serine protease inhibitors, or "serpins," characterized by their ability to inhibit proteases that possess the amino acid serine at their active site (4). Serpin molecules characteristically have a 15-residue peptide reactive loop on their surface that interacts with the active site of the target serine proteinase (5). The serpin family of proteins is large; it includes α1-antichymotrypsin (α1ACT), α2-antiplasmin, plasminogen activator inhibitors 1 and 2, antithrombin III, heparin cofactor II, active protein C inhibitor, C1 inhibitor, thyroxine-binding globulin, cortisol-

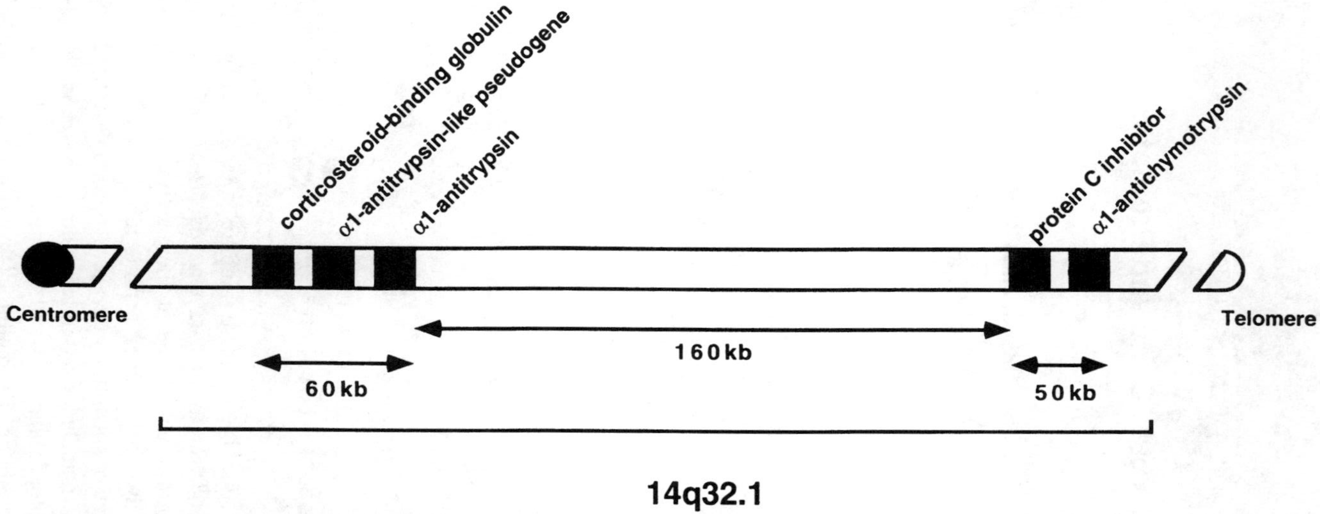


**Figure 1** Location of the human α1AT gene on chromosome 14q32.1, and the location of other serpin genes forming a cluster at this locus.

binding globulin, angiotensinogen, protease nexin-1, kallistatin, and leukocyte inhibitors.

Several of the serpin genes form a cluster on chromosome 14 at 14q32.1, including corticosteroid binding globulin, α1AT-like pseudogene, α1AT, protein C inhibitor, and α1ACT (ordered centromere to telomere) (6,7). All these genes, including the α1AT-like pseudogene, occupy a short 270 kb segment on chromosome 14 at q32.1 (Fig. 1). The genes at this locus have a similar sequence and gene organization, suggesting evolution from a common ancestor. For instance, α1AT, α1ACT, and corticosteroid-binding protein have 56% sequence homology (8) and even share one or two similar flanking restriction sites (e.g., BssH II and Sfi I) that generate restriction fragments of almost identical sizes that cross-hybridize with the same probes (6).

Similarly, the α1AT-like pseudogene has great similarity (70%) with the α1AT gene (9,10). Even the gene for corticosteroid-binding globulin (which has an entirely different function from that of the protease inhibitors) has a similar exon/intron structure, and 53% amino acid homology with α1AT (11). The fact that small changes in this basic gene structure can lead to new functions is clearly demonstrated by the α1AT mutant "Pittsburgh," in which a single amino acid change at the active site (methionine to arginine) leads to a bleeding diathesis as a consequence of the antithrombin III–like properties of the mutant molecule (12). All these features suggest that this cluster of genes on chromosome 14 has arisen by gene duplication. In addition, this group of genes is in a conserved linkage group with the immunoglobulin heavy chain gene, and this grouping is seen conserved in other species, for instance, on mouse chromosome 12.

The common α1AT deficiency Z allele has a virtually unique haplotype that encompasses the cortisol binding globulin, α1AT-like pseudogene and α1AT gene loci extending for 60kb. This suggests that the Z allele occurred as a single event, and this linkage of the Z allele to the cortisol-binding globulin (or other genes) may explain some of the disease associations with α1AT deficiency such as rheumatoid arthritis, relapsing panniculitis, asthma, immune-complex disease, and certain forms of cancer.

## III. α1AT Gene Structure

The α1AT gene encodes a protein of 418 amino acids, which includes a 24 amino acid signal peptide (Fig. 2). The protein coding region is within exons II–V (2). The reactive serine protease inhibitory site of α1AT is $Met^{358}$ in exon V (14). The two most common mutations to produce an abnormal phenotype are the Z and S alleles. The Z allele contains a G-to-A mutation within exon V that results in a change from the negatively charged glutamate (GAG) at position 342 to the positively charged lysine (AAG) within the protein. This has the effect of disrupt-

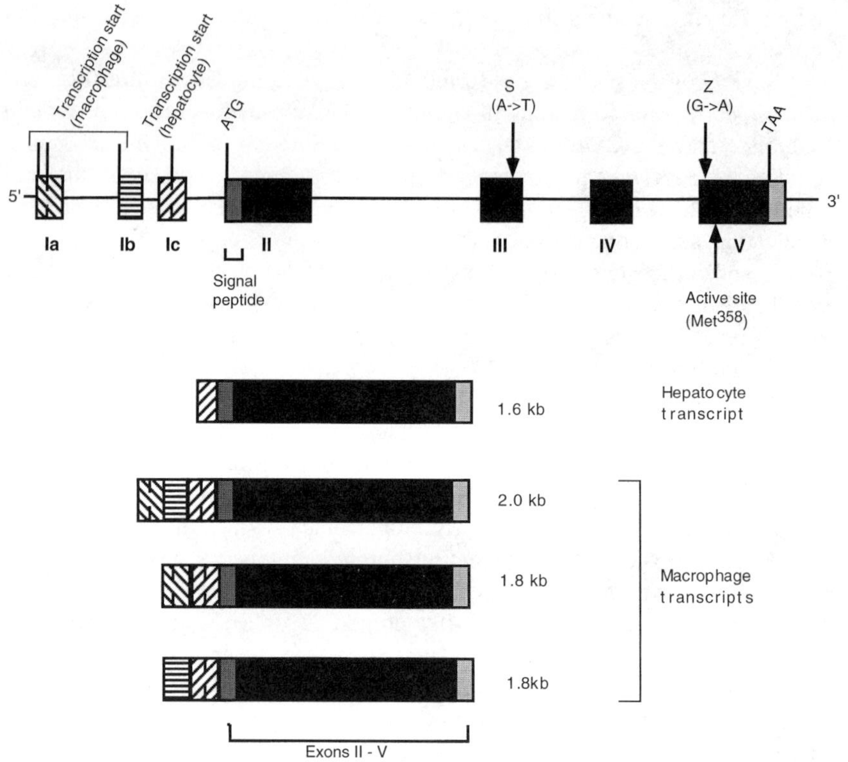


**Figure 2** Structure of the human α1AT gene. The translation start (ATG) is within exon II, and the translation termination (TAA) within exon V and the S mutation in exon III are shown. Alternative transcription initiation sites utilized by hepatocytes and mononuclear phagocytes are also shown, together with the usual transcripts generated from these sites and by alternative splicing of exon Ib.

ing the salt bridge within the molecule, leading to abnormal folding and accumulation within the endoplasmic reticulum (15). The S allele is within exon III, and is an A-to-T mutation that results in a change from glutamate (GAG) at position 264 to valine (GTG). The resulting protein has an increased susceptibility to intracellular degradation (16).

Transcription of the α1AT gene results in three major mRNA products, 1.6, 1.8, and 2.0 kb in length (Fig. 2). The shortest 1.6 kb mRNA is found exclusively in hepatocytes and enterocytes. The two longer mRNA products (1.8 and 2.0 kb) are found almost exclusively in mononuclear phagocytes. The generation of these different RNA species is a consequence of two major transcription start sites within the gene and alternative splicing (3). The transcription start site utilized by hepatocytes and enterocytes is within exon Ic; this generates the shortest mRNA product (1.6 kb) and contains just 49 bp of 5′ untranslated region. The transcription start site utilized by mononuclear phagocytes is within exon Ia (183 bp), and exon Ib (210 bp) is variably spliced out of the mature message (as suggested by the sequence of various cDNA clones). The splice site for exon Ic (invariably included) is also upstream of the transcription start site utilized by hepatocytes in exon Ic. Finally, within mononuclear phagocytes, transcription may be initiated at two sites within exon Ia, and an additional site in exon Ib (17).

The protein translation start site is within exon II, 5 kb downstream from exon Ic. The protein product from all these various RNA species is therefore the same. The importance of these different RNA species is as yet unclear, although within the longer mononuclear phagocyte transcripts, two additional open reading frames are present. This has been shown to be of importance in the regulation of other genes—for instance, the yeast GCN4 gene, which encodes a transcription factor necessary for the synthesis of biosynthetic enzymes in response to amino acid starvation, is regulated by translational events from open reading frames in the upstream region of its own mRNA (18).

The $\alpha$1AT-like pseudogene is 12 kb downstream of the authentic $\alpha$1AT gene (9,10) (Fig. 3). Exons and introns of this gene show considerable (70%) homology with the authentic gene, and one of the clones sequenced shows conservation of RNA splice sites and no premature termination codons, although exon I (which does not contain coding sequences) is not conserved (10). Another clone sequenced showed a critical mutation in the start codon (ATG→ATA), strongly suggesting that this is a pseudogene (9). This has been confirmed by the study of the deficiency mutant $\alpha 1AT_{\text{isola di procida,}}$ a mutant characterized by the deletion of a 17 kb fragment that includes exons II–V of the authentic gene. Exons Ia–c are therefore followed by exons II–V of the downstream pseudogene, yet no detectible $\alpha$1AT is found in the serum of individuals with the inheritance of this mutation and another null mutation (19).

## IV. Tissue Specificity of Expression

$\alpha$1AT is an acute phase protein, and thus the liver would be expected to be the major site of synthesis. This is the case, with hepatocytes containing 200 times more $\alpha$1AT mRNA than other cells (20). However, mononuclear phagocytes, enterocytes, and neutrophils have also been demonstrated to secrete $\alpha$1AT, although this is likely to be important only in the local milieu of these cells (21–23).

As described above, the $\alpha$1AT gene has two different transcription start sites. One (in exon Ic) directs hepatocyte specific transcription, and the other (in exon Ia) directs transcription in the other cell types. In in vitro experiments, a

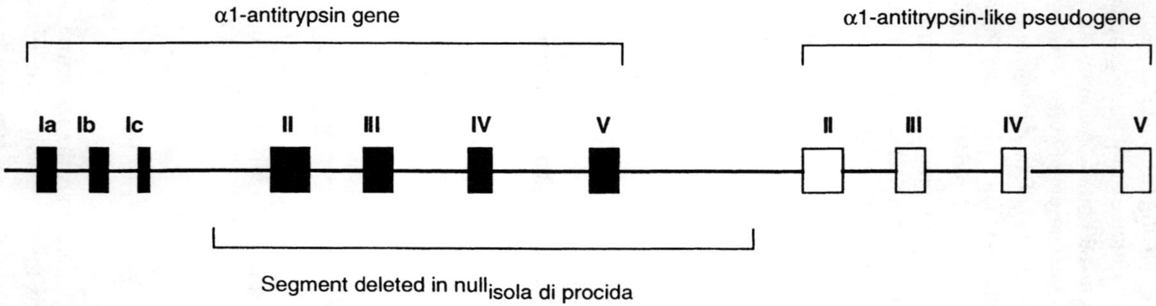


**Figure 3** α1AT gene and α1AT-like pseudogene. Also shown is the segment of DNA deleted in the α1AT deficiency mutant $\text{null}_{\text{isola di procida}}$ (19).

minimal promoter of −137 to − 2 bp from the hepatocyte transcription start nucleotide determines liver-specific transcription. An A element (−119 to −104), a B element (−77 to − 64), and a TATA-like box (TAAAT) are important for transcription; mutation of the TATA box completely inhibits transcription. The two cis elements A and B confer hepatocyte-specific transcription as shown by competition with oligonucleotides homologous to these sequences (24).

Hepatocyte extracts produce several footprints over the α1AT gene promoter. Five proteins in these liver-cell extracts have been shown to bind to the promoter; these have been labeled LF-A1, LF-A2, LF-B1, LF-B2, and LF-C. LF-A1 and LF-B1 are positive factors important for transcription and bind to the A (−104 to −119) and B (−56 to −77) elements, respectively (24). LF-B1 [also called HNF-1 (hepatocyte nuclear factor 1), HP1, and APF] has been characterized as a 90 kDa glycoprotein with structural similarities to Drosophila homeobox-encoded genes (25). This factor also plays a role in the liver-specific transcription of other genes, including albumin, C-reactive protein, α-fetoprotein, fibrinogen, pyruvate kinase, and the pre-S1 gene of the hepatitis B virus. LF-A1, also called HNF-2, is a 68 kDa protein that has recently been characterized (26,27).

## V. Modulation of Expression

In the context that α1AT is an acute phase protein that is synthesized predominantly in the liver, and that plasma levels increase fourfold in response to host injury (28), it is anticipated that the gene would be up-regulated in hepatocytes by the cytokine IL-6, which predominantly mediates the acute-phase response. IL-6 induces an increase in α1AT mRNA levels and protein synthesis in liver cell lines, although other cytokines, including TNF and IL-1, which also play a role in the acute-phase response, have no effect on α1AT transcription. The effect of IL-6 is not inhibited by corticosteroid (29,30).

IL-6 exerts its effects on gene transcription mainly through the transcription factor NF-IL6, and there are two sequences in the α1AT promoter that have partial homology to the NF-IL6 consensus sequence (Fig. 4). In primary cultures of blood monocytes, IL-6 also induces α1AT transcription and protein synthesis. It is of interest that, although transcription in hepatocytes under basal conditions is initiated in exon Ic, following IL-6 induction transcription in hepatocytes can also be detected from the transcription start sites in exon Ia (the transcription start site utilized predominantly by mononuclear phagocytes) (17).

The α1AT gene may also be regulated in mononuclear phagocytes by the serine protease neutrophil elastase and lipopolysaccharide. These two agents have an additive effect, elastase regulating the α1AT gene at the transcriptional level and LPS, by a mechanism as yet not clearly defined, by increasing translation of the gene without changes in mRNA level (31). GMC-SF has also been demon-

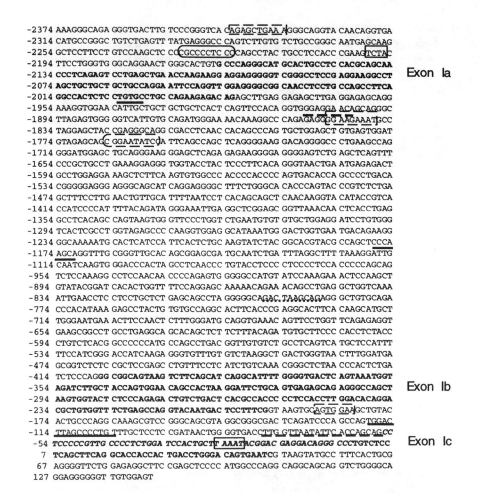

```
-2374 AAAGGGCAGA GGGTGACTTG TCCCGGGTCA CAGAGCTGAA AGGGCAGGTA CAACAGGTGA
-2314 CATGCCGGGC TGTCTGAGTT TATGAGGGCC CAGTCTTGTG TCTGCCGGGC AATGAGCAAG
-2254 GCTCCTTCCT GTCCAAGCTC CCCGCCCCTC CCCAGCCTAC TGCCTCCACC CGAAGTCTAC
-2194 TTCCTGGGTG GGCAGGAACT GGGCACTGTG CCCAGGGCAT GCACTGCCTC CACGCAGCAA
-2134 CCCTCAGAGT CCTGAGCTGA ACCAAGAAGG AGGAGGGGGT CGGGCCTCCG AGGAAGGCCT   Exon Ia
-2074 AGCTGCTGCT GCTGCCAGGA ATTCCAGGTT GGAGGGGCGG CAACCTCCTG CCAGCCTTCA
-2014 GGCCACTCTC CTGTGCCTGC CAGAAGAGAC AGAGCTTGAG GAGAGCTTGA GGAGAGCAGG
-1954 AAAGGTGGAA CATTGCTGCT GCTGCTCACT CAGTTCCACA GGTGGGAGGA ACAGCAGGGC
-1894 TTAGAGTGGG GGTCATTGTG CAGATGGGAA AACAAAGGCC CAGAGAGGGG AAGAAATGCC
-1834 TAGGAGCTAC CGAGGGCAGG CGACCTCAAC CACAGCCCAG TGCTGGAGCT GTGAGTGGAT
-1774 GTAGAGCAGC GGAATATCCA TTCAGCCAGC TCAGGGGAAG GACAGGGGCC CTGAAGCCAG
-1714 GGGATGGAGC TGCAGGGAAG GGAGCTCAGA GAGAAGGGGA GGGGAGTCTG AGCTCAGTTT
-1654 CCCGCTGCCT GAAAGGAGGG TGGTACCTAC TCCCTTCACA GGGTAACTGA ATGAGAGACT
-1594 GCCTGGAGGA AAGCTCTTCA AGTGTGGCCC ACCCCACCCC AGTGACACCA GCCCCTGACA
-1534 CGGGGGAGGG AGGGCAGCAT CAGGAGGGGC TTTCTGGGCA CACCCAGTAC CCGTCTCTGA
-1474 GCTTTCCTTG AACTGTTGCA TTTTAATCCT CACAGCAGCT CAACAAGGTA CATACCGTCA
-1414 CCATCCCCAT TTTACAGATA GGGAAATTGA GGCTCGGAGC GGTTAAACAA CTCACCTGAG
-1354 GCCTCACAGC CAGTAAGTGG GTTCCCTGGT CTGAATGTGT GTGCTGGAGG ATCCTGTGGG
-1294 TCACTCGCCT GGTAGAGCCC CAAGGTGGAG GCATAAATGG GACTGGTGAA TGACAGAAGG
-1234 GGCAAAAATG CACTCATCCA TTCACTCTGC AAGTATCTAC GGCACGTACG CCAGCTCCCA
-1174 AGCAGGTTTG CGGGTTGCAC AGCGGAGCGA TGCAATCTGA TTTAGGCTTT TAAAGGATTG
-1114 CAATCAAGTG GGACCCACTA GCCTCAACCC TGTACCTCCC CTCCCCTCCA CCCCCAGCAG
 -954 TCTCCAAAGG CCTCCAACAA CCCCAGAGTG GGGGCCATGT ATCCAAAGAA ACTCCAAGCT
 -894 GTATACGGAT CACACTGGTT TTCCAGGAGC AAAAACAGAA ACAGCCTGAG GCTGGTCAAA
 -834 ATTGAACCTC CTCCTGCTCT GAGCAGCCTA GGGGGCAGAC TAAGCAGAGG GCTGTGCAGA
 -774 CCCACATAAA GAGCCTACTG TGTGCCAGGC ACTTCACCCG AGGCACTTCA CAAGCATGCT
 -714 TGGGAATGAA ACTTCCAACT CTTTGGGATG CAGGTGAAAC AGTTCCTGGT TCAGAGAGGT
 -654 GAAGCGGCCT GCCTGAGGCA GCACAGCTCT TCTTTACAGA TGTGCTTCCC CACCTCTACC
 -594 CTGTCTCACG GCCCCCCATG CCAGCCTGAC GGTTGTGTCT GCCTCAGTCA TGCTCCATTT
 -534 TTCCATCGGG ACCATCAAGA GGGTGTTTGT GTCTAAGGCT GACTGGGTAA CTTTGGATGA
 -474 GCGGTCTCTC CGCTCCGAGC CTGTTTCCTC ATCTGTCAAA CGGGCTCTAA CCCACTCTGA
 -414 TCTCCCAGGG CGGCAGTAAG TCTTCAGCAT CAGGCATTTT GGGGTGACTC AGTAAATGGT
 -354 AGATCTTGCT ACCAGTGGAA CAGCCACTAA GGATTCTGCA GTGAGAGCAG AGGGCCAGCT   Exon Ib
 -294 AAGTGGTACT CTCCCAGAGA CTGTCTGACT CACGCCACCC CCTCCACCTT GGACACAGGA
 -234 CGCTGTGGTT TCTGAGCCAG GTACAATGAC TCCTTTCGGT AAGTGCAGTG GAAGCTGTAC
 -174 ACTGCCCAGG CAAAGCGTCC GGGCAGCGTA GGCGGGCGAC TCAGATCCCA GCCAGTGGAC
 -114 TTAGCCCCTG TTTGCTCCTC CGATAACTGG GGTGACCTTG GTTAATATTC ACCAGCAGCC
  -54 TCCCCCGTTG CCCCTCTGGA TCCACTGCTT AAATACGGAC GAGGACAGGG CCCTGTCTCC   Exon Ic
    7 TCAGCTTCAG GCACCACCAC TGACCTGGGA CAGTGAATCG TAAGTATGCC TTTCACTGCG
   67 AGGGGTTCTG GAGAGGCTTC CGAGCTCCCC ATGGCCCAGG CAGGCAGCAG GTCTGGGGCA
  127 GGAGGGGGGT TGTGGAGT
```

**Figure 4** Human α1AT gene 5′ flanking region. Exons Ia–c are shown in bold type. Several transcription factor–binding sequences are shown, including: TATA box (complete box), NFIL-6 (broken box), HNF-1 (broken underline), HNF-2 (underline), C/EBP (overline), SP1 (broken overline), EGR1 (oval), NFkB (broken oval), and AP-1 (underdots).

strated to increase transcription of the α1AT in a promonocytic cell line (32). This therefore suggests both local and systemic regulation of the α1AT gene.

In addition to the liver-specific elements in the 5′ flanking region and putative NF-IL6 sequences, there are also putative binding sequences for the transcription factors EGR1 and NFkB, both of which may mediate the host response to inflammation, and C/EBP, which is likely to be important in tissue specificity of expression (Fig. 4).

## VI. Transgenic Mice

Studies in transgenic mice have demonstrated that the 5′ flanking region of the human $\alpha$1AT gene is sufficient for tissue-specific expression of $\alpha$1AT or a marker gene, although mice express more $\alpha$1AT in the kidney than humans (33–35). In addition, the importance of the liver-specific binding elements within the promoter have been confirmed by deletion studies, and the use of alternative tissue-specific transcription initiation sites has also been confirmed (36).

## References

1. Sefton L, Kelsey G, Kearney P, Povey S, Wolfe J. A physical map of the human PI and AACT genes. Genomics 1990; 7:382–388.
2. Long GL, Chandra T, Woo SLC, Davie EW, Kurachi, K. Complete sequence of the cDNA for human $\alpha_1$-antitrypsin and the gene for the S variant. Biochemistry 1984; 23:4828–4837.
3. Perlino E, Cortese R, Ciliberto G. The human $\alpha_1$-antitrypsin gene is transcribed from two different promoters in macrophages and hepatocytes. EMBO J 1987; 6:2767–2771.
4. Carrell R, Travis J. $\alpha_1$-antitrypsin and the serpins: variation and countervariation. Trends Biochem Sci 1985; 10:20–24.
5. Johnson D, Travis J. Inactivation of human $\alpha_1$ proteinase inhibitor by thiol proteinases. Biochem J 1977; 163:639–641.
6. Billingsley GD, Walter MA, Hammond GL, Cox DW. Physical mapping of four serpin genes: $\alpha_1$-antitrypsin, $\alpha_1$-antichymotrypsin, corticosteroid-binding globulin, and protein C inhibitor, within a 280-kb region on chromosome 14q32.1. Am J Hum Genet 1993; 52:343–353.
7. Byth BC, Billingsley GD, Cox DW. Physical and genetic mapping of the serpin gene cluster at 14q32.1: allelic association and a unique haplotype associated with $\alpha_1$-antitrypsin deficiency. Am J Hum Genet 1994; 55:126–133.
8. Chandra T, Stackhouse R, Kidd VJ, Robson KJH, Woo SLC. Sequence homology between human $\alpha$1-antichymotrypsin, $\alpha$1-antitrypsin, and antithrombin III. Biochemistry 1983; 22:5055–5060.
9. Hofker MH, Nelen M, Klasen EC, Nukiwa T, Curiel D, Crystal RG, Frants RR. Cloning and characterization of an $\alpha$1-antitrypsin like gene 12 kb downstream of the genuine $\alpha$1-antitrypsin gene. Biochem Biohpys Res Comm 1988; 155:634–642.
10. Bao J-J, Reed-Fourquet L, Sifers RN, Kidd VJ, Woo SLC. Molecular structure and sequence homology of a gene related to $\alpha_1$-antitrypsin in the human genome. Genomics 1988; 2:165–173.
11. Underhill DA, Hammond GL. Organization of the human corticosteroid binding

globulin gene and analysis of its 5′-flanking region. Mol Endocrinol 1989; 3:1448–1454.

12. Owen MC, Brennan SO, Lewis JH, Carrell RW. Mutation of antitrypsin to antithrombin. $\alpha_1$-antitrypsin Pittsburgh (358 Met→Arg), a fatal bleeding disorder. N Engl J Med 1983; 309:694–698.
13. Hill RE, Shaw PH, Barth RK, Hastie, ND. A genetic locus closely linked to a protease inhibitor gene complex controls the level of multiple RNA transcripts. Mol Cell Biol 1985; 5:2114–2122.
14. Loebermann H, Tokuoka R, Deisenhofer J, Huber R. Human $\alpha_1$-proteinase inhibitor: Crystal structure analysis of two crystal modifications, molecular model and preliminary analysis of the implications for function. J Mol Biol 1984; 177:531–556.
15. Brantly M, Nukiwa T, Crystal RG. Molecular basis of alpha-1-antitrypsin deficiency. Am J Med 1988; 84(6A):13–31.
16. Curiel DT, Chytil A, Courtney M, Crystal RG. Serum α1-antitrypsin deficiency associated with the common S-type ($Glu^{264}$→Val) mutation results from intracellular degradation of α1-antitrypsin prior to secretion. J Biol Chem 1989; 264:10477–10486.
17. Hafeez W. Ciliberto G. Perlmutter DH. Constitutive and modulated expression of the human $\alpha_1$-antitrypsin gene. J Clin Invest 1992; 89:1214–1222.
18. Mueller PP, Hinnebusch AG. Multiple upstream AUG codons mediate translational control of GCN4. Cell 1986; 45:201–207.
19. Takahashi H, Crystal RG. α1-antitrypsin $null_{isola\ di\ procida}$: an α1-antitrypsin deficiency allele caused by deletion of all α1-antitrypsin coding exons. Am J Hum Genet 1990; 47:403–413.
20. Rogers J, Kalsheker N, Wallis S, Speer A, Coutelle CH, Woods D, Humphries SE. The isolation of a clone for human α1-antitrypsin and the detection of α1-antitrypsin mRNA from liver and leukocytes. Biochem Biophys Res Comm 1983; 116:375–382.
21. Carlson JA, Rogers BB, Sifers RN, Hawkins HK, Finegold MJ, Woo SLC. Multiple tissues express $alpha_1$-antitrypsin in transgenic mice and man. J Clin Invest 1988; 82:26–36.
22. Koopman P, Povey S, Lovell-Badge RH. Widespread expression of human $\alpha_1$-antitrypsin in trangenic mice revealed by in situ hybridization. Genes Devel 1989; 3:16–25.
23. Molmenti EP, Perlmutter DH, Rubin DC. Cell-specific expression of $\alpha_1$-antitrypsin in human intestinal epithelium. J Clin Invest 1993; 92:2022–2034.
24. Monaci P, Nicosia A, Cortese R. Two different liver-specific factors stimulate *in vitro* transcription from the human α1-antitrypsin promoter. EMBO J 1988; 7:2075–2087.
25. Frain M, Swart G, Monaci P, Nicosia A, Stämpfli S, Frank R, Cortese R. The liver-specific transcription factor LF-B1 contains a highly diverged homeobox DNA binding domain. Cell 1989; 59:145–157.
26. Ramji DP, Tadros MH, Hardon EM, Cortese R. The transcription factor LF-A1 interacts with a bipartite recognition sequence in the promoter regions of several liver-specific genes. Nucleic Acids Res 1991; 19:1139–1145.
27. Rangan VS, Das, GC. Purification and biochemical characterization of hepatocyte nuclear factor 2 involved in liver-specific transcription of the human $\alpha_1$-antitrypsin gene. J Biol Chem 1990; 265:8874–8879.

28. Dickson I, Alper CA. Changes in serum proteinase inhibitor levels following bone surgery. Clin Chim Acta 1974; 54:381–385.
29. Castell JV, Gómez-Lechón MJ, David M, Hirano T, Kishimoto T, Heinrich PC. Recombinant human interleukin-6 (IL-6/BSF-2/HSF) regulates the synthesis of acute phase proteins in human hepatocytes. FEBS Lett 1988; 232:347–350.
30. Perlmutter DH, May LT, Sehgal PB. Interferon β2/interleukin 6 modulates synthesis of $\alpha_1$-antitrypsin in human mononuclear phagocytes and in human hepatoma cells. J Clin Invest 1989; 84:138–144.
31. Perlmutter DH, Punsal PI. Distinct and additive effects of elastase and endotoxin on expression of $\alpha_1$ proteinase inhibitor in mononuclear phagocytes. J Biol Chem 1988; 263:16499–16503.
32. Afford SC, Burnett D, Stockley RA. Regulation of $\alpha_1$-antitrypsin synthesis by granulocyte macrophage colony-stimulating factor in the U937 promonocytic cell line. Biol Chem Hoppe-Seyler 1992; 373:219–227.
33. Sifers RN, Carlson JA, Clift SM, De Mayo FJ, Bullock DW, Woo SLC. Tissue specific expression of the human alpha-1 antitrypsin gene in transgenic mice. Nucleic Acids Res 1987; 15:1459–1475.
34. Rüther U. Tripodi M, Cortese R, Wagner EF. The human alpha-1 antitrypsin gene is efficiently expressed from two tissue-specific promoters in transgenic mice. Nucleic Acids Res 1987; 15:7519–7529.
35. Shen RF, Clift SM, DeMayo JL, Sifers RN, Finegold MJ, Woo SLC. Tissue-specific regulation of human $\alpha_1$-antitrypsin gene expression in transgenic mice. DNA 1989; 8:101–108.
36. Tripodi M, Abbott C, Vivian N, Cortese R, Lovell-Badge R. Disruption of the LF-A1 and LF-B1 binding sites in the human alpha-1-antitrypsin gene has a differential effect during development in transgenic mice. EMBO J 1991; 10:3177–3182.

# 3

# Alpha 1–Antitrypsin Gene Evolution

**TOSHIHIRO NUKIWA**

Tohoku University
Sendai, Japan

**FUMITAKA OGUSHI**

Tokushima University School of Medicine
Tokushima, Japan

**RONALD G. CRYSTAL**

The New York Hospital–Cornell Medical Center
New York, New York

## I. Closely Related Genes of Alpha 1–Antitrypsin in the Serpin Superfamily

The protein and gene of alpha 1–antitrypsin (α1AT) are the most studied members of a large family of serine protease inhibitors called serpins. α1AT and alpha 1–antichymotrypsin (α1ACT) are known to be located very close together on chromosome 14q32.1. According to recent analysis using a pulsed-field map of the surrounding region of 14q32.1, the α1AT gene is only 22 kb away from the α1ACT gene (1). Although the α1AT gene and the α1ACT gene are oriented in opposite directions, the location of the introns within these genes is identical. It seems likely that the divergence of these two loci is a relatively recent event—between 100 million (M) years and 250 M years ago (2). Also, because of the comparatively short distance, there is clearly a close genetic linkage between α1AT and α1ACT. Although these are single-copy genes in humans, they are found in mice as clusters and complexed (contrapsin is the mouse equivalent of α1ACT), indicating that species-specific duplications of these genes occurred independently.

In humans there is an α1AT-like sequence (or an α1AT-related gene; ATR) only about 10 kb downstream of the authentic α1AT gene. Although these two are located as a cluster, since there is no firm evidence that ATR gene is expressed, it is currently thought to be a pseudogene. The ATR sequence has been extensively studied because of the very strong linkage disequilibrium in a region of about 25 kb extending from 5′ of α1AT to the ATR locus. When human α1AT cDNA is used as a hybridization probe, EcoRI-treated human genomic DNA exhibits a 9.6 kb dark band and rather faint 7.7 and/or 5.8 kb bands. Bao and his colleagues (3) cloned and analyzed a 7.7 kb fragment. The nucleotide sequence revealed exten-

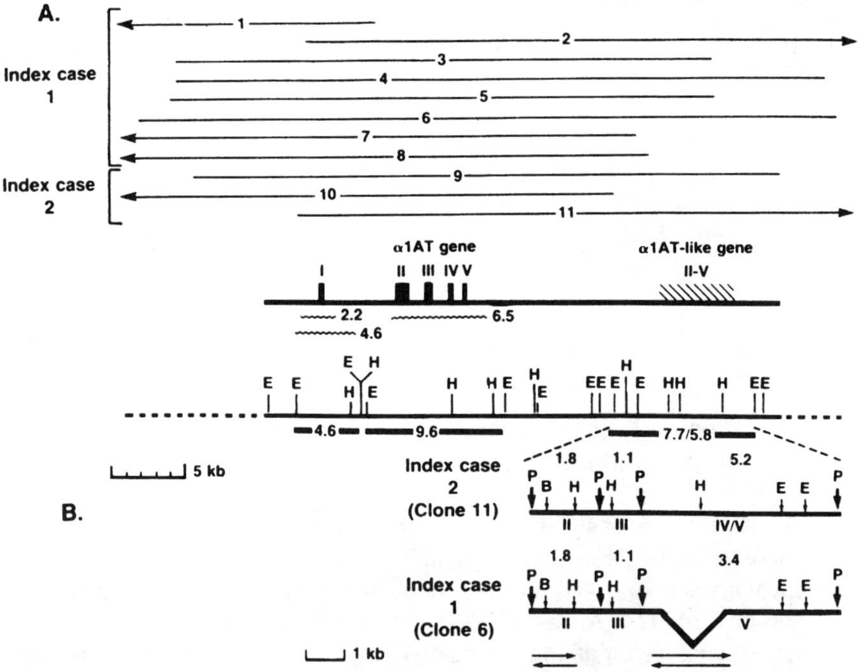


**Figure 1** Restriction map analysis of the cosmid clones covering the α1AT gene and the α1AT-like gene. (A) Restriction map of overlapping cosmid clones covering the α1AT and the α1AT-like genes (EcoRI: E, HindIII: H). The exons of the α1AT gene are indicated with filled boxes. The region of the α1AT-like gene is indicated with hatched box. The genomic probes 4.6 (and subclone 2.2) and 6.5 are indicated with broken lines. Note that clones 1–8 are from an individual with a truncated α1AT-like gene with a deletion of encompassing exon IV and parts of exon V. (B) The region containing the α1AT-like gene has been enlarged, showing the EcoRI (E), HindIII (H), and PstI (P) map. The PstI restriction fragments with homology to α1AT exons are indicated. Regions sequenced are indicated by double arrows. Clone 6 has a deletion of 1.8 kb, altering the 5.2 kb PstI fragment into a 3.4 kb fragment. (From Ref. 4.)

sive homology with the authentic α1AT gene in the possible introns as well as in the possible exons. All RNA-spliced sites were conserved and there were no internal termination codons in the exonic regions, suggesting that if the gene was expressed it could result in 420 amino acid residues, exhibiting a 70% overall homology with human α1AT. One remarkable feature of the 7.7 kb gene is the difference in the active site for proteinases. The cleaved site $Met^{358}$–$Ser^{359}$ in the α1AT gene has been changed to Try–Ser in ATR, suggesting an altered substrate specificity. Even the intronic regions in the related gene exhibit a 65% overall nucleotide homology with those of the authentic α1AT gene, indicating a recent duplication of the authentic α1AT gene some 70 M years ago. However, no transcript was detected in total RNA from human liver when an exonic DNA fragment of the α1AT-related gene was used as probe in an S1 nuclease protection assay.

Hofker and his colleagues (4) cloned and analyzed both 7.7 kb and 5.8 kb genes from different individuals. In contrast to the findings with a clone studied by Bao et al., they reported several different features of a 5.8 kb clone and concluded that the truncated α1AT-like gene is a pseudogene. First, hybridization with 4.6 kb EcoRI fragment encompassing the 5′ flanking region of the authentic α1AT yielded no additional hybridization signal, suggesting that the α1AT-like gene arose through a gene duplication, with a breakpoint in the intron between exons I and II of the authentic α1AT gene leading to a truncated gene without a normal 5′ flanking region (Fig. 1). Sequencing of a part of the pseudogene revealed that, despite 76% of overall homology, the translation initiation codon in exon II was mutated from ATG to ATA. Several additional insertions and glycosylation acceptor sites mutations were noted. Above all, a large deletion of 1795 bp encompassing exon IV to a part of exon V, including the region coding for the active site of the α1AT protein, was found in a 5.8 kb clone. The gene frequency of this deletion variant is very popular; as high as 0.3 is reported in the Dutch population (4).

## II. α1AT Gene Diversity in Mammals: Implication of Amino Acid Differences Found in Related Species

The baboon α1AT cDNA (5) was the first α1AT cDNA cloned from mammals and used as a probe to screen a human α1AT clone. To date, α1AT genes from human, baboon, sheep, mouse, rat, and rabbit have been cloned and reported (5–10). In rodents, the N-terminal regions were five amino acids shorter than those of primates. The nucleotide sequence homologies of the cDNA in the different species are 70 to 80%, while those for other serpins are 50 to 60%. In contrast, amino acids around active sites are highly conserved; all species have $Met^{358}$–$Ser^{359}$, and residues 332 to 350 and residues 380 to 394 showed 90% and 80% homologies, respectively (10).

The information on amino acid substitutions between different species provides a naturally occurring physiological substitution on both structural and functional conservedness in evolution in regard to the interpretation of the three-dimensional structure of α1AT protein. In this context, Seyama and his colleagues (11) analyzed the amino acid substitutions between human and baboon α1AT in relation to the mutational matrix number proposed by Dayhoff et al. (12) and the conservedness of residues in the serpin family (13). It is very likely that all 29 amino acid differences between human α1AT and baboon α1AT occur at less conserved residues with a positive (0 to positive) mutational matrix number, i.e., more common in amino acid substitutions in such protein families as serpins. In contrast, replacement with more negative (0 to minus) mutational matrix numbers at the positions of highly conserved residues is found in human α1AT variants of pathological importance, suggesting that evolutionally rare and functionally diverse substitutions occur at the sterically critical area in deficient α1AT variants.

## III. α1AT Gene Diversity in Higher Primates

In higher primates, such as gorillas and chimpanzees, less nucleotide difference in a gene, and hence fewer amino acid substitutions in a mature protein, are expected when compared with more distant primates. This can also be used to interpret the diversity of normal α1AT variants in humans.

In this regard, we have cloned and sequenced genomic DNAs of α1AT from gorilla and chimpanzee in the coding regions entirely containing exons II to V (Fig. 2). Between the human α1AT M1($Ala^{213}$) gene (14) and the gorilla α1AT gene, there are 19 nucleotide differences, which caused eight amino acid substitutions. Between the human α1AT M1($Ala^{213}$) gene and chimpanzee α1AT, there are 11 nucleotide differences, which corresponded to only two amino acid substitutions, $Pro^{-23}$ to Leu and $Met^{385}$ to Val. It should be noted that, because $Pro^{-23}$ to Leu occurred in the leading peptide, only one amino acid difference exists between human α1AT M1($Ala^{213}$) and chimpanzee α1AT in the secretory mature form. Utilizing the information on nucleotide substitutions in the coding sequence of the α1AT genes, Miyata and his colleagues (personal communication) calculated the divergent time of human and chimpanzee to be 6.0 M years and that of human and gorilla 8.0 M years, assuming that the divergent time of human and baboon is 30 M years.

## IV. Possible Phylogenetic Tree of Normal Human α1AT Variant Genes

Among pleomorphic variants of the α1AT proteins, at least five major normal variants have been recognized to date: M1($Ala^{213}$), M1($Val^{213}$), M2, M3, and M4

(14– 17). Although M1, M2, M3, and M4 can be discriminated on high-resolution isoelectric focusing, M1($Ala^{213}$) and M1($Val^{213}$) can be distinguished only at the DNA level (14). The phenotype frequencies of M1($Ala^{213}$), M1($Val^{213}$), M2, M3, and M4 among the U.S. Caucasian population are 20–23%, 44–49%, 14–19%, 10–11%, and about 1%, respectively. These normal variants consist of the combinations of the following three amino acid substitutions: $Arg^{101}$(CGT) to His(CAT), $Ala^{213}$(GCG) to Val(GTG), and $Glu^{376}$(GAA) to Asp(GAC). These amino acid substitutions are major substitutions in the α1AT protein. We and others (18) confirmed this through the sequencing of the exons in both normal variant α1AT genes and deficient variant α1AT genes. Through the cloning of the genomic DNA of variant α1AT genes, only certain combinations of these three substitutions have been proved to correspond to the phenotypes defined by IEF, indicating that certain combinations of these amino acid substitutions are allelic markers for haplotypes.

In this context, M1($Ala^{213}$) has the $Arg^{101}$–$Ala^{213}$–$Glu^{376}$ combination, M1($Val^{213}$) the $Arg^{101}$–$Val^{213}$–$Glu^{376}$ combination, M2 the $His^{101}$–$Val^{213}$–$Asp^{376}$ combination, M3 the $Arg^{101}$–$Val^{213}$–$Asp^{376}$ combination, and M4 the $His^{101}$–$Val^{213}$–$Glu^{376}$ combination (Fig. 3). The α1AT genes in higher primates—baboons, gorillas, and chimpanzees—all have $Arg^{101}$–$Ala^{213}$–$Glu^{376}$ combinations, although additional amino acid substitutions on the different residues exist. Ala–Val substitution is the only amino acid difference between the two most prevalent variants, M1($Ala^{213}$) and M1($Val^{213}$). Altogether, the Ala–Val substitution on residue 213 is likely the first amino acid substitution occurring in the coding sequence of the current human α1AT gene, and M1($Ala^{213}$) seems to be the oldest variant known to date. This phylogenetic tree of human normal variants starts from M1($Ala^{213}$), and the Ala–Val substitution on residue 213 resulted in a newer variant, M1($Val^{213}$) (Fig. 3). Additional substitutions of Glu–Asp on residue 376 caused M3 and of Arg-His on residue 101 yielded M4, although the gene frequency of M4 is far lower than that of M3. One more substitution of Arg–His on residue 101 of the M3 gene resulted in an M2 variant (also possibly due to Glu–Asp on residue 376 of an M4 variant).

These amino acid substitutions on three residues can be utilized as a kind of allelic marker on rare α1AT variants. For example, the classic α1AT-deficient variant type Z has a pathological mutation Glu–Lys on residue 342 on the background of the $Arg^{101}$–$Ala^{213}$–$Glu^{376}$ combination, i.e., M1($Ala^{213}$) (14). Another rare $M_{Malton}$-deficient variant has a pathological deletion of $Phe^{52}$ on the background of the $His^{101}$–$Val^{213}$–$Asp^{376}$ combination, i.e., M2 background (19).

Moreover, there is a possibility that these three amino acid substitutions are also unique to contemporary human races. When genomic DNA from 156 Japanese individuals was analyzed using PCR and restriction endonuclease BstPI, which recognizes the nucleotide sequences around residue 213, all were proved to have valine on residue 213 and none had alanine on residue 213 among 312

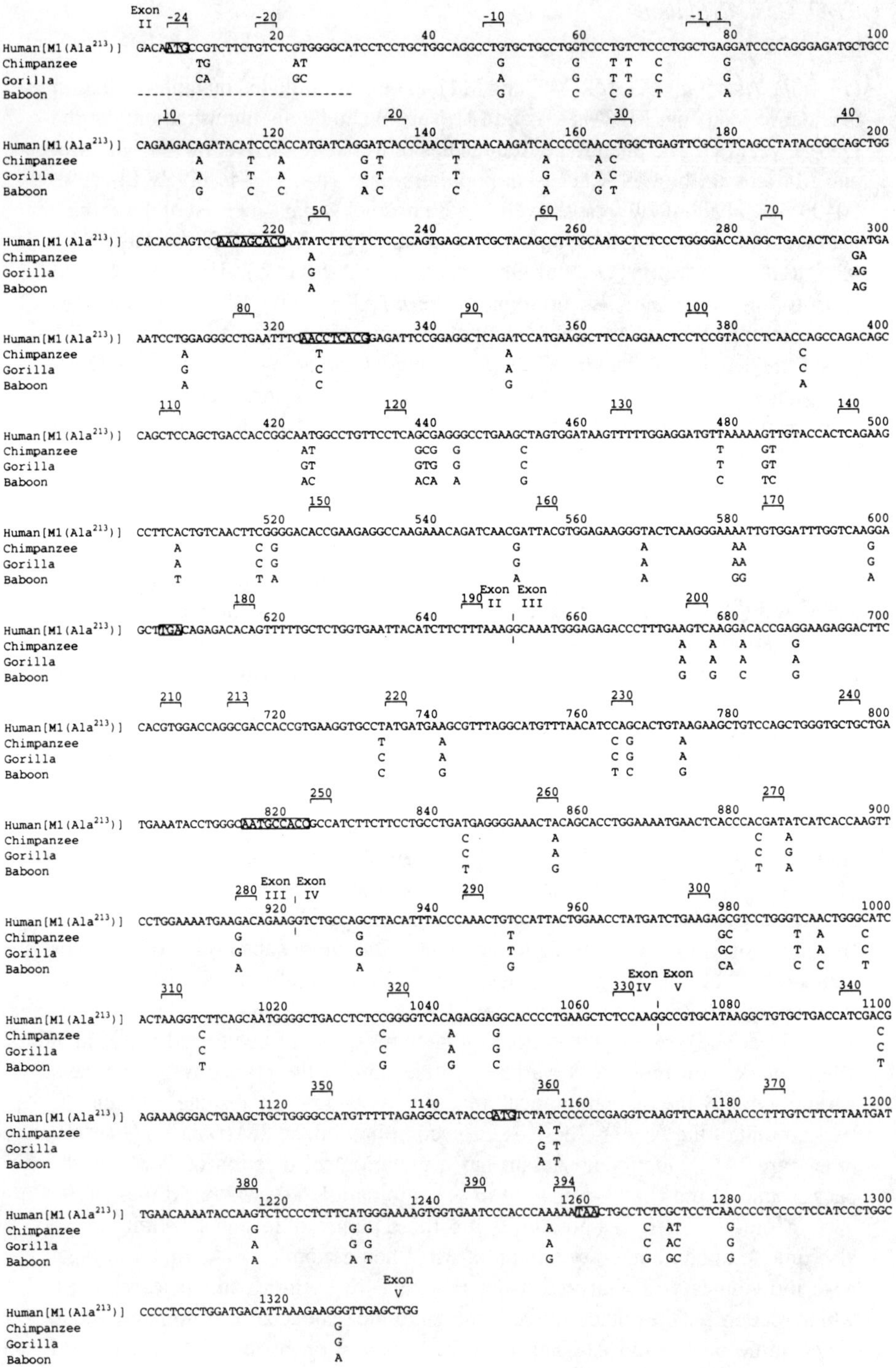

```
                Exon  -24        -20                    -10                    -1 1
                II                          20                40                60                80               100
Human[M1(Ala213)] GACAATGCCGTCTTCTGTCTCGTGGGGCATCCTCCTGCTGGCAGGCCTGTGCTGCCTGGTCCCTGTCTCCCTGGCTGAGGATCCCCAGGGAGATGCTGCC
Chimpanzee              TG        AT                   G                 G  T T      C            G
Gorilla                CA        GC                   A                 G  T T  C            G
Baboon          ---------------------------           G                 C    C G T          A

                     10                      20                      30                      40
                          120               140               160               180               200
Human[M1(Ala213)] CAGAAGACAGATACATCCCACCATGATCGGAGTCACCCAACCTTCAACAAGATCACCCCCAACCTGGCTGAGTTCGCCTTCAGCCTATACCGCCAGCTGG
Chimpanzee              A   T  A           GT          T              A      A C
Gorilla               A   T  A           GT          T              A      A C
Baboon                G   C  C           A C          C              A      G T

                          50                      60                      70
                          220               240               260               280               300
Human[M1(Ala213)] CACACCAGTCCAACAGCACCAAATATCTTCTTCTCCCCAGTGAGCATCGCTACAGCCTTTGCAATGCTCTCCCTGGGGACCAAGGCTGACACTCACGATGA
Chimpanzee                         A                                                                      GA
Gorilla                          G                                                                       AG
Baboon                           A                                                                       AG

                     80                      90                      100
                          320               340               360               380               400
Human[M1(Ala213)] AATCCTGGAGGGCCTGAATTTCAACCTCACGGAGATTCCGGAGGCTCAGATCCATGAAGGCTTCCAGGAACTCCTCCGTACCCTCAACCAGCCAGACAGC
Chimpanzee                A          T                  A                                         C
Gorilla                  G          C                  A                                         C
Baboon                   A          C                  G                                         A

                  110                      120                      130                      140
                          420               440               460               480               500
Human[M1(Ala213)] CAGCTCCAGCTGACCACCGGCAATGGCCTGTTCCTCAGCGAGGGCCTGAAGCTAGTGGATAAGTTTTTGGAGGATGTTAAAAAGTTGTACCACTCAGAAG
Chimpanzee                AT          GCG  G      C                                T   GT
Gorilla                  GT          GTG  G      C                                T   GT
Baboon                   AC          ACA  A      G                                C   TC

                     150                      160                      170
                          520               540               560               580               600
Human[M1(Ala213)] CCTTCACTGTCAACTTCGGGGACACCGAAGAGGCCAAGAAACAGATCAACGATTACGTGGAGAAGGGTACTCAAGGGAAAATTGTGGATTTGGTCAAGGA
Chimpanzee         A      C G                 G           A      AA        G
Gorilla            A      C G                 G           A      AA        G
Baboon             T      T A                 A           A      GG        A

                  180                      190 Exon Exon            200
                          620               640    II   III        680               700
Human[M1(Ala213)] GCTTGACAGAGACACAGTTTTTGCTCTGGTGAATTACATCTTCTTTAAAAGGCAAATGGGAGAGACCCTTTGAAGTCAAGGACACCGAGGAAGAGGACTTC
Chimpanzee                                                                           A  A  A        G
Gorilla                                                                             A  A  A        A
Baboon                                                                              G  G  C        G

                  210    213          220                      230                      240
                          720               740               760               780               800
Human[M1(Ala213)] CACGTGGACCAGGCGACCACCGTGAAGGTGCCTATGATGAAGCGTTTAGGCATGTTTAACATCCAGCACTGTAAGAAGCTGTCCAGCTGGGTGCTGCTGA
Chimpanzee                      T      A                  C G     A
Gorilla                        C      A                  C G     A
Baboon                         C      G                  T C     G

                  250                      260                      270
                          820               840               860               880               900
Human[M1(Ala213)] TGAAATACCTGGGCAATGCCACCGCCATCTTCTTCCTGCCTGATGAGGGGAAACTACAGCACCTGGAAAATGAACTCACCCACGATATCATCACCAAGTT
Chimpanzee                         C          A                          C  A
Gorilla                          C          A                          C  G
Baboon                           T          G                          T  A

                  280 Exon Exon            290                      300
                          920   III  IV    940               960               980              1000
Human[M1(Ala213)] CCTGGAAAATGAAGCAGAAGGTCTGCCCAGCTTACATTTACCCAAACTGTCCATTACTGGAACCTATGATCTGAAGAGCGTCCTGGGTCAACTGGGCATC
Chimpanzee         G           G             T             GC    T A    C
Gorilla            G           G             T             GC    T A    C
Baboon             A           A             G             CA    C C    T

                  310                      320                      330 Exon Exon            340
                          1020              1040              1060   IV   V    1080             1100
Human[M1(Ala213)] ACTAAGGTCTTCAGCAATGGGGCTGACCTCTCCGGGGTCACAGAGGAGGCACCCCTGAAGCTCTCCAAGGCCGTGCATAAGGCTGTGCTGACCATCGACG
Chimpanzee         C               C    A    G                                                        C
Gorilla            C               C    A    G                                                        C
Baboon             T               G    G    C                                                        T

                  350                      360                      370
                          1120              1140              1160              1180             1200
Human[M1(Ala213)] AGAAAGGGACTGAAGCTGCTGGGGCCATGTTTTTAGAGGCCATACCCATGTCTATCCCCCCCGAGGTCAAGTTCAACAAACCCTTTGTCTTCTTAATGAT
Chimpanzee                                                    A T
Gorilla                                                       G T
Baboon                                                        A T

                  380                      390      394
                          1220              1240              1260              1280             1300
Human[M1(Ala213)] TGAACAAAATACCAAGTCTCCCCTCTTCATGGGAAAAGTGGTGAATCCCACCCAAAAATAATGCTGCTCTCGCTCCTCAACCCCTCCCCTCCATCCCTGGC
Chimpanzee              GG            GG         A          C AT    G
Gorilla                 GG            GG         A          C AC    G
Baboon                  A            AT         G          G GC    G

                                    Exon
                          1320      V
Human[M1(Ala213)] CCCCTCCCTGGATGACATTAAAGAAGGGTTGAGCTGG
Chimpanzee                        G
Gorilla                          G
Baboon                           A
```

alleles, indicating that Japanese people do not have the normal variant M1 ($Ala^{213}$)—an older variant on the phylogenetic tree—or variants derived from that (20). This in turn may explain the rare occurrence of the classic Z-type deficiency variant among Japanese or Orientals, which is derived from M1($Ala^{213}$), although the entire α1AT genomic sequence needs to be evaluated to prove this concept. In this context, it is of interest that Matsunaga and his colleagues (21) compared three genomic sequences of α1AT genes (an S-deficient gene from a Caucasian, an M1($Val^{213}$) gene from a Japanese, and an $M_{nichinan}$-deficient gene from a Japanese) and found less nucleotide differences between the Japanese M1($Val^{213}$) and $M_{nichinan}$ genes compared with the S gene from a Caucasoid. They also described the incidence of the nucleotide change in the 9439 bp nonprotein coding region of the M1($Val^{213}$), $M_{nichinan}$, and S genes as being one base change per 163 bp, which

---

**Figure 2** Comparison of the nucleotide sequences of the coding exons (exons II to V) of α1AT genes from human [M1($Ala^{213}$)], chimpanzee, gorilla, and cDNA of α1AT gene from baboon. The complete α1AT nucleotide sequence (exons II to V) shown on the top is from human α1AT type M1($Ala^{213}$). Differences in the nucleotides are shown in the second (chimpanzee), third (gorilla), and fourth (baboon) lines. The exon boundaries are indicated by the broken vertical lines. The numbers on the top, corresponding to three nucleotides, indicate the deduced amino acid numbers; amino acids within the signal peptide are identified with minus numbers. The numbers of the nucleotide sequence start from the first nucleotide G of the exon II. An open box at nucleotides 5–7, ATG, indicates the open reading frame. Three open boxes at nucleotides 212–220, 323–331, and 815–823 correspond to three carbohydrate attachment sites (Asn-X-Thr). A box at 1259–1261 shows termination signal TAA. The corresponding bases of the three primates α1AT genes are indicated only at variable sites. The dashed line for baboon (nucleotides 1 to 29) indicates that the sequence is not available in the literature.

*Methods*: The nucleotide sequence of human α1AT M1($Ala^{213}$) is from the previous report (24), using the genomic DNA clones of α1AT type M1($Ala^{213}$) exons II to V. The nucleotide sequence of baboon is from the report of Kurachi et al. (5), the sequence of a cDNA pBaa1A2, cloned from a library constructed with baboon liver. The nucleotide sequence of chimpanzee and gorilla were newly analyzed. The genomic DNA library from a chimpanzee (partial EcoRI fragments inserted into Charon 32 lambda phage) was kindly provided by Dr. Slightom (Upjohn, Kalamazoo, Mich.). The genomic DNA library from a gorilla (Tomoka, of the National Zoo in Washington, D.C., partial EcoRI fragments cloned into Charon 4A lambda phage) was the gift of Dr. Scott (Johns Hopkins University, Baltimore, Md). Both libraries were screened with a human genomic DNA exon I probe (StuI fragment, 1.9 kb) and exon V probe (PstI fragment, 1.1 kb) (14). A chimpanzee clone, 10 kb, was further subcloned into three PstI fragments of 1.6 kb containing exons II, 2.4 kb encompassing exons III to IV, and 1.1 kb containing exon V, and sequenced bidirectionally using the dideoxynucleotide termination method with synthetic primers. The gorilla α1AT clone, 18 kb, was subcloned into three fragments: 2.0 kb EcoRI-PstI containing exon II, 2.4 kb PstI fragment contains exons III and IV, and 1.6 kb PstI fragment containing exon V, and sequenced as described above.

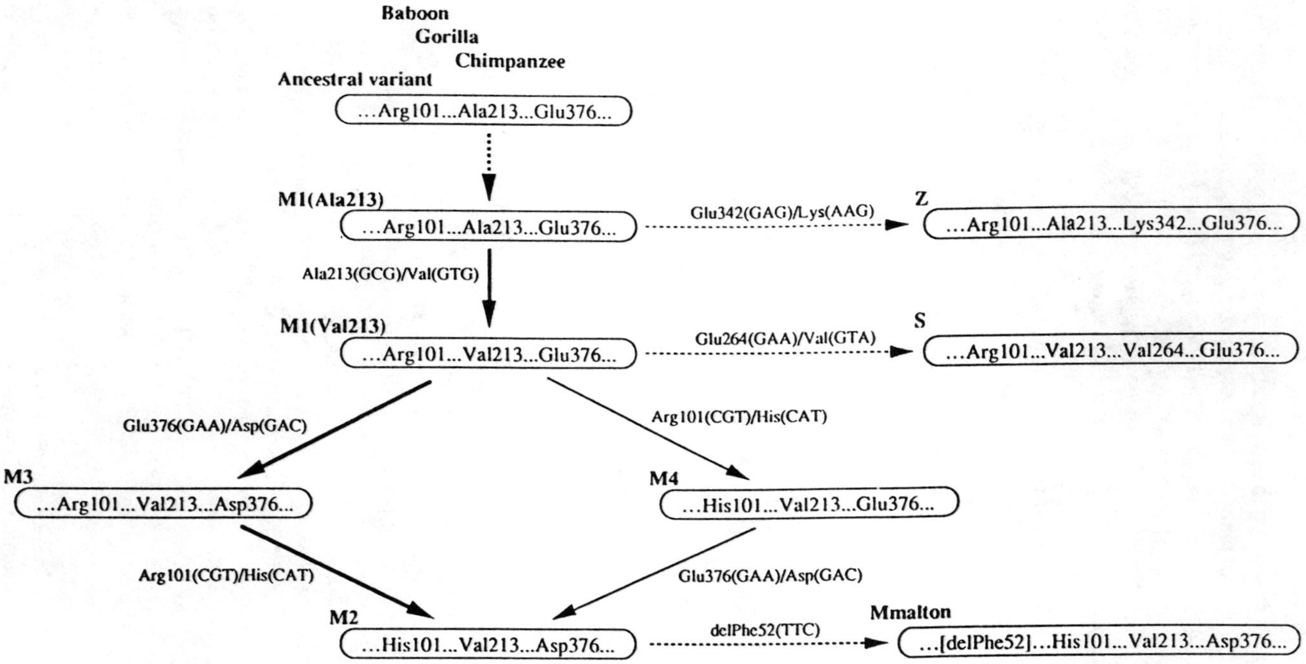


**Figure 3** Possible phylogenetic tree based on the allelic mutations in the coding exons of the α1AT gene. Major amino acid substitutions of normal variants on residues 101, 213, and 376 correspond to exons II, III, and V of the α1AT genomic structure, respectively—(specifically, these correspond to the mutation at nucleotide numbers, 5738, 7524, and 10093 of the reported sequence of

is higher than that estimated in human genome sequences by Cooper et al. (22) (one change per 200 or 300 bp), thereby suggesting that the α1AT gene is relatively susceptible to mutations.

There are exceptions, however, to this phylogenetic tree. When the rare deficient variant Zaugusburg is sequenced (23), it has pathological mutation of $Glu^{342}$ to Lys on a background of M2 ($His^{101}$–$Val^{213}$–$Asp^{376}$ combination). The sequence around the $Glu^{342}$ has a number of AG repetitions, suggesting an area of possible increased mutational activity. Alternately, the Zaugusburg variant could have arisen via genetic recombination in an M2Z heterozygote. Probably similar mechanisms might have worked in the formation of the M4 variant (17) because of its very low incidence among the major normal variants.

## V. Summary

There is abundant information on evolution concerning both variations within the serpin superfamily and differences between α1AT genes among mammalian species. Resemblance between the exon–intron structures of α1AT and α1ACT and their proximity on chromosome 14q31 indicate relatively recent divergence of these genes. Although two kinds of high homologous α1AT-like genes exist about 10 kb downstream of the authentic gene, these seem to be truncated pseudogenes. Coding exons (exons II to V) of chimpanzee and gorilla were recently sequenced. Only one amino acid difference has been shown between human α1AT M1($Ala^{213}$) and chimpanzee α1AT. Cloning of normal and deficient α1AT variants revealed the existence of three major amino acid substitutions—$Arg^{101}$–His, $Ala^{213}$–Val, and $Glu^{376}$–Asp—and certain combinations of these mutations correspond to the phenotypes defined on IEF. Utilizing these substitutions as haplotype markers, a possible phylogenetic tree of current major normal variants is as follows: M1($Ala^{213}$)–M1($Val^{213}$)–M3–M2 (or M4–M2). Some of these markers may correspond to the differences in the α1AT genes found in contemporary human races.

---

α1AT genomic DNA by Long et al. (6). Certain combinations of these allelic mutations have been proved to correspond to serum phenotypes by cloning of phenotype-determined α1AT genomic DNAs. (Left) the possible tree structure of the major normal variants. The dotted arrow at the top suggests the existence of the ancestral variant of the human α1AT gene. Five major variants—M1($Ala^{213}$), M1($Val^{213}$), M2, M3, and M4—are shown with amino acid and nucleotide substitutions added along the arrows. Variant M4 is connected with thin arrows because of low incidence and the possibility of genetic recombination. (Right) some examples of the deficient variants possibly derived from the major normal variants connected with thin dotted arrows. Pathological mutations or deletion of these deficient variants are shown along the dotted arrows.

## References


1. Sefton L, Kelsey G, Kearney P, Pove S, Wolfe J. A physical map of the human PI and AACT genes. Genomics 1990; 7:382–388.
2. Bao J-J, Sifers RN, Kidd VJ, Ledley FD, Woo SLC. Molecular evolution of serpins: homologous structure of the human α1-antichymotrypsin and α1-antitrypsin genes. Biochemistry 1987; 26:7755–7759.
3. Bao J-J, Reed-Fourquet L, Sifers RN, Kidd VJ, Woo SLC. Molecular structure and sequence homology of a gene related to α1-antitrypsin in the human genome. Genomics 1988; 2:165–173.
4. Hofker MH, Nelen M, Klasen EC, Nukiwa T, Curiel D, Crystal RG, Frants RR. Cloning and characterization of an α1-antitrypsin gene 12 kb downstream of the genuine α1-antitrypsin gene. Biochem Biophys Res Commun 1988; 155:634–642.
5. Kurachi K, Chandra T, Degen SJF, White TT, Marchioro TL, Woo SLC. Cloning and sequence of cDNA coding for alpha-antitrypsin. Proc Natl Acad Sci USA 1981; 78:6826–6830.
6. Long GL, Chandra T, Woo SLC, Davie EW, Kurachi K. Complete sequence of the cDNA for human alpha-1-antitrypsin and the gene for the S variant. Bichemistry 1984; 23:4828–4837.
7. Brown WM, Dziegielewska KM, Foreman RC, Saunders NR, Wu Y. Nucleotide and deduced amino acid sequence of sheep α1-antitrypsin. Nucl Acids Res 1989; 17: 6398.
8. Sifers RN, Ledley FD, Reed-Fourquet L, Ledbetter DH, Ledbetter SA, Woo SLC. Genebank, Accession M25529, 1989.
9. Chao S, Chai KX, Chao L, Chao J. Molecular cloning and primary structure of rat α1-antitrypsin. Biochemistry 1990; 29:323–329.
10. Saito A, Sinohara H. Cloning and sequencing of cDNA coding for rabbit α-1-antiproteinase F: aminoacid sequence comparison of α-1-antiproteinases of six mammals. J Biochem 1991; 109:158–162.
11. Seyama K, Nukiwa T, Takabe K, Takahashi H, Miyake K, Kira S. Siiyama (serine 53 (TCC) to phenylalanine 53 (TTC)): a new α1-antitrypsin deficient variant with mutation on a predicted conserved residue of the serpin backbone. J Biol Chem 1991; 266:12627–12632.
12. Dayhoff MO, Schwartz RM, Orcutt BC. Atlas of protein sequence and structure. Washington, DC: National Biochemical Foundation, 1987:345–352.
13. Carrell RW, Travis J. α1-antitrypsin and the serpins: variation and countervariation. Trends Biochem Sci 1985; 10:20–24.
14. Nukiwa T, Satoh K, Brantly ML, Ogushi F, Fells GA, Courtney M, Crystal RG. Identification of a second mutation in the protein-coding sequence of the Z type alpha 1-antitrypsin gene. J Biol Chem 1986; 261:15989–15994.
15. Nukiwa T, Brantly ML, Ogushi F, Fells GA, Crystal RG. Characterization of the gene and protein of the common α1-antitrypsin normal M2 allele. Am J Hum Genet 1988; 43:322–330.
16. Curiel D, Laubach V, Vogeimeier C, Wurts L, Crystal RG. Characterization of the

sequence of the normal alpha-1-antitrypsin M3 allele and function of the M3 protein. Am J Respir Cell Mol Biol 1989; 1:471–477.
17. Okayama H, Holmes MD, Brantly ML, Crystal RG. Characterization of the coding sequence of the normal M4 α1-antitrypsin gene. Biochem Biophys Res Commun 1989; 162:1560–1570.
18. Graham A, Kalsheker NA, Newton CR, Bamforth FJ, Powell SJ, Markham AF. Molecular characterisation of three alpha-1-antitrypsin deficiency variants: proteinase inhibitor (Pi) nullcardiff (Asp256—Val); PiMmalton (Phe51—deletion) and PiI (Arg39—Cys). Hum Genet 1989; 84(1):55–58.
19. Curiel DT, Holmes MD, Okayama H, Brantly ML, Vogelmeier C, Travis WD, Stier LE, Perks WH, Crystal RG. Molecular basis of the liver and lung disease associated with the α1-antitrypsin deficiency allele $M_{malton}$. J Biol Chem 1989; 264:13938–13945.
20. Nukiwa T, Seyama K, Takahashi H, Takahashi K, Ohwada A, Matsuda K, Kira S. Why is Z type α1-antitrypsin deficiency not found in Japan? Jap J Thoracic Soc 1991; 29(suppl):371.
21. Matsunaga E, Shiokawa S, Nakamura H, Maruyama T, Tsuda K, Fukumaki Y. Molecular analysis of the gene of the α1-antitrypsin deficiency variant, $M_{nichinan}$. Am J Hum Genet 1990; 46:602–612.
22. Cooper DN, Smith BA, Cooke HJ, Niemann S, Schmidtke J. An estimate of unique DNA sequence heterozygosity of the human genome. Hum Genet 1985; 69:201–205.
23. Faber J-P, Weidinger S, Olek K. Sequence data of the rare deficient alpha 1-antitrypsin variant PI Zaugusburg. Am J Hum Genet 1990; 46:1158–1162.
24. Nukiwa T, Brantly M, Ogushi F, Fells G, Satoh K, Stier L, Courtney M, Crystal RG. Characterization of the M1($Ala^{213}$) type of α1-antitrypsin, a newly recognized, common "normal" α1-antitrypsin haplotype. Biochemistry 1987; 26:5259–5267.

# 4

# Alpha 1–Antitrypsin Genotypes and Phenotypes

**MARK BRANTLY**

Pulmonary–Critical Care Medicine Branch
National Heart, Lung, and Blood Institute
National Institutes of Health
Bethesda, Maryland

## I. Introduction

Our understanding of the inheritance of normal and abnormal alpha 1–antitrypsin ($\alpha$1AT) genes began with the observation that emphysema and the absence of alpha 1–globulin were transmitted to more than one generation (1). The variant X was the first $\alpha$1AT variant of normal identified (2). The very rare X variant, characterized on agrose-gel electrophoresis as a slow migrating doublet, was not associated with the disease or a low $\alpha$1AT level. This observation, in combination with the already identified deficient and common normal variants, led Axelsson and Laurell (2) to propose that $\alpha$1AT was a three-allele system that was codominantly inherited. At about the same time, Fagerhol and Braend (3), utilizing the new technique of starch-gel electrophoresis to evaluate serum electrophoretic polymorphism, determined that variation in the prealbumin region was the result of electrophoretic variants of $\alpha$1AT. Together these variants constituted an allelic system that early investigators called the Pi (protease inhibitor) system. Variants, initially named according to their migration rates in a starch-gel electrophoresis system, were divided into three groups: medium (M), fast (F), and slow (S). The very slow (Z) variant was later added to the allelic system (4).

The number of newly identified α1AT variants increased with each incremental advance to electrophoresis technology. Because variants were identified based on their pI differences, it was presumed that most of these differences were due to substitutions of differently charged amino acids. Early investigators believed that the Z variant was the result of a substitution of a negatively charged amino acid for a positively charged one. The molecular nature of the Z variant was confirmed using protolytic digestion, two-dimensional electrophoresis, and peptide sequencing of the Z variant demonstrating a glutamine-to-lysine substitution in an abnormally migrating tryptic fragment (5).

In the early 1980s our understanding of the molecular basis of α1AT variation made a substantial advance following the cloning and sequencing of the α1AT cDNA and, later, the α1AT genomic segment (6,7). Initially, novel variants were cloned and sequenced. However, the development of the polymerase chain reaction allowed for direct sequencing of DNA as an alternative to labor-intensive screening and cloning of α1AT variants prior to sequencing (8).

## II. Nomenclature and Definitions

α1AT variants are now named according to their migration characteristics in a pH 4–5 isoelectric focusing gel. The most anodal variants are assigned letters from the beginning of the alphabet; the most cathodal migrating variants are assigned letters from the end of the alphabet. Isoelectric focusing of the α1AT demonstrates both pleomorphism among variants and microheterogeneity with a single variant (Fig. 1). Assignment of the numbers corresponding to the banding patterns of α1AT is based on crossed immunoelectrophoresis, and some bands seen in crossed immunoelectrophoresis are not seen on IEF. Bands not seen on IEF included the 1, 3, and 5 bands. The major bands of α1AT are the 4 and 6 bands, and the minor bands are the 2, 7, and 8 bands. The 2, 4, and 6 bands migrate differently from one another because of differences in the degree of carbohydrate side-chain branching. The 7 and 8 bands are similar in carbohydrate composition to the 4 and 6 bands, but differ in their migration pattern because 5 amino acids have been cleaved from the N-terminus of both bands (Fig. 1) (9). There are many normal alleles and at least four (M1–M4) common middle migrating M variants (Fig. 1). Designations for the rarer new alleles are, by convention, a combination of the letter of the most closely migrating variant and the city of the oldest living carrier of the variant (10,11). The α1AT allelic system, formally abbreviated Pi for protease inhibitor, now uses PI* to designate the gene locus, in keeping with the international convention of identifying genetic loci by capital letters. Null α1AT variants—variants that do not have detectable serum α1AT—are now designated QO.

For clinical classification purposes, α1AT variants may be divided into at least four different categories: normal variants—with normal α1AT levels and not

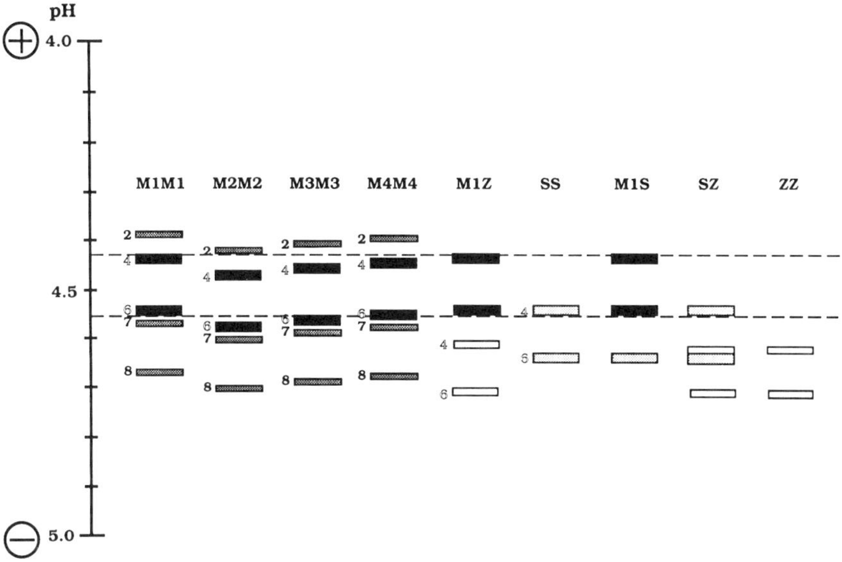


**Figure 1** Schematic of α1-antitrypsin PI types separated according their isoelectric point. Isoelectric focusing of α1AT on a thin-layer polyacrylamide gel. In a pH gradient of 4–5, α1AT variants migrate as two major bands designated 4 and 6; additionally, three minor bands—2, 7, and 8—contribute to the microheterogeneity of α1AT (9). Major variation in the migration of α1AT alleles is the result of amino acid substitutions that alter the net charge of the protein and hence the isoelectric point of the protein. The normal allele is M (black bands); the M variant has at least four subtypes: M1, M2, M3, and M4. The most common deficiency allele is Z (white bands). The Z variant bands are located near the cathode (−) and are significantly fainter because of the low serum α1AT concentration. The S variant bands (gray bands) migrate in a position intermediate to M and Z. Serum from heterozygous individuals, such as MZ, MS, and SZ, demonstrate a more complex pattern due to the individual contribution of each allele to the total α1AT serum concentration and phenotype.

associated with a risk of lung or liver disease; deficient variants—associated with reduced but detectable serum α1AT and with lung and/or liver disease; dysfunctional variants—associated with altered function, e.g., α1AT Pittsburgh; and null variants—which contribute no α1AT to the serum concentration and are associated with an increased risk of lung disease (Tables 1–3) (12,13). While deficiency of α1AT may be a relative term, the serum level of 11 μM was chosen as the upper limit for the category of deficiency based primarily on serum α1AT level of borderline deficient individuals with the PI*SZ phenotype, individuals who have an increased risk of emphysema (14,15).

**Table 1** Normal α1 AT Alleles

| Allele | Base allele | Exon[a] | Mutation |
|---|---|---|---|
| M1(Ala213) | | | |
| M1(Val213) | M1(Ala213) | III | Ala213 GCG→Val GTG |
| M3 | M1(Val213) | V | Glu376 GAA→Asp GAC |
| M2 | M3 | II | Arg101 CGT→His CAT |
| $M2_{obernburg}$ | M1(Ala213) | II | Gly148 GGG→Trp TGG |
| M4 | M1(Val213 | II | Arg101 CGT→His CAT |
| $M5_{karlsruhe}$ | M1(Val213) | II | Ala34 GCCT→Thr ACC |
| $M5_{berlin}$ | M1(Val213) | II | Pro88 CCG→Thr ACC |
| M6 | M1(Val213) | II | Ala60 GCC→Thr ACC |
| $L_{frankfurt}$ | M2 | II, III | Gln156 CAG→Glu GAG/Pro255 CCT→Thr ACT |
| $L_{offenbach}$ | M1(Val213) | V | Pro362 CCC→Thr ACC |
| V | M1(Val213) | II | Gly148 GAC→Asn AAC |
| $V_{donauworth}$ | M1(Val213) | V | Asp341 GAC→Asn AAC |
| $P_{st.\ albans}$ | M1(Val213) | III, V | Asp341 GAC→Asn AAC/Asp256 GAT→Asp GAC |
| X | M1(Val213) | III | Glu204→Lys |
| $X_{christchurch}$ | Unknown | V | Glu363→Lys |
| $V_{munich}$ | M1(Val213) | II | Asp2 GAT→ Ala GCT |
| $B_{alhambra}$ | Unknown | Unknown | Lys→Asp |
| $P_{st.\ louis}$ | M2 | III | Met221 ATG→Thr ACG |

[a]Exon in which the mutation is located.

Although the terms *phenotype* and *genotype* are sometimes used interchangeably to denote the PI type of individuals, *phenotype* refers specifically to the protein variant determined by IEF and based on a charge difference and *genotype* implies the specific identification of both parental alleles. The difference between these terms can best be illustrated by considering the heterozygous null individual. When an individual has the phenotype of PI*M1 determined by IEF and a level of 20 μM, the identity of the second allele is unconfirmed without an informative family study or specific DNA typing. This is because the other allele could be either a null allele expressing no α1AT or a second M1 allele giving rise to a serum α1AT level at the lower limit of normal.

## III. The Relationship of α1AT PI Type to α1AT Serum Concentration

The α1AT PI type dictates the serum α1AT concentration. Both alleles contribute to the α1AT serum concentration in proportion to their ability to express, synthesize, and secrete α1AT. Therefore, the combination of the profoundly deficient Z

**Table 2** Deficiency and Dysfunctional α1AT Alleles

| Allele | Base allele | Exon[a] | Mutation |
|---|---|---|---|
| Deficient | | | |
| F | M1(Val213) | III | Arg223 CGT→Cys TGT |
| Z | M1(Ala213) | V | Glu342 GAG→Lys AAG |
| T | M2 | III | Glu264 GAA→Val GTA |
| S | M1(Val213) | III | Glu264 GAA→Val GTA |
| $M_{heerlen}$ | M1(Ala213) | V | Pro369 CCC→Leu CTC |
| $M_{malton}$ | M2 | II | Phe52 TTC→delete |
| $M_{mineral\ springs}$ | M1(Ala213) | II | Gly67 GGG→Glu GAG |
| $M_{procida}$ | M1(Val213) | II | Leu41 CTG→Pro CCG |
| $W_{bethesda}$ | M1(Ala213) | V | Ala336 GCT→Thr ACT |
| I | M1(Val213) | II | Arg39 CGC→Cys TGC |
| $M_{palermo}$ | M1(Val213) | II | Phe51 TTC→delete |
| $M_{nichinan}$ | M1(Val213) | II | Phe52 TTC→delete/Gly148 GGG→Arg AGG |
| $P_{lowell}$ | M1(Val213) | III | Asp256 GAT→Val GTT |
| $P_{duarte}$ | M4 | III | Asp256 GAT→Val GTT |
| $S_{iiyama}$ | M1(Val213) | II | Phe53 TTC→Ser TCC |
| $Z_{ausburg}$ | M2 | V | Glu342 GAG→Lys AAG |
| Dysfunctional | | | |
| Pittsburgh | Unknown | V | Met358→Arg |

[a]Exon in which the mutation is located.

variant and the normal M1 variant will result in an intermediate α1AT serum concentration (Fig. 2) (16). Because the α1AT gene is responsive to acute-phase stimuli, there can be substantial variation in the serum concentration, depending on whether the individual has an inflammatory condition, is pregnant, or is taking a drug that mimics the acute-phase response. In this context there is substantial overlap in the total serum α1AT level among different combinations of α1AT variants.

## IV. Inheritance of α1AT Alleles

The clinical phenotypes for emphysema and liver disease are inherited in a recessive fashion; i.e., two deficient or null alleles are required to substantially increase the risk of disease. The "biochemical" phenotype (the α1AT level and IEF pattern) is the result of autosomal and codominant inheritance of both parental genes' α1AT alleles. Transmission of α1AT alleles follows basic mendelian

**Table 3** Null α1AT Alleles

| Allele | Base allele | Exon[a] | Mutation |
|---|---|---|---|
| $QO_{\text{granite falls}}$ | M1(Ala213) | II | Tyr 160 TAC→ delete C → 5′ shift → stop 160 TAG |
| $QO_{\text{bellingham}}$ | M1(Val213) | III | Lys217 AAG → stop 217 TAG |
| $QO_{\text{mattawa}}$ | M1(Val213) | V | Leu 353 TTA → insert T → 3′ shift → stop 376 TGA |
| $QO_{\text{bolton}}$ | M1(Val213) | V | Pro 362 CCC → delete C → 5′ shift → stop 373 TAA |
| $QO_{\text{hong kong}}$ | M2 | IV | Leu 318 CTC → delete TC → 5′ shift → stop 334 TAA |
| $QO_{\text{ludwigshafen}}$ | M2 | II | Ile 92 ATC → Asn AAC |
| $QO_{\text{isola di procida}}$ | Unknown | II–V | 10 kb deletion of exons II–V, ΔII–V |
| $QO_{\text{clayton}}$ | M1(Val213) | V | Pro 362 CCC → insert C → 3′ → stop376 TGA |
| $QO_{\text{bonny blue}}$ | M1(Val213) | [b] | ΔG deletion at position 1 of intron II splice acceptor |
| $QO_{\text{new hope}}$ | M1(Ala213) | IV, V | Gly320 GGG → Glu GAG/Glu 342 GAG → Lys AAG |
| $QO_{\text{trastevere}}$ | M1(Val213) | III | Trp194 TGG→ stop TGA |
| $QO_{\text{kowloon}}$ | M1(Val213) | II | Tyr38 TAC → stop TAA |
| $QO_{\text{saarbruecken}}$ | M1(Ala213) | V | Pro 362 CCC → insert C → 3′ shift → stop376 TGA |
| $QO_{\text{lisbon}}$ | M1(Val213) | II | Thr68 ACC→Ile ATC |
| $QO_{\text{reidenburg}}$ | Unknown | II–V | Deletion of exons II–V, ΔII–V |
| $QO_{\text{west}}$ | M1(Val213) | [b] | G→T position 1 of intron II splice donor substitution |

[a]Exon in which the mutation is located.
[b]Mutation in a noncoding portion of the α1AT gene.

genetics, and the probability that any one individual will receive two deficient or null alleles from parents who are carriers is 25% (Fig. 3).

## V. Genetic Variation at the α1AT Locus

There are at least 49 α1AT gene allelic variations characterized by DNA sequencing (Tables 1–3) (5,8,17–52). The α1AT gene, located on the long arm of chromosome 14 near the immunoglobulin locus, encompasses 12 kb (53). Approximately 11% of the nucleotide sequence codes for α1AT protein sequence and, not surprisingly, most of the characterized mutations are found within the protein-coding exons since screening for mutations is most often initiated based on protein variation (Figs. 4 and 5) (6,7). Among the mutations within the protein-coding regions, the mutations are relatively evenly dispersed. Two exceptions to this are the codon 51–53 region and the codon 361–363 region (Fig. 5). The most likely explanation for the concentration of variants in these locations is that these regions represent mutational "hot spots." Analysis of the nucleotide sequence in both areas reveals reiterated DNA sequences that may be sites of slippage misalignment (Fig. 5) (54).

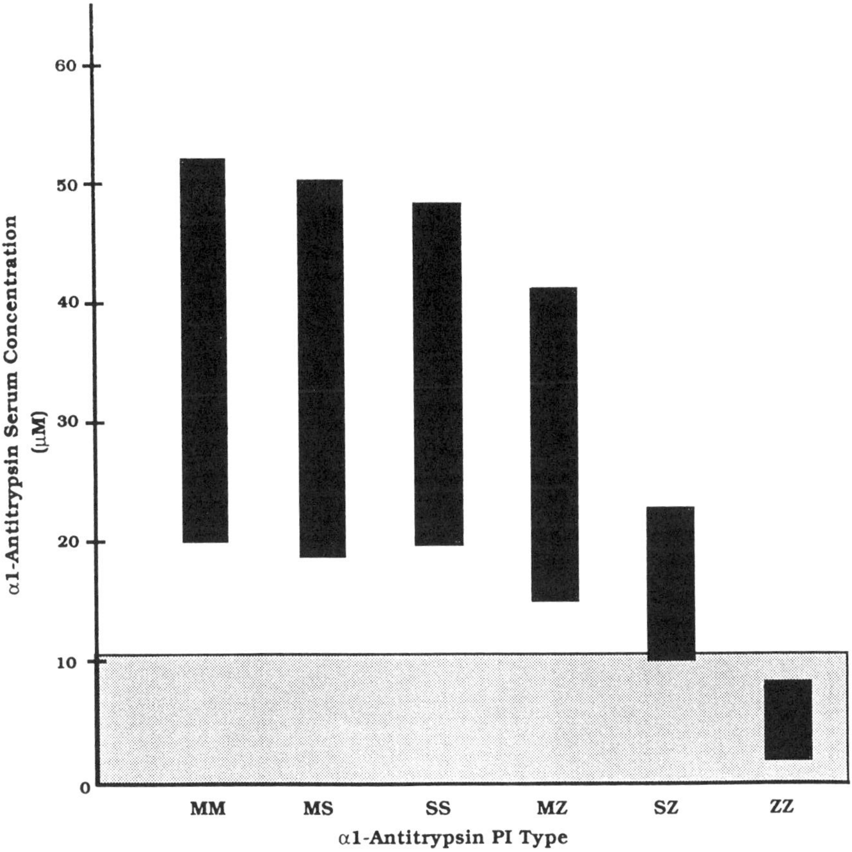


**Figure 2** Range of α1AT serum levels by protease inhibitor type. Abscissa: six α1AT phenotypes representing all possible combinations of the normal M allele (all subtypes combined), the mildly deficient S allele, and the profoundly deficient Z allele. α1AT serum concentrations in the shaded area are below 11 μM and are associated with an increased risk for liver and lung disease. α1AT serum concentration ranges: MM = 20–53 μM; MS = 18–52 μM; SS = 20–48 μM; MZ = 15–42 μM; SZ = 10–23 μM; ZZ = 3.4–7.0 μM (16).

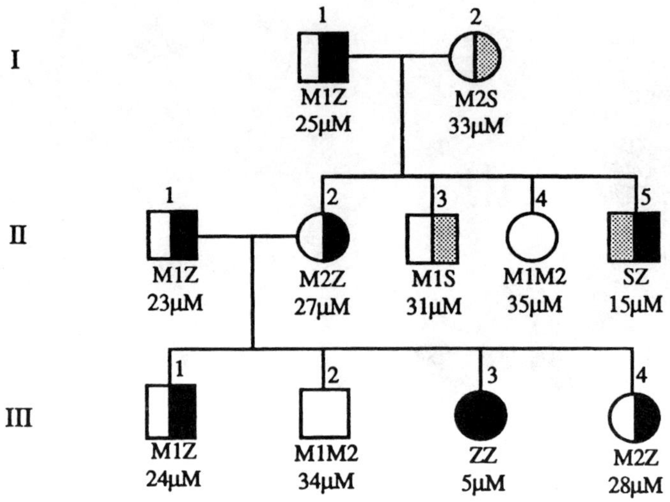


**Figure 3** Example of a three-generation pedigree with α1AT deficiency. PI types are shown below each α1AT; serum levels are shown below the PI types. Autosomal codominant inheritance of normal α1AT alleles M1 and M2 (white symbols) is associated with normal serum α1AT levels (II-4 and III-2). Inheritance of a normal M allele in combination with the deficient Z allele (black symbols) yields intermediate serum levels (I-1, II-1, II-2, III-1, and III-4). Inheritance of a normal M allele with the mildly deficient S allele (shaded symbols) yields near-normal serum α1AT levels (I-2 and II-3). Inheritance of the S allele is associated with a significant reduction in α1AT concentration when found in combination with the Z allele (II-5). A profound reduction in serum α1AT results from the inheritance of two Z alleles (III-3).

---

**Figure 4** Organization of the α1-antitrypsin gene. Top (5′) to bottom (3′), the boxes denote coding regions (exons) of the α1AT gene; lines between the boxes are intervening sequences (introns). Exons Ia, Ib, and Ic are regulatory elements essential for normal α1AT expression. Ia and Ib are macrophage-specific regulatory elements and Ic has both macrophage- and hepatocyte-specific regulatory elements. Four kilobases (kb) 3′ to exon Ic are the exons responsible for encoding the amino acid backbone of α1AT. Exon II encodes the start codon (ATG), signal peptide (hatched box), and two of the three carbohydrate attachment sites (N46-CHO and N83-CHO). Exon III encodes the third carbohydrate attachment site (N247-CHO). Exon V encodes the active site (M358), the stop codon (TAA), and the polyadenylation signal (ATTAA) (7). Right, reference distance of 500 bp.

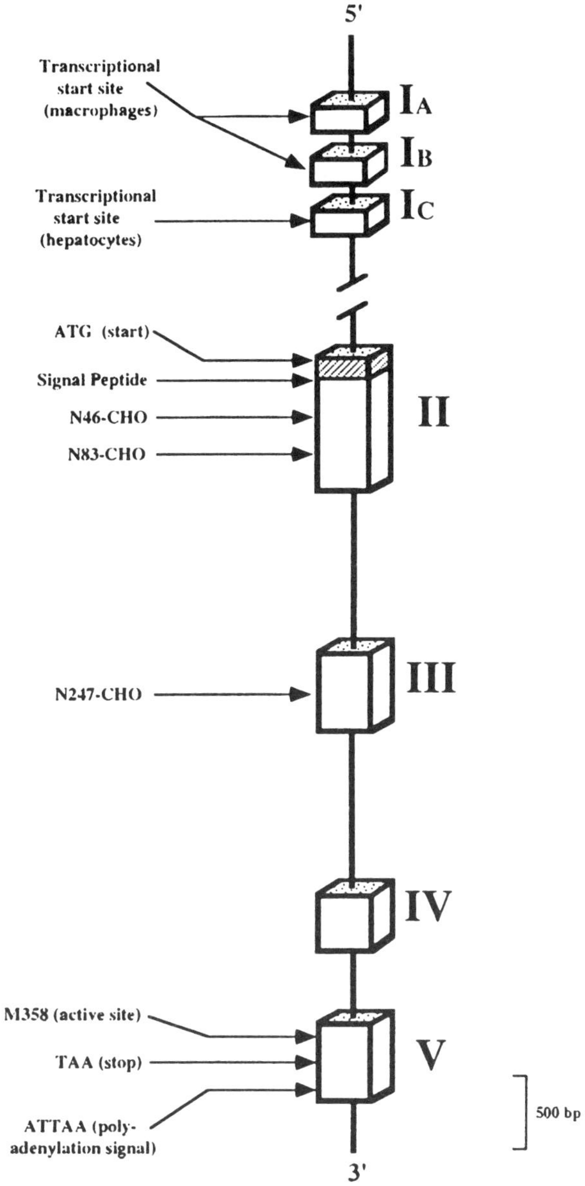
5'
Transcriptional start site (macrophages)
IA
IB
Transcriptional start site (hepatocytes)
IC
ATG (start)
Signal Peptide
N46-CHO
N83-CHO
II
N247-CHO
III
IV
M358 (active site)
TAA (stop)
ATTAA (poly-adenylation signal)
V
500 bp
3'

Figure 4

```
-24         -20                                     -10                                     -1  +1                                      10
ATG CCG TCT TCT GTC TCG TGG GGC ATC CTC CTG CTG GCA GGC CTG TGC TGC CTG GTC CCT GTC TCC CTG GCT GAG GAT CCC CAG GGA GAT GCT GCC CAG AAG ACA GAT
Met Pro Ser Ser Val Ser Trp Gly Ile Leu Leu Leu Ala Gly Leu Cys Cys Leu Val Pro Val Ser Leu Ala Glu Asp Pro Gln Gly Asp Ala Ala Gln Lys Thr Asp

                            20                                      30                                      40
ACA TCC CAC CAT GAT CAG GAT CAC CCA ACC TTC AAC AAG ATC ACC CCC AAC CTG GCT GAG TTC GCC TTC AGC CTA TAC CGC CAG CTG GCA CAC CAG TCC AAC AGC ACC
Thr Ser His His Asp Gln Asp His Pro Thr Phe Asn Lys Ile Thr Pro Asn Leu Ala Glu Phe Ala Phe Ser Leu Tyr Arg Gln Leu Ala His Gln Ser Asn Ser Thr

    50                                      60                                      70                                      80
AAT ATC TTC TTC TCC CCA GTG AGC ATC GCT ACA GCC TTT GCA ATG CTC TCC CTG GGG ACC AAG GCT GAC ACT CAC GAT GAA ATC CTG GAG GGC CTG AAT TTC AAC CTC
Asn Ile Phe Phe Ser Pro Val Ser Ile Ala Thr Ala Phe Ala Met Leu Ser Leu Gly Thr Lys Ala Asp Thr His Asp Glu Ile Leu Glu Gly Leu Asn Phe Asn Leu

                    90                                      100                                     110                                     120
ACG GAG ATT CCG GAG GCT CAG ATC CAT GAA GGC TTC CAG GAA CTC CTC CGT ACC CTC AAC CAG CCA GAC AGC CAG CTC CAG CTG ACC ACC GGC AAT GGC CTG TTC CTC
Thr Glu Ile Pro Glu Ala Gln Ile His Glu Gly Phe Gln Glu Leu Leu Arg Thr Leu Asn Gln Pro Asp Ser Gln Leu Gln Leu Thr Thr Gly Asn Gly Leu Phe Leu

                                    130                                     140                                     150
AGC GAG GGC CTG AAG CTA GTG GAT AAG TTT TTG GAG GAT GTT AAA AAG TTG TAC CAC TCA GAA GCC TTC ACT GTC AAC TTC GGG GAC ACC GAA GAG GCC AAG AAA CAG
Ser Glu Gly Leu Lys Leu Val Asp Lys Phe Leu Glu Asp Val Lys Lys Leu Tyr His Ser Glu Ala Phe Thr Val Asn Phe Gly Asp Thr Glu Glu Ala Lys Lys Gln

                                                                                                                                  Exon II | Exon III
            160                                     170                                     180                                     190
ATC AAC GAT TAC GTG GAG AAG GGT ACT CAA GGG AAA ATT GTG GAT TTG GTC AAG GAG CTT GAC AGA GAC ACA GTT TTT GCT CTG GTG AAT TAC ATC TTC TTT AAA GGC
Ile Asn Asp Tyr Val Glu Lys Gly Thr Gln Gly Lys Ile Val Asp Leu Val Lys Glu Leu Asp Arg Asp Thr Val Phe Ala Leu Val Asn Tyr Ile Phe Phe Lys Gly

                        200                                     210                                     220
AAA TGG GAG AGA CCC TTT GAA GTC AAG GAC ACC GAG GAA GAG GAC TTC CAC GTG GAC CAG GTG ACC ACC GTG AAG GTG CCT ATG ATG AAG CGT TTA GGC ATG TTT AAC
Lys Trp Glu Arg Pro Phe Glu Val Lys Asp Thr Glu Glu Glu Asp Phe His Val Asp Gln Val Thr Thr Val Lys Val Pro Met Met Lys Arg Leu Gly Met Phe Asn

    230                                     240                                     250                                     260
ATC CAG CAC TGT AAG AAG CTG TCC AGC TGG GTG CTG CTG ATG AAA TAC CTG GGC AAT GCC ACC GCC ATC TTC TTC CTG CCT GAT GAG GGG AAA CTA CAG CAC CTG GAA
Ile Gln His Cys Lys Lys Leu Ser Ser Trp Val Leu Leu Met Lys Tyr Leu Gly Asn Ala Thr Ala Ile Phe Phe Leu Pro Asp Glu Gly Lys Leu Gln His Leu Glu

                                                                  Exon III | Exon IV
                        270                                     280                                     290                                     300
AAT GAA CTC ACC CAC GAT ATC ATC ACC AAG TTC CTG GAA AAT GAA GAC AGA AGG TCT GCC AGC TTA CAT TTA CCC AAA CTG TCC ATT ACT GGA ACC TAT GAT CTG AAG
Asn Glu Leu Thr His Asp Ile Ile Thr Lys Phe Leu Glu Asn Glu Asp Arg Arg Ser Ala Ser Leu His Leu Pro Lys Leu Ser Ile Thr Gly Thr Tyr Asp Leu Lys

                                                                                                                     Exon IV | Exon V
                                    310                                     320                                     330
AGC GTC CTG GGT CAA CTG GGC ATC ACT AAG GTC TTC AGC AAT GGG GCT GAC CTC TCC GGG GTC ACA GAG GAG GCA CCC CTG AAG CTC TCC AAG GCC GTG CAT AAG GCT
Ser Val Leu Gly Gln Leu Gly Ile Thr Lys Val Phe Ser Asn Gly Ala Asp Leu Ser Gly Val Thr Glu Glu Ala Pro Leu Lys Leu Ser Lys Ala Val His Lys Ala

            340                                     350                                     360                                     370
GTG CTG ACC ATC GAC GAG AAA GGG ACT GAA GCT GCT GGG GCC ATG TTT TTA GAG GCC ATA CCC ATG TCT ATC CCC CCC GAG GTC AAG TTC AAC AAA CCC TTT GTC TTC
Val Leu Thr Ile Asp Glu Lys Gly Thr Glu Ala Ala Gly Ala Met Phe Leu Glu Ala Ile Pro Met Ser Ile Pro Pro Glu Val Lys Phe Asn Lys Pro Phe Val Phe

                        380                                     390             394
TTA ATG ATT GAA CAA AAT ACC AAG TCT CCC CTC TTC ATG GGA AAA GTG GTG AAT CCC ACC CAA AAA TAA CTGCCTCTCGCTCCTCAACCCCTCCCCTCCATCCCTGGCCCCCTCCCTGGATG
Leu Met Ile Glu Gln Asn Thr Lys Ser Pro Leu Phe Met Gly Lys Val Val Asn Pro Thr Gln Lys ***
```

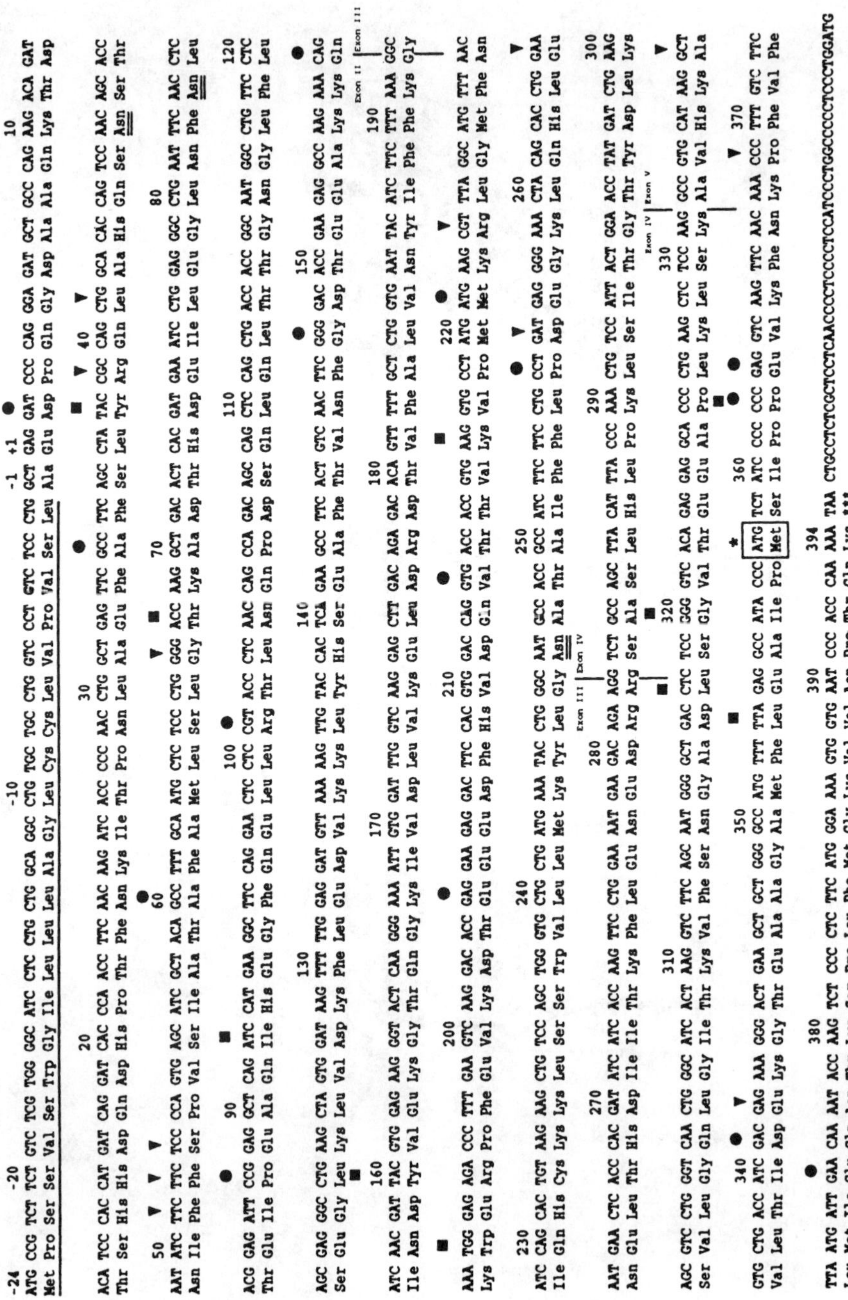

Figure 5

## VI. α1AT Mutations and Risk for Emphysema or Liver Disease

Although there are at least 32 alleles associated with altered, reduced, or absent serum α1AT, 96% of all individuals with lung disease and α1AT deficiency are PI*Z (55). In this context α1AT deficiency is a monogenetic disease. The predominance of a single α1AT allele associated with disease contrasts with that of cystic fibrosis, in which the transmembrane regulator (CFTR) gene is associated with hundreds of mutations and the predominant disease-associated mutation (Δ508) constitutes only 60–70% of the CFTR alleles. Because the Z variant is the only "common" allele associated with α1AT deficiency, genetic screening of α1AT deficiency is more feasible than screening for cystic fibrosis.

While disease risk is a complex issue, certain observations regarding specific variants have emerged. The risk of emphysema appears to correlate with variants associated with significant reductions in serum α1AT. Those α1AT variants associated with the greatest risk of lung disease in the homozygous form or in the heterozygous form with another deficient or null allele include all deficient and null variants (Tables 2 and 3). Risk for liver disease is somewhat more controversial, but at least four alleles in the homozygous form or associated with the Z allele have been reported in association with liver disease including PI*Z, S, F, and $M_{malton}$ (Table 2).

## VII. Molecular Mechanisms of α1AT Deficiency

The molecular mechanisms responsible for α1AT deficiency include errors in the expression, translation, and intercellular processing of α1AT. Two variants, $QO_{iso\ di\ procida}$ and $QO_{riedenburg}$ are associated with the deletion of most of the coding region of α1AT (26,46). $QO_{west}$, $QO_{trastevere}$, and probably $QO_{bonny\ blue}$ are associated with abnormalities in mRNA splicing or stability (51,56). $QO_{hong\ kong}$, $OQ_{trastevere}$, $OQ_{clayton}$, and Z are associated with retention in the rough endoplasmic reticulum and intracellular degradation (51,57–59).

**Figure 5** Location of mutations in α1AT and coding exons and the corresponding normal α1AT amino acid sequence. Numbers −24 to 394 above DNA codons correspond to the amino acid. Below each DNA triplet is the amino acid encoded by the codon. Vertical bars indicate the boundary between exons. Double horizontal lines under Asn residues denote the location of carbohydrate attachment sites. The boxed residue is the active site. The stop codon is indicated by (***). Filled arrow denotes site of a deficiency variant mutation, filled circle site of a normal variant mutation, filled square site of a null mutation, asterisk site of the dysfunctional variant mutation Pittsburgh. (See Tables 1–3 for details.)

## VIII. Conclusion

While there are a number of variants associated with $\alpha 1$AT deficiency, the PI*Z variant represents the allele predominantly responsible for $\alpha 1$AT deficiency–related emphysema and liver disease. In this context, population-based genetic screening for $\alpha 1$AT deficiency is feasible and may have significant public health benefits.

## References

1. Laurell C, Eriksson S. The electrophoretic $\alpha 1$-globulin pattern of serum in $\alpha 1$-antitrypsin deficiency. Scand J Clin Lab Invest 1963; 15:132–140.
2. Axelsson U, Laurell CB. Hereditary variants of serum alpha-1-antitrypsin. Am J Hum Genet 1965; 17(6):466–472.
3. Fagerhol M, Braend M. Serum prealbumin: polymorphism in man. Science 1965; 419:986–987.
4. Fagerhol MK, Laurell CB. The Pi system–inherited variants of serum alpha 1-antitrypsin. Prog Med Genet 1970: 7(96):96–111.
5. Yoshida A, Lieberman J, Gaidulis L, Ewing C. Molecular abnormality of human alpha 1-antitrypsin variant (Pi-ZZ) associated with plasma activity deficiency. Proc Natl Acad Sci USA 1976; 73(4):1324–1328.
6. Kurachi K, Chandra T, Degen SJ, et al. Cloning and sequence of cDNA coding for alpha 1-antitrypsin. Proc Natl Acad Sci USA 1981; 78(11):6826–6830.
7. Long GL, Chandra T, Woo SL, Davie EW, Kurachi K. Complete sequence of the cDNA for human alpha 1-antitrypsin and the gene for the S variant. Biochemistry 1984; 23(21):4828–4837.
8. Okayama H, Holmes MD, Brantly ML, Crystal RG. Characterization of the coding region of the normal M4 alpha-1-antitrypsin gene. Biochem Biophys Res Comm 1989; 162(3):1560–1570.
9. Jeppsson JO, Lilja H, Johansson M. Isolation and characterization of two minor fractions of alpha 1-antitrypsin by high-performance liquid chromatographic chromatofocusing. J Chromatogr 1985; 327(173):173–177.
10. Cox DW, Nakamura Y, Gedde DTJ. Report of the committee on the genetic constitution of chromosome 14. Cytogenet Cell Genet 1990; 55(1–4):183–188.
11. Cox DW, Johnson AM, Fagerhol MK. Report of nomenclature meeting for alpha 1-antitrypsin, INSERM, Rouen/Bois-Guillaume–1978. Hum Genet 1980; 53(3) 429–433.
12. Brantly M, Nukiwa T, Crystal RG. Molecular basis of alpha-1-antitrypsin deficiency. Am J Med 1988; 84(6A):13–31.
13. Crystal RG. The alpha 1-antitrypsin gene and its deficiency states. Trends Genet 1989; 5(12):411–417.
14. Gadek J, Crystal R. $\alpha 1$-Antitrypsin deficiency. In: Stanbury JB, Fredrickson D, Wyngaarden IB, Goldstein J, Brown M, eds. The Metabolic Basis of Inherited Disease. 5th ed. New York: McGraw-Hill, 1982:1450–1467.

15. Wewers M, Casolaro M, Sellers S, et al. Replacement therapy for alpha-1-antitrypsin deficiency associated with emphysema. N Engl J Med 1987; 316:1055–1062.
16. Brantly ML, Wittes JT, Vogelmeier CF, Hubbard RC, Fells GA, Crystal RG. Use of a highly purified alpha 1-antitrypsin standard to establish ranges for the common normal and deficient alpha 1-antitrypsin phenotypes. Chest 1991; 100(3):703–708.
17. Billingsley G, Cox D. Rare deficiency alpha-1-antitrypsin variants: current status and SSCP analysis. Am J Hum Gen 1994; 55(3):A212.
18. Brantly M, Hildeshiem J, Laubach V, Rundquist B, Paul L. Alpha-1-antitrypsin $null_{new\ hope}$: Natural conversion of the alpha-1-antitrypsin deficiency Z variant into a null variant by the addition of second amino acid substitution. Clin Res 1992; 40:A328.
19. Brennan SO, Carrell RW. Alpha 1-$antitrypsin_{chistchurch}$, 363 Glu–Lys: mutation at the P′5 position does not affect inhibitory activity. Biochim Biophys Acta 1986; 873(1):13–19.
20. Curiel D, Brantly M, Curiel E, Steir L, Crystal RG. Alpha-1-antitrypsin deficiency caused by the alpha-1-antitrypsin $null_{mattawa}$ gene. J Clin Invest 1989; 83:1144–1152.
21. Curiel D, Laubach V, Vogelmeier C, Wurts L, Crystal RG. Characterization of the sequence of the normal alpha-1-antitrypsin M3 allele and function of the M3 protein. Am J Respir Cell Mol Biol 1989; 1(6):471–477.
22. Curiel D, Holmes MD, Okayama H, et al. Molecular basis of the liver and lung disease associated with the alpha 1-antitrypsin deficiency allele $M_{malton}$. J Biol Chem 1989; 264(23):13938–13945.
23. Curiel DT, Vogelmeier C, Hubbard RC, Stier LE, Crystal RG. Molecular basis of alpha 1-antitrypsin deficiency and emphysema associated with the alpha 1-antitrypsin $M_{mineral\ springs}$ allele. Mol Cell Biol 1990; 10(1):47–56.
24. Faber JP, Weidinger S, Olek K. Sequence data of the rare deficient alpha 1-antitrypsin variant PI Zaugsburg. Am J Hum Genet 1990; 46(6):1158–1162.
25. Faber JP, Weidinger S, Goedde HW, Olek K. The deficient alpha-1-antitrypsin phenotype PI P is associated with an A-to-T transversion in exon III of the gene [letter]. Am J Hum Genet 1989; 45(1):161–163.
26. Faber JP, Poller W, Weidinger S, et al. Identification and DNA sequence analysis of 15 new alpha 1-antitrypsin variants, including two PI*QO alleles and one deficient PI*M allele. Am J Hum Genet 1994; 55(6):1113–1121.
27. Fraizer GC, Harrold TR, Hofker MH, Cox DW. In-frame single codon deletion in the $M_{malton}$ deficiency allele of alpha 1-antitrypsin. Am J Hum Genet 1989; 44(6): 894–902.
28. Fraizer GC, Siewertsen M, Harrold TR, Cox DW. Deletion/frameshift mutation in the alpha 1-antitrypsin null allele, PI*$QO_{bolton}$. Hum Genet 1989; 83(4):377–382.
29. Frazier GC, Siewertsen MA, Hofker MH, Brubacher MG, Cox DW. A null deficiency allele of alpha 1-antitrypsin, $QO_{ludwigshafen}$, with altered tertiary structure. J Clin Invest 1990; 86(6):1878–1884.
30. Hofker MH, Nukiwa T, van PH, et al. A Pro→Leu substitution in codon 369 of the alpha-1-antitrypsin deficiency variant PI MHeerlen. Hum Genet 1989; 81(3): 264–268.
31. Holmes M, Curiel D, Brantly M, Crystal RG. Characterization of the intracellular

mechanism causing the alpha-1-antritrypsin null$_{granite\ falls}$ deficiency state. Am Rev Respir Dis 1989; 140(6):1662–1667.
32. Holmes MD, Brantly ML, Crystal RG. Molecular analysis of the heterogeneity among the P-family of alpha-1-antitrypsin alleles. Am Rev Respir Dis 1990; 142(5):1185–1192.
33. Holmes MD, Brantly ML, Curiel DT, Weidinger S, Crystal RG. Characterization of the normal alpha 1-antitrypsin allele V$_{munich}$: a variant associated with a unique protein isoelectric focusing pattern. Am J Hum Genet 1990; 46(4):810–816.
34. Holmes MD, Brantly ML, Fells GA, Crystal RG. Alpha 1-antitrypsin W$_{bethesda}$: molecular basis of an unusual alpha 1-antitrypsin deficiency variant. Biochem Biophys Res Commun 1990; 170(3):1013–1020.
35. Jeppsson JO, Laurell CB. The amino acid substitutions of human alpha 1-antitrypsin M3, X and Z. Febs Lett 1988; 231(2):327–330.
36. Nukiwa T, Brantly M, Ogushi F, et al. Characterization of the M1(Ala213) type of alpha 1-antitrypsin, a newly recognized, common "normal" alpha 1-antitrypsin haplotype. Biochemistry 1987; 26(17):5259–5267.
37. Nukiwa T, Brantly ML, Ogushi F, Fells GA, Crystal RG. Characterization of the gene and protein of the common alpha 1-antitrypsin normal M2 allele. Am J Hum Genet 1988; 43(3):322–330.
38. Nukiwa T, Satoh K, Brantly ML, et al. Identification of a second mutation in the protein-coding sequence of the Z type alpha 1-antitrypsin gene. J Biol Chem 1986; 261(34):15989–15994. Published erratum appears in J Biol Chem 1987; 262(21): 10412.
39. Nukiwa T, Takahashi H, Brantly M, Courtney M, Crystal RG. Alpha 1-antitrypsin null$_{granite\ falls}$, a nonexpressing alpha 1-antitrypsin gene associated with a frameshift to stop mutation in a coding exon. J Biol Chem 1987; 262(25):11999–12004.
40. Okayama H, Brantly M, Holmes M, Crystal RG. Characterization of the molecular basis of the alpha 1-antitrypsin F allele. Am J Hum Genet 1991; 48(6):1154–1158.
41. Owen MC, Brennan SO, Lewis JH, Carrell RW. Mutation of antitrypsin to antithrombin alpha 1-antitrypsin Pittsburgh (358 Met leads to Arg), a fatal bleeding disorder. N Engl J Med 1983; 309(12)694–698.
42. Owen MC, Carrell RW. Alpha-1-antitrypsin: sequence of the Z variant tryptic peptide. Febs Lett 1977; 79(2):245–247.
43. Owen MC, Carrell RW. Alpha-1-antitrypsin: molecular abnormality of the S variant. Br Med J 1976; 17:130–131.
44. Owen MC, Carrell RW, Brennan SO. The abnormality of the S variant of human alpha-1-antitrypsin. Biochim Biophys Acta 1976; 453(1)257–261.
45. Poller W, Faber JP, Weidinger S, Olek K. DNA polymorphisms associated with a new alpha 1-antitrypsin PIQO variant (PIQO$_{riedenburg}$). Hum Genet 1991; 86(5):522–524.
46. Takahashi H, Crystal RG. Alpha 1-antitrypsin null (isola di procida): an alpha 1-antitrypsin deficiency allele caused by deletion of all alpha 1-antitrypsin coding exons. Am J Hum Genet 1990; 47(3):403–413.
47. Takahashi H, Nukiwa T, Satoh K, et al. Characterization of the gene and protein of the alpha-1-antitrypsin "deficiency" allele M$_{procida}$. J Biol Chem 1988; 263(30):15528–15534.

48. Yoshida A, Ewing C, Wessels M, Lieberman J, Gaidulis L. Molecular abnormality of PI S variant of human alpha 1-antitrypsin. Am J Hum Genet 1977; 29(3):233–239.
49. Yoshida A, Chillar R, Taylor JC. An alpha 1-antitrypsin variant, Pi B Alhambra (Lys to Asp, Glu to Asp), with rapid anodal electrophoretic mobility. Am J Hum Genet 1979; 31(5):555–563.
50. Yoshida A, Taylor JC, Brock van den, WG. Structural difference between the normal PiM1 and the common PiM2 variant of human alpha 1-antitrypsin. Am J Hum Genet 1979; 31 (5):564–568.
51. Lee J, Novoradskaya N, Saltini C, Ong S, Brantly M. $QO_{trastevere}$: An alpha-1-antitrypsin null variant associated with reduced mRNA expression and intracellular protein degradation. Resp Crit Care Med 1995; 151:A533.
52. Hildesheim J, Kinsley G, Bissell M, Pierce J, Brantly M. Genetic diversity from a limited repertoire of mutations on different common allelic backgrounds: α1-antitrypsin deficiency variant $P_{duarte}$. Hum Mutation 1993; 2:221–228.
53. Lai EC, Kao FT, Law ML, Woo SL. Assignment of the alpha 1-antitrypsin gene and a sequence-related gene to human chromosome 14 by molecular hybridization. Am J Hum Genet 1983; 35(3):385–392.
54. Streisinger G, Owen JE. Mechanisms of spontaneous and induced frameshift mutation in bacteriophage T4. Genetics 1985; 109:633–659.
55. Brantly ML, Paul LD, Miller BH, Falk RT, Wu M, Crystal RG. Clinical features and history of the destructive lung disease associated with alpha-1-antitrypsin deficiency of adults with pulmonary symptoms. Am Rev Respir Dis 1988; 138(2):327–336.
56. Laubach V, Ryan J, Brantly M. Characterization of a human α1-antitrypsin null allele involving aberrant mRNA splicing. Hum Mol Genet 1993; 2:1001–1005.
57. Le A, Graham KS, Sifers RN. Intracellular degradation of the transport-impaired human PiZ alpha 1-antitrypsin variant: Biochemical mapping of the degradative event among compartments of the secretory pathway. J Biol Chem 1990; 265(23):14001–14007.
58. Le A, Ferrel GA, Dishon DS, Le QQ, Sifers RN. Soluble aggregates of the human PiZ alpha 1-antitrypsin variant are degraded within the endoplasmic reticulum by a mechanism sensitive to inhibitors of protein synthesis. J Biol Chem 1992; 267(2): 1072–1080.
59. Sifers RN, Brashears MS, Kidd VJ, Muensch H, Woo SL. A frameshift mutation results in a truncated alpha 1-antitrypsin that is retained within the rough endoplasmic reticulum. J Biol Chem 1988; 263(15):7330–7335.

# 5

# Structure and Expression of the Human Neutrophil Elastase Gene

**KUNIHIKO YOSHIMURA**

Daisan Hospital
The Jikei University School of Medicine
Tokyo, Japan

## I. Introduction

Human neutrophil elastase (NE; EC 3.4.21.37) is a 29 kDa, 220-residue single-chain glycoprotein that functions as a powerful serine protease. It is stored in the azurophilic (primary) granules of mature neutrophils and released when the neutrophil is activated or disintegrates (1–5). NE is capable of destroying a broad range of substrates, including cross-linked elastin, the major forms of collagen, the protein components of proteoglycans, fibronectin, laminin, components of the complement, coagulation cascades, and the cell walls of gram-negative bacilli such as *Escherichia coli* (1–5). In this regard, NE is considered a two-edged sword: it is required for normal tissue turnover and host defense yet is potentially harmful in its ability to destroy normal tissues simultaneously. For example, NE plays a central role in the pathogenesis of pulmonary emphysema by destroying the alveolar walls of the lung (6). Although natural substances with antiprotease activity in the lung, such as alpha 1–antitrypsin ($\alpha$1AT) or secretory leukoprotease inhibitor, could protect the lung from NE in the normal human body, the conditions in which the normal $\alpha$1AT molecule is inactivated—e.g., cigarette smoking or $\alpha$1AT deficiency caused by mutations of the $\alpha$1AT gene—would result in excess burden of NE in the lung, causing pulmonary emphysema (6). Because of its essential role in health and disease, it is important to understand the structure and expression of the gene that codes for the NE protein. Furthermore, elucidation of the mechanism that regulates expression of the NE gene in bone marrow cell differentiation is also crucial to develop the therapeutic strategy for such diseases as pulmonary emphysema.

## II. Structure of the Human NE Gene

### A. Chromosomal Localization

In the original article by Takahashi et al. (7) describing genomic organization of the NE gene, it was postulated that the gene was a single-copy gene and was localized to the region of the long arm of chromosome 11 at q14 by in situ hybridization using a $^{3}$H-labeled cDNA probe. In this report, the authors observed that 20% of total grains accumulated to that region. However, Zimmer et al. (8) recently reported that the human NE gene, along with other two genes coding for serine proteases, proteinase 3 and azurocidin, was organized as a single genetic locus on the 19pter using the fluorescence in situ hybridization technique. Thus the chromosome localization of the NE gene is still controversial. Further study is needed to elucidate this particular question. Interestingly, the other cluster of genes coding hematopoietic serine proteases cathepsin G, granzyme B (CGL-1), and granzyme H (CGL-2) has been localized to 14q11.2 (9).

### B. Genomic Organization

Irrespective of the chromosomal localization, the NE gene spans the 6 kb segment of the genome including the 5′ flanking region, five exons, four introns, and the 3′ flanking region (7,10,11) (Fig. 1). The five exons range in length from 93 bp (exon I), 157 bp (exon II), 142 bp (exon III), 231 bp (exon IV), to more than 270 bp (exon V). The intervening sequences are 480 bp in length (intron I), 231 bp (intron II), approximately 2160 bp (intron III), and 163 bp (intron IV). The major transcription initiation site defined by the primer extension analysis is 26 bp upstream of the ATG translation start codon (Met$^{-29}$) (7,11). The start codon for translation is located in exon I, and the stop codon (TGA) is located in exon V. In exon V, there is a typical polyadenylation signal (AATAAA) 58 bp downstream of the stop codon (7,11).

Interestingly, there are at least three direct repetitive sequences in the NE gene (7,11). First, in the 5′ flanking region 1032 bp upstream of the cap site, there start six tandem direct repeats of a 53 bp element (REP53; see below). Second, in intron I, there are three repeats of a 23 bp sequence containing a *Bam*HI restriction site in itself. Finally, in intron III, there are 10 direct repeats of a 41 bp sequence. The sequence of each element is tandemly aligned and directly repeated. However, they are unrelated and no high homology is seen among them. Further, at

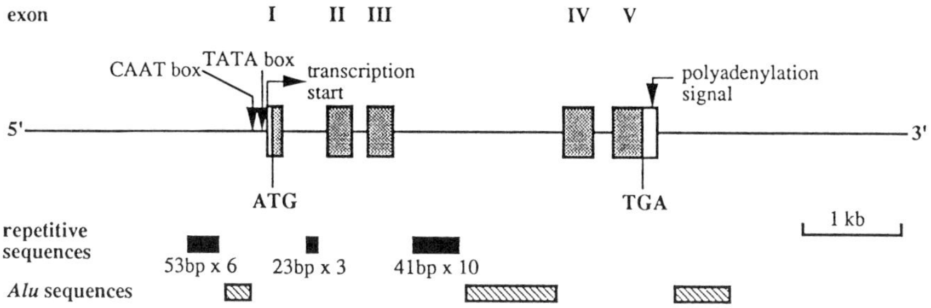


**Figure 1** Structure of the human neutrophil elastase (NE) gene (7,11). The protein coding regions (gray boxes) and 5′ and 3′ untranslated regions (white boxes) in exons (labeled I–V) and the introns and flanking regions (horizontal line) are depicted. Also shown are promoter consensus sequences such as the CAAT box (GGGCAATGC) and the TATA box (TATAAGA) 5′ to exon I, the transcription start site (defined as +1), the start codon (ATG, $Met^{-29}$) in exon I, the stop codon (TGA), and the putative polyadenylation signal in exon V. The codons for N-terminal ($Ile^{1}$) and C-terminal ($Ser^{220}$) amino acid residues of mature NE protein reside in exon II and exon V, respectively. Three distinct repetitive sequences (six repeats of a 53 bp sequence in the 5′ flanking region, three repeats of a 23bp sequence in intron I, and 10 repeats of a 41bp sequence in intron III) are indicated by black boxes. Three regions of full or partial *Alu*-related sequences are shown by hatched boxes.

least three full or partial *Alu* sequences are present in the entire genomic structure of the NE gene: the first in the 5′ flanking region, the second in intron III, and the last in the 3′ untranslated region (7,11). Little is known about function of these repetitive sequences except for the REP53 in the 5′ flanking region (see below). These sequences are probably unique since no other nucleotide sequence is detected with an identity of higher than 85% in the GenBank database (7).

### C. Promoter and Enhancer Elements in the 5′ Flanking Region

In the 5′ region of the NE gene, there are preserved consensus sequences for promoter elements, including a CAAT box (GGGCAATGC, −61 to −53 relative to the major transcription start) and a TATA box flanked with G+C rich sequences (TATAAGA, −31 to −25) (7,11). Besides these elements, sequences homologous to the putative binding sites for known transcription factors such as Sp1 (GC box; GGGCGG, −18 to −13) or NF-1 (AGCCAAT, −89 to −83) are found (12).

As stated previously, there are six direct repeats of a 53 bp motif from −1032 to −716 of the gene (Fig. 2A) (7,11). The consensus nucleotide sequence of the repeat (REP53) is also shown. In each 53 bp motif, there is one potential recognition site for the basic helix-loop-helix (bHLH) protein family (CAGCTG; +6 to +11 relative to the start of repeat sequence), which is considered a critical

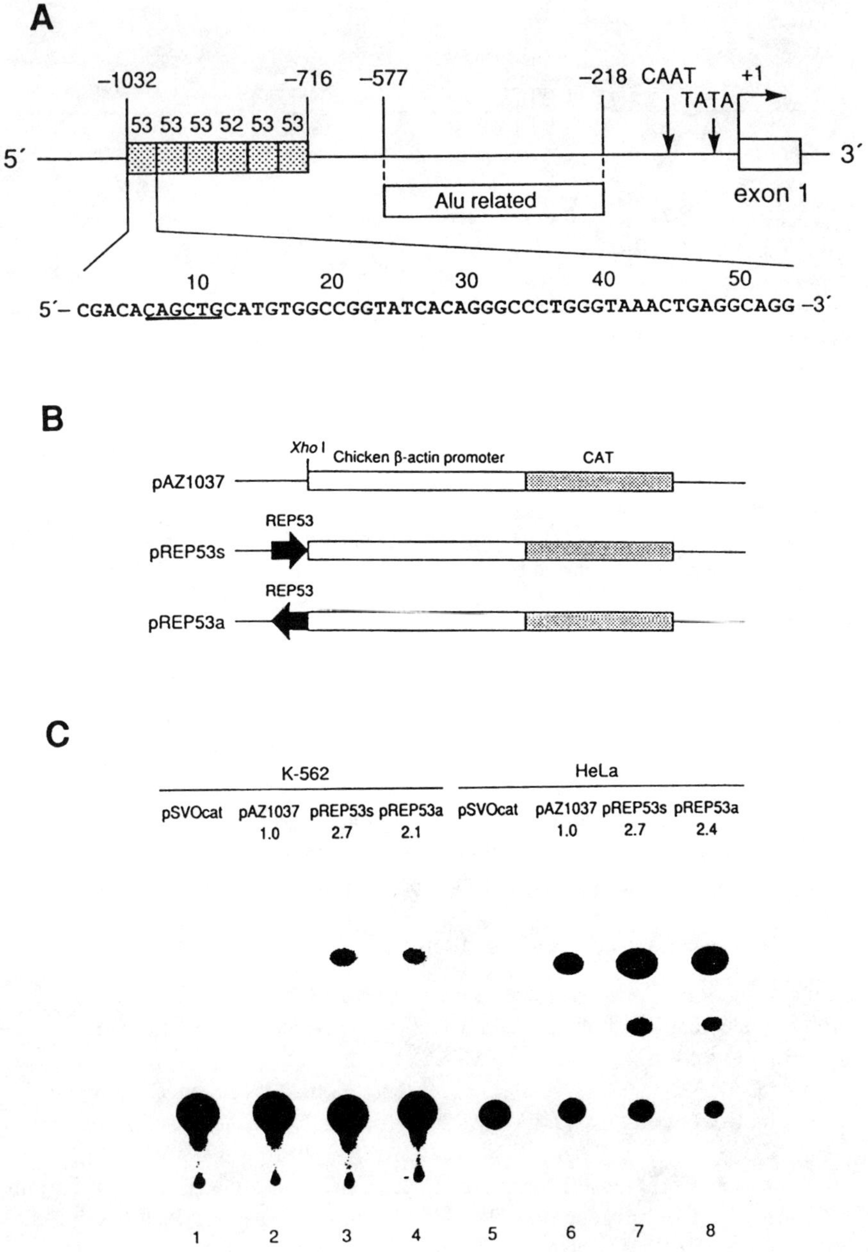
A
–1032
–716
–577
–218
CAAT
+1
TATA
53 53 53 52 53 53
5´
3´
Alu related
exon 1
10
20
30
40
50
5´– CGACACAGCTGCATGTGGCCGGTATCACAGGCCCTGGGTAAACTGAGGCAGG –3´
B
Xho I
Chicken β-actin promoter
CAT
pAZ1037
REP53
pREP53s
REP53
pREP53a
C
K-562
HeLa
pSVOcat
pAZ1037
pREP53s
pREP53a
pSVOcat
pAZ1037
pREP53s
pREP53a
1.0
2.7
2.1
1.0
2.7
2.4
1
2
3
4
5
6
7
8

transcription factor related to the differentiation and development of eukaryotic cells (13–16), although the REP53 motif is not present in the 5′ flanking region of other genes, such as myeloperoxidase or cathepsin G, genes whose expression is also limited to the early stage of myeloid differentiation (17–20). Interestingly, the single REP53 motif exhibits enhancer function even in cells that normally do not express the NE gene (21). For example, when human cervical carcinoma HeLa cells or HFL1 human lung fibroblasts were transfected with plasmids containing the single REP53 motif in front of the chicken β-actin promoter linked with the bacterial chloramphenicol acetyltransferase (CAT) gene, cells exhibited three- to fourfold higher CAT activity compared to cells transfected with the control plasmid pAZ1037 without containing the REP53 element (Fig. 2B and C) (21). Importantly, the orientation of the repeat was not critical in enhancing activity of the plasmid: the plasmid with the REP53 motif in either normal or reversed orientation exhibited the same enhancing activity (Fig. 2C). However, the function of the element in NE gene expression in myelocytic lineage bone marrow cell differentiation is undetermined because transfection with plasmids containing the chimera genes was hardly achieved in promyelocytic leukemia HL-60 cells, which normally epress the NE gene (22–24). Overall, the REP53 is capable of functioning as an enhancer in cells that normally do not express the NE gene (21). Although the effect of multiple copies of the REP53, either additive or synergistic, is undetermined, it is possible that the REP53 element may be crucial in de novo transcription of the NE gene in bone marrow cells during myelocytic-lineage differentiation.

---

**Figure 2** The 53 bp repetitive element in the 5′ flanking sequence of the NE gene functioning as an enhancer for the heterologous promoter (21). (A) Top: structure of the NE 5′ flanking region (7). Bottom: nucleotide sequence of the 53 bp repeat (REP53). The nucleotide sequence homologous to the E-box consensus motif is underlined. (B) Schematics of plasmids pAZ1037, pREP53s, and pREP53a. pREP53s and pREP53a were constructed from pAZ1037 by inserting a single REP53 element at the *Xho*I site in front of the chicken β-actin sequences [including the promoter, exon 1, intron 1, and partial exon 2 (50)] in either normal or inverted orientation. (C) Examples of CAT assay data from K-562 erythroleukemia cells and HeLa cells tranfected with 10 μg of pSV0cat (negative control), pAZ1037, pREP53s, or pREP53a. K-562 cells were transfected by electroporation, and HeLa cells were transfected with cationic liposomes (51–53). After 48 hr, cells were recovered and CAT activity was quantified in cell lysates by phosphorimaging of thin-layer chromatography sheets and normalized using luciferase expression directed by cotransfection of the pRSVL plasmid vector (51,54). Numbers above the columns indicate the average relative CAT activity compared to that of the parental pAZ1037 (K-562, $n = 4$; HeLa, $n = 2$). Lane 1: K-562 cells transfected with pSV0cat; lane 2: same as 1, but with pAZ1037; lane 3: same as lane 1, but with pREP53s; lane 4: same as lane 1, but with pREP53a; lane 5: HeLa cells transfected with pSV0cat; lane 6: same as lane 5, but with pAZ1037; lane 7: same as lane 5, but with pREP53s; lane 8: same as lane 5, but with pREP53a.

### D. Protein Product Coded by the NE Gene

The protein sequence derived from the genomic DNA and mRNA (cDNA) sequences predicts that NE is initially synthesized as a 267 amino acid precursor protein, including a 29-residue N-terminal portion and a 18-residue C-terminal portion flanking the 220-residue mature protein (5,7,11). In the 29-residue peptide N-terminal to the $Glu^{-1}$ of the mature protein, a high proportion of hydrophobic amino acids, typical of a signal sequence, is observed (7). Further, a typical consensus signal peptidase cleavage signal (Ala–Leu–Ala) ends at $Ala^{-3}$, suggesting that the N-terminal extension represents a 27-residue "pre-" signal peptide ($Met^{-29}$–$Ala^{-3}$) followed by a two-residue "$pro_N$" peptide ($Ser^{-2}$–$Glu^{-1}$) (7). This structural characteristic places NE in the group of proteinases that includes cathepsin G, rat mast cell proteinase II, and other serine proteases found in cytotoxic T lymphocytes, such as CSP-B, whose activation is thought to involve cleavage of a Glu–Ile bond in a manner similar to zymogen activation of the pancreatic serine proteinases (11,25–27). The $pro_N$ dipeptide of NE would allow the enzyme to be transported and stored before being packaged in the azurophilic granule, where it is stored in an active form without the danger of proteolysis for protein components of the cell itself (2,5,11).

The sequences coding for the mature protein are spread out over exons II–V, with the sequence of the N-terminal $Ile^1$ close to the 5′ end of exon II and the sequence for the C-terminal $Ser^{220}$ in the middle of exon V (7,11). The three amino acid components of the catalytic active site $His^{41}$–$Asp^{88}$–$Ser^{173}$ are found in these different exons (II, III, and V, respectively). The two N-linked glycosylation acceptor sites ($Asp^{95}$ and $Asp^{144}$) used for the mature protein are coded by the nucleotide sequences in exon IV. Beyond the $Ser^{220}$ C-terminus of the mature protein, the nucleotide sequence in exon V codes for a 18-residue "$pro_C$" extension. The $pro_C$ peptide is composed of a mixture of hydrophobic, acidic, and basic residues (7).

## III. Expression of the Human NE Gene

### A. Cell-Specific Expression of the NE Gene

Despite its name and the fact that human neutrophils carry large amounts of NE (1,2,28), the NE gene is not expressed in mature neutrophils (24). In this regard, NE mRNA transcripts are not detectable by Northern hybridization analysis or RNase protection assay in mature neutrophils recovered from normal individuals. However, NE transcripts were detected in bone marrow cells, particularly in the fraction enriched for precursor cells (24). Fouret et al. (17), using the in situ hybridization technique, have demonstrated that NE mRNA transcripts were present only in bone marrow myelocytic precursor cells, mostly promyelocytes. With these data, it seems obvious that the NE gene is turned off prior to the time at which neutrophils leave the bone marrow. The mature neutrophils merely utilize the stored enzyme or export NE when neutrophil is stimulated (24).

Consistent with these observations, NE mRNA transcripts are abundantly present in HL-60 promyelocytic leukemia cells or, to a lesser extent, U-937 histiocytic lymphoma cells. Both cell lines exhibit the characteristics of early myelocytic lineage bone marrow cells (22–24,29,30). However, like mature blood neutrophils, other hematopoietic cells such as K-562 erythroleukemia cells, mature monocytes, macrophages, or T lymphocytes do not express the NE gene, although all these cells contain similar amounts of control gene mRNA transcripts such as β-actin (24,29).

Bone marrow cell-specific expression of the NE gene is regulated primarily at the level of gene transcription. In this context, nuclear run-on analysis demonstrated that HL-60 cells actively transcribed the NE gene, in contrast to cells such as K-562, human blood monocytes, human T lymphocytes, HeLa cervical carcinoma cells, or WI-26VA4 human lung fibroblasts, in which no transcription was observed although active transcription of the control β-actin gene was observed in all cell types (29). However, compared to the β-actin gene, the NE gene was transcribed at a lower level (24% of the β-actin gene) in undifferentiated HL-60 cells.

### B. Differentiation-Specific Expression of the NE Gene

#### *Mononuclear Phagocytic Lineage Differentiation*

To study differentiation-specific expression of the NE gene, HL-60 cells were used as a model for bone marrow precursor cells (29). HL-60 cells are known to be induced to differentiate toward the mononuclear phagocytic lineage with phorbol 12-myristate 13-acetate (PMA) or vitamin $D_3$ (31,32). For example, when these cells were treated with PMA, NE mRNA levels declined rapidly and became undetectable after 36 hr (Fig. 3A) (29). The decline of the NE transcript level appeared to be due primarily to the decrease in NE transcription rate (29). In this regard, the transcription rate of the NE gene declined after induction with PMA in a time-dependent manner (Fig. 3B; after 2 hr, 54% of control level; 15 hr, 47%; 48 hr, 17%). While the changes in transcription rate of the NE gene induced by PMA paralleled the decrease in NE mRNA transcript level, the NE transcripts remained stable (29). The half-life ($T_{1/2}$) of NE mRNA transcripts in undifferentiated HL-60 cells was 10.1 hr (29). Although the NE mRNA $T_{1/2}$ transiently increased up to 15.1 hr when HL-60 cells were induced to differentiate toward the mononuclear phagocytic lineage with stimulation by PMA for 2 hr, after 15 hr of PMA the $T_{1/2}$ returned to the basal level (10.4 hr). These data indicate that at least a significant proportion of the down-regulation of NE gene expression in the HL-60 model of bone marrow precursor cells during mononuclear phagocytic lineage differentiation is controlled at the transcriptional level (29).

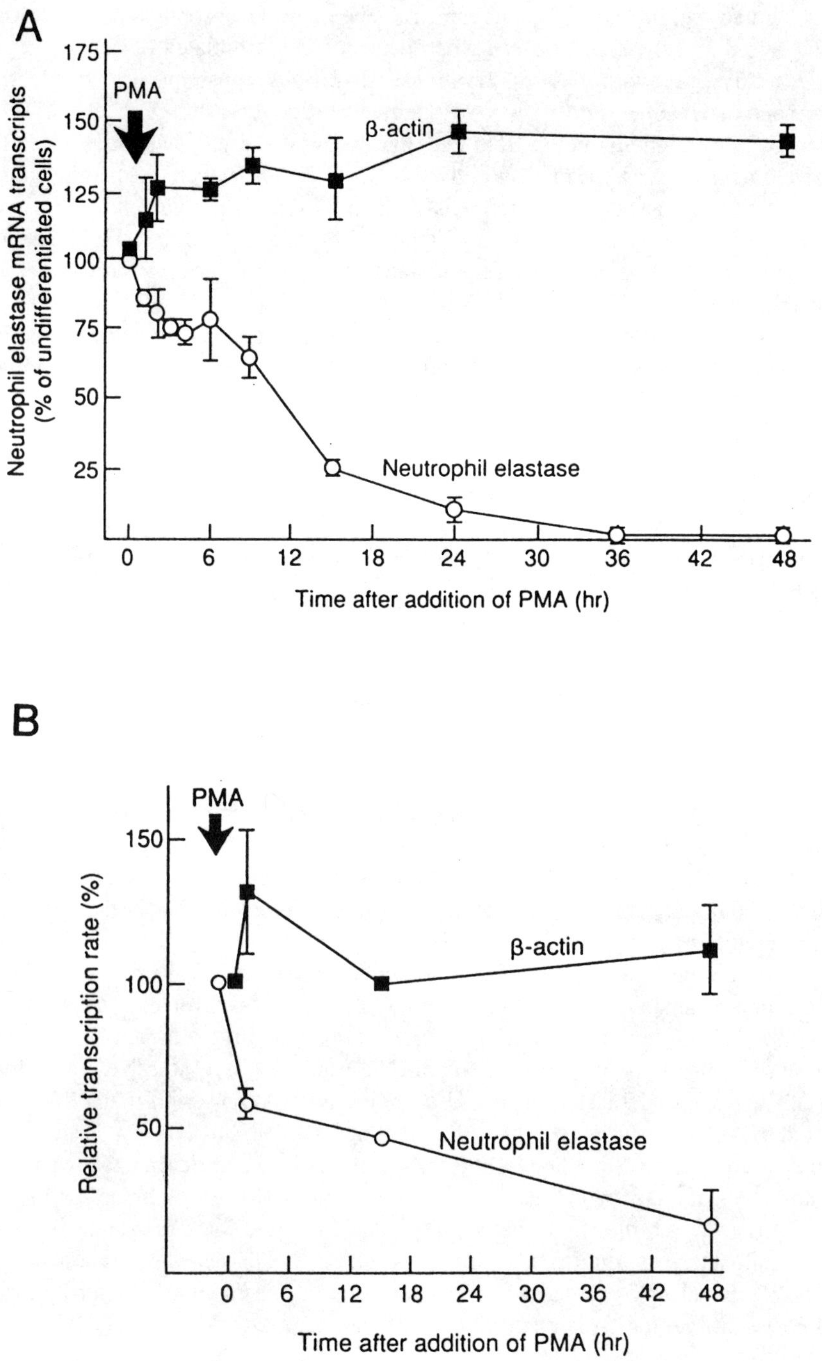
A
175
150
125
100
75
50
25
PMA
β-actin
Neutrophil elastase
Neutrophil elastase mRNA transcripts
(% of undifferentiated cells)
0
6
12
18
24
30
36
42
48
Time after addition of PMA (hr)
B
PMA
150
100
50
β-actin
Neutrophil elastase
Relative transcription rate (%)
0
6
12
18
24
30
36
42
48
Time after addition of PMA (hr)

### *Myelocytic Lineage Differentiation*

In contrast to the mononuclear phagocytic lineage differentiation, NE mRNA transcript levels increased when HL-60 cells were induced to differentiate toward the myelocytic lineage with dimethyl sulfoxide ($Me_2SO$) (24,29,32–34). That is, following a small decrease at 24 hr, NE mRNA transcript levels increased up to 188% (3 days) and 211% (5 days) of the initial level and remained elevated even after 7 days (Fig. 4A) (29). As with the changes in NE transcript levels following differentiation toward the mononuclear phagocytic lineage, the changes in NE mRNA levels following myelocytic lineage differentiation appeared to be modulated by NE gene transcription, but in a direction opposite to that following mononuclear phagocytic differentiation (29). In this regard, during myeloctyic lineage differentiation with $Me_2SO$, although the NE gene transcription rate first showed a mild decrease to 72% of the basal level at 18 hr, there was a marked increase up to 208% after 3 days which remained elevated at 191% after 5 days of incubation (Fig. 4B). Interestingly, in contrast to the changes in NE mRNA $T_{1/2}$ following mononuclear phagocytic differentiation, the $T_{1/2}$ of NE mRNA transcripts showed a marked decrease from the baseline value of 10.1 hr after the induction of HL-60 cells to differentiate toward the myelocytic lineage with $Me_2SO$ (4.1 hr at 18 hr; 4.5 hr at 3 days; 5.1 hr at 5 days) (29). Thus, as with mononuclear phagocytic differentiation, the changes in NE mRNA levels were modulated primarily at the level of transcription despite the decline in NE transcript stability. Thus, opposing regulatory forces appear to be functioning during myelocytic differentiation, with the transcriptional processes dominating as evidenced by the marked increase in NE mRNA transcript levels (29).

Expression of the NE gene remains active in the HL-60 cell model as late as 7 days during incubation with $Me_2SO$, whereas normal mature neutrophils do not contain detectable NE mRNA transcripts (24). Although it has been well established in the literature that HL-60 cells are capable of differentiating toward the myelocytic lineage after 6–7 days of $Me_2SO$ treatment and the majority of cells could differentiate to mature myeloid cells (32–34), some populations of HL-60 cells still remain undifferentiated at the stage of promyelocytes (33,34) and thus keep expressing the NE gene. In this context, HL-60 cells may deviate from

---

**Figure 3** Expression of the NE gene during differentiation of HL-60 cells toward the mononuclear phagocytic lineage induced by PMA (29). (A) NE mRNA transcript levels evaluated by Northern analysis. Relative levels of NE and, as a control, β-actin mRNA transcripts after addition of PMA, are shown. The NE and β-actin mRNA levels in undifferentiated HL-60 cells were defined as 100%. Each data point represents the average of three independent experiments. (B) Relative transcription rate of the NE and β-actin genes after incubation of HL-60 cells with PMA compared to that of undifferentiated cells defined as 100%. Each point represents the average of two separate determinations.

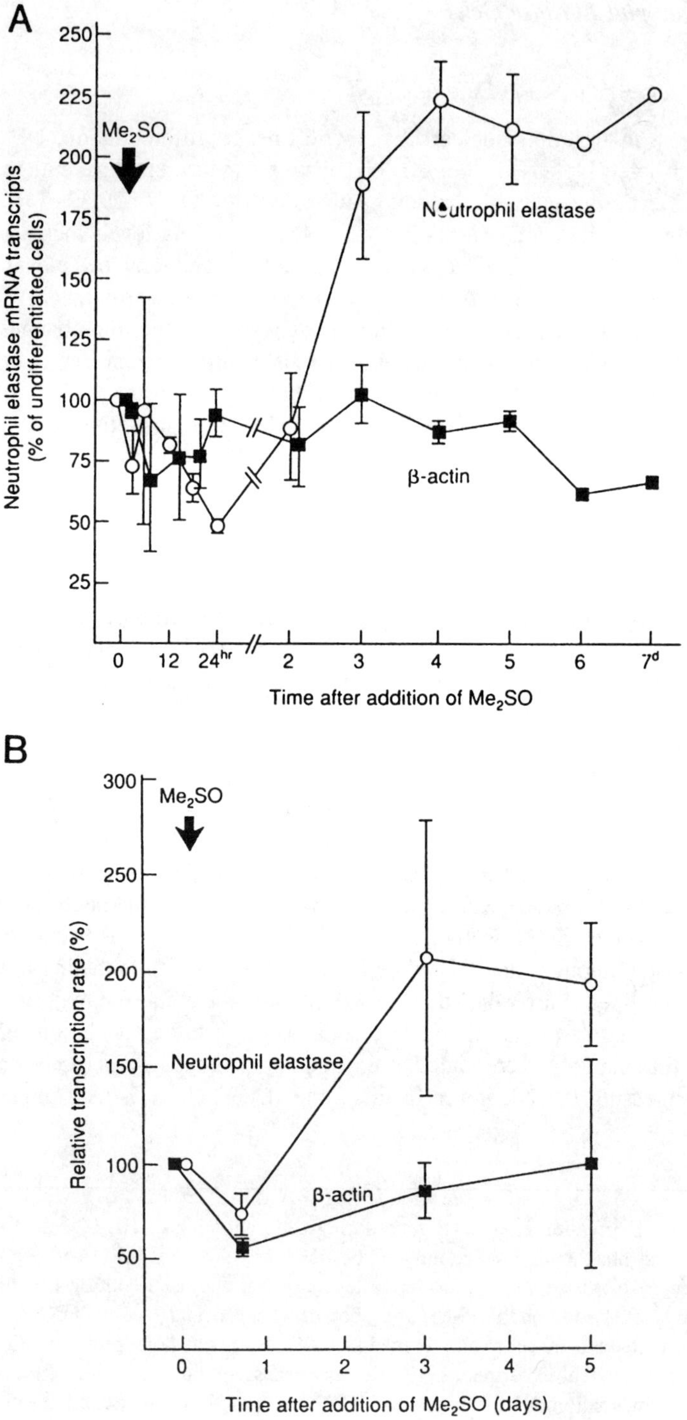
A
Me2SO
Neutrophil elastase mRNA transcripts (% of undifferentiated cells)
250
225
200
175
150
125
100
75
50
25
Neutrophil elastase
β-actin
0
12
24hr
2
3
4
5
6
7d
Time after addition of Me2SO
B
Me2SO
Relative transcription rate (%)
300
250
200
150
100
50
Neutrophil elastase
β-actin
0
1
2
3
4
5
Time after addition of Me2SO (days)

normal myeloid maturation in some aspects, and the discrepancy of NE mRNA levels between $Me_2SO$-treated HL-60 cells and normal neutrophils may be one of the examples.

### C. Regulation of NE Gene Expression

The transcriptional and posttranscriptional modulation of NE gene expression during bone marrow differentiation is of interest in comparison to that of the genes coding for other enzymes stored in the azurophilic granules of neutrophils such as myeloperoxidase (MPO) and cathepsin G (2,18,20,27,28,35–39). The MPO gene, like the NE gene, is expressed in the limited period of the early stage of myelocytic differentiation, although MPO mRNA transcripts disappear earlier than do NE mRNA transcripts during myelocytic differentiation in bone marrow (17,18). As for the NE gene, the expression of the MPO gene in HL-60 cells is modulated during differentiation at both the transcriptional and posttrantscriptional levels (40,41). In this regard, the relative transcription rate of the MPO gene in HL-60 cells is higher than that of the NE gene (24% vs. 62% relative to that the β-actin gene) (29). Interestingly, NE mRNA transcripts in undifferentiated HL-60 cells are relatively stable, with a half-life of 10 hr, in contrast to the much shorter half-life (4.5 hr) of MPO mRNA transcripts (29,40). The relative stability of NE mRNA transcripts is consistent with the fact that they do not contain an AUUUA sequence in the 3′ untranslated regions (7,10,11), a destabilizing signal that modulates the half-life of mRNA transcripts of some cytokines and proto-oncogenes (42–44), whereas MPO mRNA transcripts have three motifs of this sequence (40,41). This may also be true for gene expression of cathepsin G, another serine protease of neutrophils (19,20). Although not much is known about differentiating-specific expression of the cathepsin G gene toward the myelocytic lineage, there is evidence that PMA causes transcriptional down-regulation of the gene in the U-937 cells along with differentiation toward the mononuclear phagocytic lineage (20). The NE gene and the MPO gene share a 19 bp highly homologous (90%) sequence in their 5′ flanking regions (7), and a similar pyrimidine-rich motif is also found in the 5′ flanking region of the cathepsin G gene, starting at the position of −53 (19). Since the first part of this sequence (CCCCTTC) is identical in these three genes, it is conceivable that these genes

---

**Figure 4** Expression of the NE gene during differentiation of HL-60 cells toward the myelocytic lineage induced by $Me_2SO$ (29). (A) NE mRNA transcript levels evaluated by Northern analysis. Relative levels of NE and, as a control, β-actin mRNA transcripts after addition of $Me_2SO$, are shown. The NE and β-actin mRNA levels in undifferentiated HL-60 cells were defined as 100%. Each data point represents the average three independent experiments except at 6 and 7 days. (B) Relative transcription rate of the NE and β-actin genes after incubation of HL-60 cells with $Me_2SO$ compared to that of undifferentiated cells defined as 100%. Each point represents the average of two separate determinations.

may be transcriptionally regulated, at least in part, in a related manner during myeloid differentiation.

## IV. Future Direction of Research on the NE Gene and Its Product

These observations of the modulation of lineage-specific NE gene expression in bone marrow cell differentiation could offer possible clinical applications. First, for human disorders in which a relative excess of NE plays a central role, such as pulmonary emphysema associated with $\alpha$1AT deficiency (6,45,46), one therapeutic strategy to modulate the amount of NE in the target organ could be directed at suppressing expression of the NE gene in bone marrow in the early stages of myeloid differentiation by developing agents that would mimic the down-regulating effect of PMA. However, such an approach may carry risks if NE serves functions critical for normal biological activities. Second, the fact that NE gene expression is tightly controlled and limited to the promyelocytic stage of myeloid differentiation provides a possible marker for the subclassification of acute leukemias based on the identification of the stage of arrest of myeloid cells during their differentiation (47). Third, by virtue of progress in science and modern technology, it is now possible to elucidate the biological function of NE using transgenic animals overexpressing the NE gene, or animals that are disrupted at the NE gene locus by gene targeting (48). Finally, the transfer of the normal NE gene using a viral or plasmid vector to the local site may prove an effective therapeutic approach for disease conditions such as prolonged superficial infection or excess scar formation (49).

## References

1. Janoff A, Scherer J. Mediators of inflammation in leukocyte lysosomes: IX. elastinolytic activity in granules of human polymorphonuclear leukocytes. J Exp Med 1968; 128:1137–1155.
2. Travis J, Giles PJ, Porcelli L, Reilly CF, Bauch R, Powers J. Human leucocyte elastase and cathepsin G: structural and functional characteristics. In Evered D, Whelan J, eds. Protein Degradation in Health and Disease. Amsterdam: Ciba Foundation Symposium 75, 1980:51–68.
3. Heck LW, Darby WL, Hunter FA, Brown A, Miller EJ, Bennett JC. Isolation, characterization, and amino-terminal amino acid sequence analysis of human neutrophil elastase from normal donors. Ann Biochem 1985; 149:153–162.
4. Bieth JG. Elastase: catalytic and biological properties. In: Mecham R, ed. Regulation of Matrix Accumulation. New York: Academic Press, 1986:217–320.
5. Sinha S, Watorek W, Karr S, Giles J, Bode W, Travis J. Primary structure of human neutrophil elastase. Proc Natl Acad Sci USA 1987; 84:2228–2232.

6. Janoff A. Elastase in tissue injury. Ann Rev Med 1985; 36:207–216.
7. Takahashi H, Nukiwa T, Yoshimura K, Quick CD, States DJ, Holmes MD, Whang-Peng J, Knutsen T, Crystal RG. Structure of the human neutrophil elastase gene. J Biol Chem 1988; 263:14739–14747.
8. Zimmer M, Medcalf RL, Fink TM, Mattmann C, Lichter P, Jenne DE. The human elastase-like genes coordinately expressed in the myelomonocyte lineage are organized as a single genetic locus on 19pter. Proc Natl Acad Sci USA 1992; 89:8215–8219.
9. Heusel JW, Hanson RD, Silverman GA, Ley TJ. Structure and expression of a cluster of human hematopoietic serine protease genes found on chromosomes 14q11.2. J Biol Chem 1991; 266:6152–6158.
10. Nakamura H, Okano K, Aoki Y, Shimizu H, Naruto M. Nucleotide sequence of human bone marrow serine protease (medullasin) gene. Nucleic Acids Res 1987; 15: 9601–9602.
11. Farley D, Travis J, Salvesen G. The human neutrophil elastase gene: analysis of the nucleotide sequence reveals three distinct classes of repetitive DNA. Biol Chem Hoppe-Seyler 1989; 370:737–744.
12. Mitchell PJ, Tjian R. Transcriptional regulation in mammalian cells by sequence-specific DNA binding proteins. Science 1989; 245:371–378.
13. Murre C, McCaw PS, Baltimore D. A new DNA binding and dimerization motif in immunoglobulin enhancer binding, *daughterless, MyoD*, and *myc* proteins. Cell 1989; 56:777–783.
14. Murre C, McCaw PS, Vaessin H, Caudy M, Jan LY, Jan N, Cabrera CV, Buskin JN, Hauschka SD, Lassar AB, Weintraub H, Baltimore D. Interactions between heterologous helix-loop-helix proteins generate complexes that bind specifically to a common DNA sequence. Cell 1989; 58:537–544.
15. Chakraborty T, Brennan TJ, Li L, Edmondson D, Olson EN. Inefficient homo-oligomerization contributes to the dependence of myogenin on E2A products for efficient DNA binding. Mol Cell Biol 1991; 11:3633–3641.
16. Roy AL, Carruthers C, Gutjahr T, Roeder RG. Direct role for Myc in transcription initiation mediated by interactions with TFII-I. Nature 1993; 365:359–361.
17. Fouret P, du Bois RM, Bernaudin J-F, Takahashi H, Ferrans VJ, Crystal RG. Expression of the neutrophil elastase gene during human bone marrow cell differentiation. J Exp Med 1989; 169:833–845.
18. Yamada M, Kurahashi K. Regulation of myeloperoxidase gene expression during differentiation of human myeloid leukemia HL-60 cells. J Biol Chem 1984; 259: 3021–3025.
19. Hohn P, Popescu NC, Hanson RD, Salvesen G, Ley TJ. Genomic organization and chromosomal localization of the human cathepsin G gene. J Biol Chem 1989; 264: 13412–13419.
20. Hanson RD, Connolly NL, Burnett D, Campbell EJ, Senior RM, Ley TJ. Developmental regulation of the human cathepsin G gene in myelomonocytic cells. J Biol Chem 1990; 265:1524–1530.
21. Yoshimura K, Chu C-S, Crystal RG. Enhancer function of a 53-bp repetitive element in the 5′ flanking region of the human neutrophil elastase gene. Biochem Biophys Res Commun 1994; 204:38–42.

22. Collins SJ, Gallo RC, Gallagher RE. Continuous growth and differentiation of human myeloid leukemic cells in suspension culture. Nature 1977; 270:347–349.
23. Collins SJ. The HL-60 promyelocytic leukemia cell line: proliferation, differentiation, and cellular oncogene expression. Blood 1987; 70:1233–1244.
24. Takahashi H, Nukiwa T, Basset P, Crystal RG. Myelomonocytic cell lineage expression of the neutrophil elastase gene. J Biol Chem 1989; 263:2543–2547.
25. Lobe CG, Finlay BB, Paranchych W, Paetkau VA, Bleackley RC. Novel serine proteases encoded by two cytotoxic T-lymphocyte-specific genes. Science 1986; 232:858–862.
26. Klein JL, Shows TB, Dupont B, Trapani JA. Genomic organization and chromosomal assignment for a serine protease gene (CSPB) expressed by human cytotoxic lymphocytes. Genomics 1989; 5:110–117.
27. Salvesen G, Farley D, Shuman J, Przybyla A, Reilly C, Travis J. Molecular cloning of human cathepsin G: structural similarity to mast cell and cytotoxic T lymphocyte proteinases. Biochemistry 1987; 26:2289–2293.
28. Falloon J, Gallin JI. Neutrophil granules in health and disease. J Allergy Clin Immunol 1986; 77:653–662.
29. Yoshimura K, Crystal RG. Transcriptional and posttranscriptional modulation of human neutrophil elastase gene expression. Blood 1992; 79:2733–2740.
30. Han J, Unlap T, Rado TA. Expression of the human neutrophil elastase gene: positive and negative transcriptional elements in the 5′ flanking region. Biochem Biophys Res Commun 1991; 181:1462–1468.
31. Rovera G, O'Brien TG, Diamond L. Induction of differentiation in human promylocytic leukemia cells by tumor promoters. Science 1979; 204:868–870.
32. Harris P, Ralph P. Human leukemia models of myelomonocytic development: a review of the HL-60 and U937 cell lines. J Leukocyte Biol 1985; 37:407–422.
33. Collins SJ, Ruscetti FW, Gallagher RE, Gallo RC. Terminal differentiation of human promyelocytic leukemia cells induced by dimethyl sulfoxide and other polar compounds. Proc Natl Acad Sci USA 1978; 75:2458–2462.
34. Collins SJ, Ruscetti FW, Gallagher RE, Gallo RC. Normal functional characteristics of cultured human promyelocytic leukemia cells (HL-60) after induction of differentiation by dimethylsulfoxide. J Exp Med 1979; 149:969–974.
35. Morishita K, Kubota N, Asano S, Kaziro Y, Nagata S. Molecular cloning and characterization of cDNA for human myeloperoxidase. J Biol Chem 1987; 262:3844–3851.
36. Weil SC, Rosner GL, Reid MS, Chisholm RL, Farber NM, Spitznagel JK, Swanson MS. cDNA cloning of human myeloperoxidase: decrease in myeloperoxidase mRNA upon induction of HL-60 cells. Proc Natl Acad Sci USA 1987; 84:2057–2061.
37. Yamada M, Hur S-J, Hashinaka K, Tsuneoka K, Saeki T, Nishio C, Sakiyama F, Tsunasawa S. Isolation and characterization of a cDNA coding for human myeloperoxidase. Arch Biochem Biophys 1987; 255:147–155.
38. Morishita K, Tsuchiya M, Asano S, Kaziro Y, Nagata S. Chromosomal gene structure of human myeloperoxidase and regulation of its expression by granulocyte colony-stimulating factor. J Biol Chem 1987; 262:15208–15213.
39. Johnson KR, Nauseef WM, Care A, Wheelock MJ, Shane S, Hudson S, Koeffler HP,

Selsted M, Miller C, Rovera G. Characterization of cDNA clones for human myeloperoxidase: predicted amino acid sequence and evidence for multiple mRNA species. Nucleic Acids Res 1987; 15:2013–2028.
40. Tobler A, Miller CW, Johnson KR, Selsted ME, Rovera G, Koeffler HP. Regulation of gene expression of myeloperoxidase during myeloid differentiation. J Cell Physiol 1988; 136:215–225.
41. Sagoh T, Yamada M. Transcriptional regulation of myeloperoxidase gene expression in myeloid leukemia HL-60 cells during differentiation into granulocytes and macrophages. Arch Biochem Biophys 1988; 262:599–604.
42. Caput D, Beutler B, Hartog K, Thayer R, Brown-Shimer S, Cerami A. Identification of a common nucleotide sequence in the 3′-untranslated region of mRNA molecules specifying inflammatory mediators. Proc Natl Acad Sci USA 1986; 83:1670–1674.
43. Shaw G, Kamen R. A conserved AU sequence from the 3′ untranslated region of GM-CSF mRNA mediates selective mRNA degradation. Cell 1986; 46:659–667.
44. Wilson T, Treisman R. Removal of poly(A) and consequent degradation of c-fos mRNA facilitated by 3′ AU-rich sequences. Nature 1988; 336:396–399.
45. Hubbard RC, Brantly ML, Crystal RG. Proteases. In: Crystal RG, West JB, eds. The Lung. New York: Scientific Foundations, Raven, 1991:1763–1774.
46. Hubbard RC, Crystal RG. Susceptibility of the lung to proteolytic injury. In: Crystal RG, West JB, eds. The Lung. New York: Scientific Foundations, Raven, 1991:2059–2072.
47. Kramps JA, Van der Valk P, Van der Sandt MM, Lindeman J, Meijer CJLM. Elastase as a marker for neutrophilic myeloid cells J Histochem Cytochem 1984; 32:389–394.
48. Capecchi MR. The new mouse genetics: altering the genome by gene targeting. TIG 1989; 5:70–76.
49. Anderson WF. Human gene therapy. Science 1992; 256:808–813.
50. Schmidt A, Setoyama C, De Crombrugghe B. Regulation of a collagen gene promoter by the product of viral *mos* oncogene. Nature 1985; 314:286–289.
51. Gorman C, Moffat LF, Howard BH. Recombinant genomes which express chloramphenicol acetyltransferase in mammalian cells. Mol Cell Biol 1982; 2:1044–1051.
52. Potter H, Weir L, Leder P. Enhancer-dependent expression of human κ immunoglobulin genes introduced into mouse pre-B lymphocytes by electroporation. Proc Natl Acad Sci USA 1984; 81:7161–7165.
53. Felgner PL, Gadek, TR, Holm M, Roman R, Chan HW, Wenz M, Northrop JP, Ringold GM, Danielsen M. Lipofection: a highly efficient, lipid-mediated DNA-transfection procedure. Proc Natl Acad Sci USA 1987; 84:7413–7417.
54. De Wet JR, Wood KV, DeLuca M, Helinski RD, Subramani S. Firefly luciferase gene: structure and expression in mammalian cells. Mol Cell Biol 1987; 7:725–737.

# 6

# The Three-Dimensional Structure of α1AT

**RICHARD A. ENGH and WOLFRAM BODE**

Max-Planck-Institut für Biochemie
Martinsried, Germany

## I. Introduction

The first x-ray structure determination of a serpin was of a reactive-site-modified form of the normal (M variant) human alpha 1–antitrypsin (α1AT*), also called alpha 1–proteinase inhibitor (1). After cleavage at the reactive site Met358–Ser359 by chymotrypsinogen A, α1AT* formed crystals that diffracted to a resolution of 3.0Å (2). The three-dimensional structure revealed that a major conformational rearrangement took place upon cleavage, since the residues at the cleavage site were separated by 69Å in the cleaved structure but are covalently bonded in the uncleaved inhibitor. The structure of the similarly cleaved S variant (a1AT-S*), along with the refinement of the normal cleaved M variant α1AT*, was subsequently reported (3). These structures provided the basis for evaluation of serpin function (4), but still failed to provide a detailed structure of the active inhibitor form. To date, no such structure has been reported. The recently solved structures of noninhibitory conformations of other serpins (for a summary, see Table 1), including ovalbumin (5,6), the latent, noninhibitory form of plasminogen activator inhibitor 1 (7), unmodified antichymotrypsin (8), and antithrombin dimers (9,10), and a variety of experimental studies (11) provide clues for modeling aspects of the active form (12).

**Table 1** X-Ray Structures of Serpins

| Serpin | Resolution | R-factor | Description |
|---|---|---|---|
| Modified α1AT, tetragonal form I (1,3) | 0.30 | 0.19 | First structure, obviated structural transition |
| Modified α1AT, hexagonal form (3) | 0.31 | 0.22 | Allowed averaging of crystal forms for improved refinement |
| Modified α1AT, tetragonal form II (3) | 0.30 | 0.21 | Allowed averaging of crystal forms for improved refinement |
| Modified α1AT, variant (3) | 0.31 | 0.22 | Very similar to normal M variant |
| Modified ovalbumin (plakalbumin) (5) | 0.28 | 0.19 | Five-stranded beta sheet A, model for intact serpins |
| Ovalbumin (6) | 0.20 | 0.17 | High-resolution, showed flexible alpha-helical conformation of binding loop |
| Modified horse leukocyte elastase inhibitor (37) | 0.20 | 0.18 | High-resolution structure, localization of internal solvent positions |
| Modified α1ACT (30) | 0.27 | 0.18 | Different conformation in the beta ribbon of sheet C, at DNA-binding site |
| Latent plasminogen activator inhibitor 1 (7) | 0.26 | 0.18 | Completely inserted beta strand s4A, flexible beta sheet C |
| Antichymotrypsin (8) | 0.25 | 0.20 | Intact inhibitory serpin, reactive loop forms distorted helix |
| Antithrombin III (9) | 0.32 | 0.18 | Modeled as a dimer of cleaved/intact inhibitor |
| Antithrombin III (10) | 0.30 | 0.21 | A latent/active dimer with some evidence for partial insertion of s4A |

## II. The X-Ray Structure of Cleaved α1AT

Two cleavages occur during the proteolytic modification of α1AT (2), namely, at Thr11–Asp12 and at Met358–Ser359. The 11-residue N-terminus is thereby eliminated, leaving 383 of the inhibitor's original 394 residues. The cleaved α1AT* is folded into a highly ordered structure, with almost all of its residues found in three beta sheets (A–C), nine alpha helices (A–I), and six helical turns (Fig. 1 and Table 2; the nomenclature of the secondary structure elements is based on the following abbreviations: h = helix; s = beta sheet; and t = turn between the elements following it). Beta sheets A and B are the most extensive structures of the

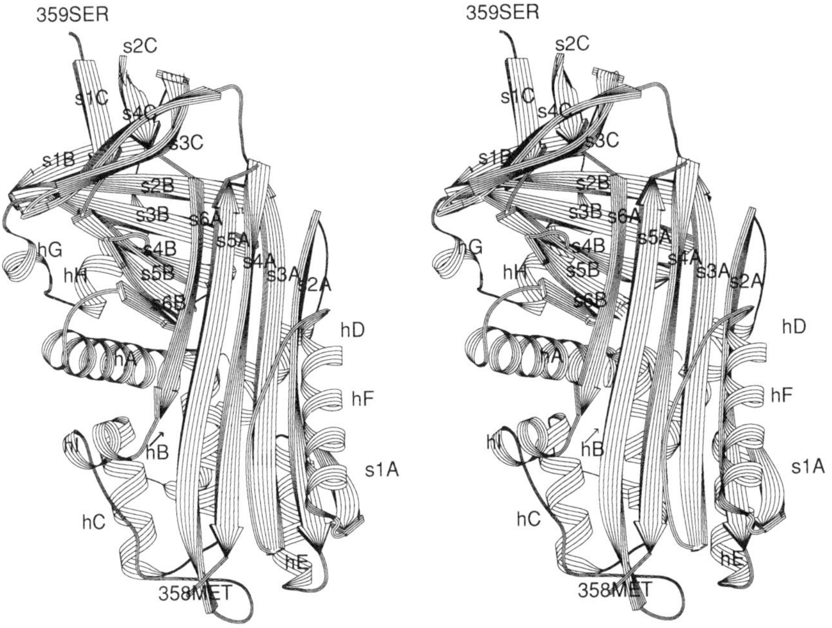


**Figure 1** Ribbon-type stereo representation of α1AT. (From Ref. 55.)

molecule. Each consists of six beta strands. Eleven of these are in an antiparallel orientation; the first short strand in sheet A (s1A in Fig. 1) is parallel to the adjacent s2A strand.

The following description refers approximately to the orientation of Fig. 1. The lower three strands (s4B, s5B, and s6B) of beta sheet B, and below them the vertically oriented helix B, form a highly conserved hydrophobic core. The planar beta sheet A is packed perpendicular to the orientation of beta sheet B in front of this core. Helix F and the following residues form a kind of flap, which is found in front of the lower part of sheet A. Beta sheet C is found on top of beta sheet B. The lower rear of the molecule consists of helices A, C, D, and E, while helices G and H are found under and behind beta sheet B. The residues at the cleavage site, Met358 and Ser359, are fixed at opposite poles of the molecule by sheets A and C; the segment that forms the new intermediate carboxy-terminus (s4A) after cleavage at Met358–Ser359 is incorporated into the middle of sheet A, and the segment forming the new intermediate amino-terminus is incorporated onto the end of sheet C (sheet s1C).

One reactive cysteine residue in the molecule was used for the preparation of heavy-metal derivatives for the multiple isomorphous replacement solution of

**Table 2** Secondary Structure Designations

| Helices and helical turns | Beta strands | Turns | Bulges |
|---|---|---|---|
| hA: 20–44 | s6B: 49–53 | thAs6B: 45–48 | 169–172 |
| hB: 53–68 | s5B: 380–389 | thBhC: 68–70 | 171–174 |
| hC: 69–81 | s4B: 369–378 | thChD: 81–88 (lh: 81) | 173–176 |
| hC1: 83–87 | s3B: 247–255 | thDs2A: 105–110 | bs5B: 382–385 |
| hD: 88–105 | s2B: 236–245 | ts2AhE: 122–127 | bs5A: 329–332 |
| hE: 127–139 | s1B: 228–233 | thEs1A: 130–140 (lh: 139) | |
| hF: 149–166 | s6A: 290–299 | ts1AhF: 146–149 | |
| hF1: 200–203 | s5A: 326–342 | thFs3A: 166–181 (lh: 166) | |
| hF2: 232–236 | s4A: 343–356 | ts3AhF1: 194–199 | |
| hG: 259–264 | s3A: 181–194 | ts4Cs3C: 211–214 | |
| hH: 268–278 | s2A: 109–121 | ts3Cs1B: 226–228 | |
| hI: 299–306 | s1A: 140–146 | ts1Bs2B: 233–236 (lh: 236) | |
| hI1: 309–312 | s4C: 203–212 | ts2Bs3B: 244–248 | |
| hI2: 376–380 | s3C: 213–226 | ts3BhG: 256–259 | |
| hI3: 390–393 | s2C: 283–289 | tsHs2C: 278–283 | |
| | s1C: 362–367 | thIls5A: 318–325 | |
| | | ts5As4A: 341–344 | |
| | | ts4Bs5B: 377–380 (lh: 380) | |
| | | ts5Bc-ter: 389–394 | |

the structure. It makes a disulfide bridge to an exogenous cysteine residue. There are no other disulfide bridges, although they are found among other serpins, either at positions corresponding to neighboring residues in α1AT or at sites of insertions or deletions.

### A. Helices and Turns

Most of the helices are grouped together behind the lower part of sheet A, with helix F the prominent exception. They are mostly regular alpha helices; helices A, B, and C have $3_{10}$ geometry at their N- and C-termini, and helix A is kinked at Pro28. Helices hF2 and hI2 are helical turns between beta strands. Helix F, together with the following "turn" segment, makes a "flap" partially covering sheet A.

Five nonglycine residues (Asn81, His139, Gln166, Ser236, and Lys380) are consistently found in a left-handed alpha-helical conformation. They occur at the C-terminal ends of helices or helical turns. Ala70, found in the three-residue turn thBhC, is well defined in a high-energy conformation. The turn region designated thFs3A is a series of overlapping bulges or turns stabilized by hydrophobic and polar interactions with helix F and sheet A residues. In particular, residues Ile169, Leu172, and Val173 of this bulge region make hydrophobic side-chain contacts to other parts of the molecule which are conserved in all serpins with only one exception. Polar interactions are similarly conserved (Lys168 to Thr339, Asp171 to Lys335).

### B. Beta Sheets

Beta sheet A dominates the overall structure of cleaved α1AT. The upper portion is almost devoid of twist. The first strand is short, with a right-handed twist when viewed along the strand, and is parallel to the second. Strands 2–5 are similar in length and antiparallel. Strands 4 and 5 are connected by a short turn segment. Strand 6, also antiparallel, is somewhat shorter than strands 2 to 5 and provides the edge of the flat upper face. The sheet has a large number of conserved hydrophobic interactions and several hydrogen bonds with the mostly hydrophobic core, comprising approximately strands 4 to 6 of sheet B and helix B. Several conserved hydrophobic contacts exist between strands 1 to 3 of sheet A and helix F, while strands 4 and 5 have many contacts to the series of bulges following helix F. These bulges form the left-hand half of the "flap" that partially covers sheet A. Glu342 of the turn between strands 4 and 5 anchors sheet A to beta sheet C via a hydrogen bond to the conserved Thr203.

Beta sheet B has a strong right-handed twist, as viewed along the strands. Most of the sheet is buried in the protein interior; strands 4–6 are hydrophobic and especially conserved among the serpins. Strands 1–3 are much more polar and exposed. Strands 1–4 form a barrel-like structure together with strands 1–3 of sheet C. The funnel-like opening to this barrel is lined with conserved hydrophobic residues and is thought to be the attachment site for the substrates of carrier serpins such as thyroxin-binding globulin and corticol-binding globulin.

Beta sheet C has four strands, and two parts can be distinguished: a three-stranded beta sheet formed by strands 1–3 and a two-stranded beta ribbon formed by strands 3 and 4. Strands 2–4 are antiparallel. Strand 1 is formed by the residues immediately following the cleavage site at Ser359 and is parallel to strand 2. Sheet C is exposed to the solvent on one side and on the other is packed with hydrophobic contacts to sheet B in the three-stranded region. The absolutely conserved Phe208 of strand 4 fixes the center of the beta-ribbon region to a hydrophobic patch defined by the very highly conserved Val218, Phe370, Pro391, and Val388, situated at the edge of sheet B near the N-terminus. The outer several residues at the beta hairpin ts4Cs3C at the end of the beta ribbon make no significant contacts with the main body of the molecule, but have two hydrogen bonds with the saccharides modeled at the Asn46 glycosylation site. Despite the dearth of intramolecular contacts to the loop, temperature factors do not indicate significantly higher mobility.

### C. Surface Properties and Glycosylation

As expected, charged and polar residues are found mostly at the surface of the molecule. A few polar residues, especially serine, are buried but typically have hydrogen bonds to main-chain peptide groups. Glu264 is mostly buried, but is near the surface and is rendered inaccessible to solvent partially through its salt-bridge partner Lys387. Similarly, Glu354, located in strand s4A under the bulge region of the helix F flap, is buried by its salt-bridge partner Lys331. This residue presumably becomes accessible to solvent in the intact form. Glu376 is mostly buried, with hydrogen bonds to the main chain and to Thr379. The distribution of the charges is not uniform; acidic residues predominate at the base of sheet A and helix F, and basic residues predominate in the region of sheet C, creating a significant dipole moment.

Three glycosylation sites could be verified by the presence of electron density. However, packing disorder, chemical heterogeneity of the carbohydrate (13) (see also the review of Travis and Salveson, Ref. 14) and high mobility precluded determination of the carbohydrate structure. The coordinates (3) available from the Brookhaven Protein Data Bank (15,16) include model coordinates based on the expected sequence Asn–NAG–NAG–MAN–branch, where NAG represents N-acetylglucosamine and MAN represents mannose, which branches to form a bi- or triantennary side chain, but the modeled three-dimensional structure is not uniquely determined by the electron density. Crystal packing allows more carbohydrate to be present than is shown by the electron density.

### D. Crystal Packing, Solvent, and Disordered Regions

Both crystal forms have similar main crystal contacts, dominated by head (the Ser359 end) to tail (the Met358 end) packing. A salt bridge between the Ser359 N-terminus of the head end and Glu324 of the tail end is included among these interactions. A side-by-side packing interaction forms an antiparallel sheet between a short strand of the beta ribbon of sheet C (Val213–Val216) and the same strand in the neighboring molecule. A third interaction including salt bonds between the segment from Lys310 to Asp314, with the C-terminus Met358, and the segment from Glu279 to Arg281 of the neighbor molecule occurs in the tetragonal crystal form. The different crystal forms have very similar structures. The entire molecules of the tetragonal and hexagonal forms could be fit with an r.m.s. deviation of 0.46 Å including all atoms and an r.m.s. deviation of 0.33 Å including only alpha carbons.

The first eight residues (Asp12–Asp19) were not resolved in any of the crystal forms, nor was the side chain of the last residue, Lys394. The side chain of His20 was not resolved in the tetragonal form. The nine N-terminal residues are located in a solvent-filled cavity in the unit cell and are disordered. The hexagonal crystal form had the lowest temperature factors. Areas with high temperature factors correlate clearly with turn regions. The greatest exception to this is the N-terminal side of helix hA, which has very large temperature factors for the main-chain atoms, especially residues His20, Pro21, and Thr22.

In the hexagonal form, 159 water molecule positions were determined. Three water molecules were found that form bridges between side-chain atoms. The turn thAs6B is stabilized through a solvent molecule. The end of helix D (His139CO) is hydrogen-bonded via a water molecule to the center of strand s2A (Gly116NH). The amine groups of residues 174 and 175 in the bulge region following helix F are bridged through a water molecule. Fifteen other hydrogen bonds are found between water molecules and main-chain atoms in turn regions. The ordered solvent molecules in the areas of highest concentration are generally conserved in both crystal forms.

### E. The Cleaved α1AT Structure and α1AT Deficiency Variants

Of the more than 75 alleles identified for variants of α1AT, some 20 variants associated with risk of α1AT deficiency have been sequenced (17–19). One of these, the Pittsburgh variant, differs at the P1 reactive site (in the notation of Schechter and Berger, Ref. 20) and shows altered inhibitor specificity. The substitution of an arginine for methionine at position 358 renders it a potent thrombin inhibitor, as expected for serine proteinase inhibition by the standard mechanism (21,22), and leads to a fatal bleeding disorder (23). The other pathological variants are associated with decreased plasma levels of α1AT and an increased risk of emphysema, and liver disease in cases of normal expression but faulty secretion of α1AT.

#### *The S Variant*

The most common deficiency variant, the S variant, occurs with the mutation of Glu264 to Val (24). Its crystal structure does not differ significantly from the native structure except at the mutation site (3). Glu264 is found in helix G, mostly buried, and is hydrogen-bonded to $O^{\eta}$ of Tyr38 in helix A and $N^{\zeta}$ of Lys387 of s5B. The mutation to valine eliminates these interactions and increases the mobility of the nearby residues. The temperature factors of the valine side chain are 33 $Å^2$, versus 7 $Å^2$ for the Glu264 side chain in the hexagonal form. The temperature factors of the Tyr38 side chain also increase. Tyr38 and Lys387 do not make hydrogen bonds in either structure, but are closer together in the mutant (3.6 Å vs. 4.0 Å). These residues are partially accessible to solvent in the native structure, and slightly more so in the mutant, so solvent may moderate the electrostatic and hydrogen-bonding effects of the change. An ordered solvent molecule is found close to the previous position of $O^{\epsilon 1}$ of Glu264. The loss of the polar interactions offers an explanation for the lower thermodynamic stability of the mutant. The S variant inhibits trypsin normally in vitro, and also inhibits elastase relatively well, and the half-life in circulation also seems normal (25). This, and the observation that there are no dramatic differences in the variant structure, indicates that slower folding and increased aggregation and degradation of the mutant might be the causes of the α1AT deficiency in SS homozygotes.

### The Z Variant

Like the S variant, the Z variant (Glu342→Lys) (26) involves the loss of a conserved salt bridge, and results in reduced plasma levels. Its structure was not determined crystallographically. Glu342 makes a conserved hydrogen bond to Thr203 and a salt bridge to the conserved positive charge of Lys290, thereby linking sheet A with sheet C. The importance of this salt bridge is confirmed by the observation that a second mutation of Lys290→Glu can partially correct the defect (27). Unlike the S variant, the Z variant apparently inhibits elastase much less efficiently than normal variants (28). Wu and Foreman (17) review the effects of various charge substitutions at sites 290 and 342 on the secretion of α1AT.

### Other Mutants

Most of the deficiency mutants involve the replacement of a conserved residue or property such that a disruption of the inhibitor may be rationalized on structural grounds. However, it is in general not possible to predict exactly what effect point mutations will have. For example, the highly conserved Gly67 in helix B makes close contacts with the similarly conserved Phe/Tyr130 of helix E and Gly320. Replacement by large and polar glutamic acid in the Mineral Springs deficiency variant (29) must disrupt this structure. A less clearly understood disruption, the Null Newport or Null Devon variant, involves the mutation of Gly115→Ser (30). Residue 115 is not conserved among serpins, has a backbone conformation compatible with any residue type, and is accessible to solvent, so replacement by the small, polar serine residue is not obviously detrimental. Other variants are summarized together with structural considerations in reviews (4,19).

## III. X-Ray Structures Related to the Intact Form

Certain features of the postcleavage structural transformation, and thus of the intact structure, were clear from the original α1AT structure. At least one of the beta strands (s4A or s1C) surrounding the cleavage site in the cleaved structure would have to adopt a different conformation in the intact structure. Because Ala350 in s4A of α1AT is buried in the hydrophobic interior but is a cleavage site for a metalloprotease (31), and because its cognate residue in ovalbumin, a serine, is phosphorylated (32), Loebermann et al. (1) proposed that the strand s4A is incorporated into sheet A only after cleavage. They suggested that sheet A is in a destabilized state prior to cleavage. The reactive site would be positioned somewhere near the barrel end of the molecule, probably in a conformation similar to that found in the small serine proteinase inhibitors (33,34). This transition was called the S→R transition, denoting the uncleaved conformation as strained and the cleaved conformation as relaxed (1,35). This very general model of serpin behavior is consistent with the x-ray structures of other serpins determined since α1AT.

### A. α1ACT and Leukocyte Elastase Inhibitor

The structures of cleaved alpha 1–antichymotrypsin (α1ACT) (36) and cleaved horse leukocyte elastase inhibitor (37) showed similar structures and reinforced the earlier conclusions at 2.0 Å resolution. In addition, the antichymotrypsin structure showed an altered but well-defined conformation of the beta ribbon in sheet C, at the DNA-binding site. This has ramifications for models of the intact α1AT (see the description of the PAI-1 structure, and the models, below). The high resolution of the leukocyte elastase inhibitor structure allowed the determination of 17 internal solvent molecules, in positions likely related to α1AT.

### B. Plakalbumin

Ovalbumin was recognized as a serpin with the identification of the serpin family (38), although it had no recognized inhibitory function. Later studies showed that dephosphorylated ovalbumin does not undergo the S→R transition (39,40). Plakalbumin, which is ovalbumin modified by the excision of the hexapeptide (P6-P1, or 353–358 in α1AT nomenclature) by subtilisin cleavage of ovalbumin, was therefore considered a possible model for the overall folding of uncleaved serpins, especially sheet A. It also reproducibly formed large, plaque-like crystals, giving it the name plakalbumin (41).

As expected, the structure of plakalbumin (5) differs from that of α1AT primarily at sheet A. Strand s4A of cleaved a1AT is absent in sheet A, as predicted by Loebermann et al. (1). The beta sheet was found to have a nearly ideal five-stranded beta-sheet geometry (see Fig. 2), with antiparallel interactions between strand pairs s5A–s6A and s2A–s3A, and parallel interactions between s4A–s5A and s1A–s2A. By aligning the conserved hydrophobic core regions of α1AT and plakalbumin, it became apparent that the conformational transition involves a translation of strands s1A–s3A relative to the rest of the molecule; strands s5A and s6A had nearly identical conformations and positions. Helix F is apparently translated in parallel with strands s1A–s3A. The flatness of sheet A may be a prerequisite for this reformation of sheet A to occur.

In plakalbumin, at the turn between s4A and s5A, the remaining residues up to the cleavage site emerge from the sheet and lie along the protein surface. Strand s3A is found mostly at the position corresponding to s4A in cleaved α1AT*, and strand s2A mostly at α1AT's s3A position. However, the upper segments of these

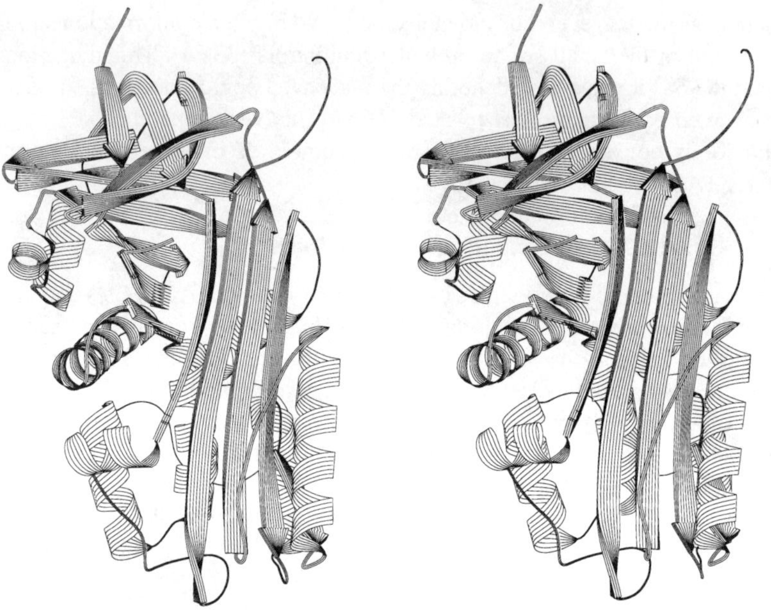

**Figure 2** Ribbon-type stereo representation of plakalbumin. Removal of a hexapeptide from strand s4A, and especially the occurrence of an arginine at the P14 position, prevents insertion of the strand into sheet A after cleavage. Sheet A is five-stranded, with parallel interactions between strands s3A and s5A (compare with Figure 1). (From Ref. 5.)

strands have identical positions as in α1AT*, leaving a small opening that in α1AT* contains the first residues of s4A but here is filled with ordered water molecules. Residue 345, following the turn between strands s5A and s4A, is an arginine in ovalbumin and the angiotensinogens, but is otherwise conserved as Thr, Val, or Ala among all inhibitory serpins. Wright et al. (5) pointed out that a small hydrophobic residue at this site is a prerequisite for the insertion of strand s4A into sheet A.

### C. Ovalbumin

The 1.9 Å structure of intact ovalbumin, solved with molecular replacement using the plakalbumin coordinates, followed soon after (6). In three of the four crystallographically independent ovalbumin molecules, the strand from P9 to P1′ unambiguously adopted an alpha-helix structure. This was contrary to expectations based on the canonical structure of small serine proteinase inhibitors, but is consistent with a strong alpha-helix propensity predicted for this region (42). Superposition of the independent structures showed deviations in the position of this new helix of 2–3 Å. Since helical residues are not accessible to cleavage by serine proteinases, the helix was supposed to unfold prior to or during proteinase binding. The similarity between the structure of the ovalbumin-reactive loop and an intact α1AT structure is uncertain, especially since ovalbumin is not an inhibitor and does not undergo the postcleavage structural rearrangement, and since all known structures of "standard mechanism" serine proteinase inhibitors adopt stable canonical conformations. However, the ovalbumin structure does corroborate the strong secondary structure predictions for an alpha helix in the binding loop of α1AT, and especially reinforces the view that the binding loop is uniquely flexible.

### D. Latent PAI

The motility of the serpins was dramatically demonstrated with the 2.6 Å resolution structure of the latent form of human plasminogen activator inhibitor-1 (PAI-1) (7). PAI-1 was known to spontaneously and reversibly adopt a "latent" and noninhibitory conformation (43). The crystal structure showed that strand s4A was completely inserted into sheet A, with only one fewer hydrogen bond than in α1AT*, and that the residues C-terminal to the cleavage site, comprising strand s1C in α1AT*, were no longer part of sheet C. Instead, this strand approaches strand s5B of sheet B from below the beta ribbon of sheet C, rather than from above as in the α1AT* and ovalbumin structures. If the inhibitory conformation of PAI-1 is to resemble that suggested by the plakalbumin and ovalbumin structures, strands s3C and s4C of the beta ribbon must move to accommodate the transition to the latent form. These were found to be disordered in latent PAI-1.

As with ovalbumin, the relevance of this structure to the structure of intact α1AT is unclear. Only PAI-1 is known to spontaneously adopt a latent conformation, although latent states have been artificially induced in antithrombin-III (44). The conserved hydrophobic residues that tether the beta ribbon of sheet C to the rest of the molecule are also present in PAI-1. PAI-1 has little homology to α1AT in the region corresponding to sheet s1C. In any case, the PAI-1 structure dramatically demonstrates the motility not only of sheet A and strand s4A, but also of sheet C.

### E. Antichymotrypsin

The first published crystal structure of an uncleaved, inhibitory serpin not in a latent state was that of antichymotrypsin (8). Extensive crystallization trials produced crystals of an inhibitory cross-linked dimer of an antichymotrypsin variant showing an alpha-helical structure of the reactive loop, similar to ovalbumin. The beta sheet A was also similar to the ovalbumin and plakalbumin structures, with a gap available for insertion of strand s4A. The alpha-helical structure is not consistent with proteinase binding, but may represent a physiological conformation of the inhibitor at some point prior to binding. The occurrence of an alpha helix in two serpin structures and the secondary structure prediction (42) support the view that α1AT may also adopt the conformation.

### F. Antithrombin III

Two groups independently reported medium-resolution crystal structures for dimers of antithrombin III (9,10). Although some ambiguity remains regarding the identity of a noninhibitory species in the dimer (cleaved or latent), the other species shows evidence of partial insertion into sheet A at position P14 (see below). Further, the reactive-site loop is in an extended conformation more suitable to proteinase binding, although it is involved in extensive crystal contacts with its dimerization partner. These structures may be particularly relevant to considerations of structures of serpins, including α1AT, as they occur during proteinase binding.

## IV. Models for the Inhibitory Form

The inhibitory state (nonlatent state of an inhibitory serpin) may involve a variety of conformations, including the helical or extended forms seen in the x-ray structures of antichymotrypsin (8) or antithrombin (9,10). This is in contrast to the small serine proteinase inhibitors (21), which apart from small local changes in cleaved forms are unchanged upon complexation. The crystallographic and other experimental evidence for serpins indicates, rather, a picture of an inhibitor with a flexible binding loop that may be induced to adopt a canonical confirmation either by complexation or prior to it, although it is not clear whether a canonical conformation must be retained after initial binding. In addition, partial insertion of the loop into sheet A must be possible for inhibitory activity; whether the stable complex occurs before or after generation of an acyl intermediate is not known.

Possibilities for a bound conformation have been examined in modeling studies (45), in which the postcleavage structural rearrangements of sheet A were investigated by computer simulations that modeled the reverse of the natural process: sheet s4A was removed from sheet A, and the structure was relaxed using molecular dynamics. The simulations showed the relaxation of the structure by the formation of a five-stranded beta sheet A. The subsequent determination of the structure of plakalbumin (5) confirmed this result and also showed that the simulations correctly predicted the translation of the strands s1A, s2A, and s3A relative to the rest of the molecule. In other work (46), the character of this transition and the relationship to the structure of ovalbumin were analyzed in further detail.

With the assumptions that the loop acquires the canonical conformation for the standard mechanism of serine proteinase inhibition (21) and that sheet C is at least as extensive in the intact structure as in the cleaved structure, two basic models for general positioning of the binding strands were created. These were further refined by the requirement that the inhibitory conformation be able to bind serine proteinases elastase (47) and, especially, thrombin (48). Thrombin forms weak complexes with α1AT, but also quite stable complexes with the Pittsburgh variant (17) (Met359→Arg at P1), which imposes very restrictive constraints on possible positions of the binding loop because of thrombin's particularly deep and narrow cleft. The strand from P14 to P5 was not sufficiently constrained by these assumptions to be modeled. The assumption of an unchanged sheet C is especially critical, since P4′ is part of sheet C and P4′ and P3′ are both proline residues, with very restricted conformational possibilities. This links the region of the likewise restricted canonical conformation (approximately P2 to P3′) to sheet C. The unknown features of the intact inhibitory form remain, however, the conformation of the whole segment defined by residues P14 to P10′, its position relative to the rest of the molecule, and details of any rearrangements of the rest of the molecule (especially sheet A).

Peptide-annealing experiments demonstrated that a peptide identical in sequence to P1–P14 could stably induce the S–R conformational transition without cleavage; by incubating at elevated temperatures, the peptide is incorporated into beta sheet A (49). The resulting binary complex is not a stable complex but instead leads to substrate-like cleavage and dissociation. In another experiment, replacement of Thr345 with Arg in α1AT by site-directed mutagenesis, done to prevent incorporation of s4A into sheet A, also renders α1AT a substrate with denaturation stability similar to that of ovalbumin (50). These two experiments, and the fact that the ability to insert s4A into sheet A is conserved among the inhibitory serpins, indicate that strand s4A in the intact, inhibitory form of α1AT is neither completely removed from sheet A as in ovalbumin nor completely inserted into sheet A as in cleaved α1AT or latent PAI-1, but is partially inserted into sheet A in inhibitory α1AT, perhaps similar to the crystal structures of antithrombin (9,10).

The extent of this insertion remains uncertain, although several recent experiments have narrowed the possibilities. Based on studies of naturally occurring mutants of the C1 inhibitor—in particular, mutations at the P12 and P10 sites that render the C1 inhibitor a substrate—Skriver et al. (51) proposed that the insertion includes residues from P14 to approximately the P10 position. Mast et al. (52) have used several enzymes to cleave the reactive site at different sites. Aggregation of the cleaved species, assumed to be by insertion of the reactive-site loop of one inhibitor into sheet A of the other, indicated a partial insertion to no more than P13. Schulze et al. (53) investigated the inhibitory properties of α1AT complexed with active-site loop mimics of incrementally varying length. The onset of inhibitory behavior with peptides corresponding to P1–P12 or shorter indicate that the partial insertion of the inhibitory form includes only the key residue Thr345 (P14). Such a minimal insertion leaves open the possibility that sheet A is essentially five-stranded in the intact inhibitor in a structure similar to that seen in plakalbumin. However, since the appropriate peptide–inhibitor binary complexes are still inhibitory, either the inhibition is relatively insensitive to (peptide-induced) rearrangements in sheet C or the inhibitory form has an open and unstable sheet A, unlike plakalbumin.

A partial insertion of strand s4A into sheet A requires the removal of beta-strand S1C residues from sheet C if the insertion includes residues beyond approximately Thr345. The PAI-1 structure indicates the possibility for large-scale structural transitions including sheet C. Considering the results of Schulze et al. (53), a possible model for the intact and inhibitory form of α1AT includes a partial insertion of strand s4A into sheet A to the Thr345 position, followed by a turn segment connecting to the binding loop in the canonical conformation, and finally leading into sheet C as modeled by Engh et al. (45). This model can be built such that it may bind to elastase or thrombin without adjustment, a further requirement for a binding model. Such a model (Fig. 3) is necessarily speculative, but provides a possibility for testable predictions.

In a model complex with elastase, most contacts between α1AT and elastase are the usual contacts of the canonical conformation (see Chapter 7 for relevant discussions of elastase and inhibitors in the canonical conformation) and are therefore largely independent of other aspects of the model. Predictions of these contacts may be derived from the structure of the complex between human leukocyte elastase and the ovomucoid third-domain inhibitor (47). Contacts between the rest of α1AT and elastase are also possible, however, and predicting these contacts depends on the model. Predicted long-range electrostatic interactions are similarly model-dependent. Besides the binding-loop interactions, the most likely contacts with elastase are (in chymotrypsinogen numbering) from 143–151, especially 146Arg and 147Asn, and with 192Phe. These regions of elastase also make contacts to the main body of the ovomucoid inhibitor. If the assumptions of the model described above are correct, these regions of elastase would be nearest to the top of sheet C (214Leu, e.g.) and the helical turn hF1 (not pictured in Fig. 1) between s3A and s4C of α1AT.

Although much indirect experimental evidence is available (11), crystallization of a stable proteinase–serpin complex is necessary to unambiguously define further details of the serpin inhibitory mechanism, especially questions of "inhibitory structure(s)." The remarkable mobilities of beta sheets C and A, demonstrated in the various crystal structures available, indicate the difficulties in inferring inhibitory properties from a limited set of structures. Another indicator of the potential pitfalls of seeking a static inhibitory structure may be found in the

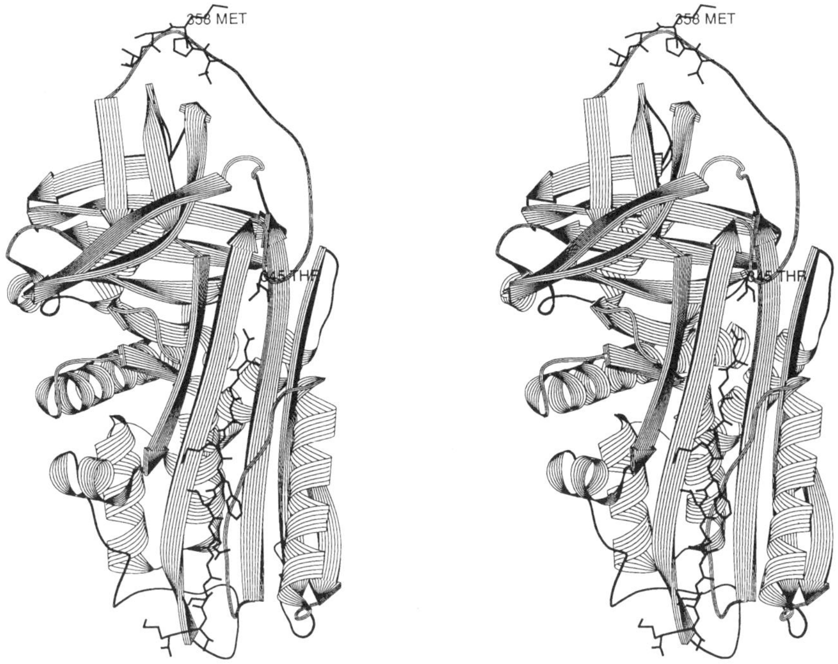


**Figure 3** Ribbon-type stereo representation of a model of intact inhibitory α1AT. The reactive site has been modeled by assuming an insertion of strand s4A to 345Thr, a canonical conformation at the reactive site (the P1 residue 358Met is labeled) in an orientation that may be docked to serine proteases, and an identical composition of sheet C as in the cleaved inhibitor. Sheet A is in the extended (six-stranded) conformation, identical to the cleaved form, as presumably induced by complexation with a peptide identical in sequence to strand s4A (see text).

property of alpha 2–antiplasmin, which is reported to inhibit trypsin and chymotrypsin at adjacent reactive sites (54). This would require sufficient flexibility to allow the inhibitor to adopt (at least) two distinct inhibitory forms with the appropriate "canonical conformation" for each enzyme.

## Acknowledgments

Discussions with Andreas Schulze and Paul Frohnert were essential for the production of this chapter, as were the ideas and assistance of Professor Robert Huber.

## References

1. Loebermann H, Tokuoka R, Deisenhofer J, Huber R. Human alpha-1 proteinase inhibitor: Crystal structure analysis of two modifications. Molecular model and preliminary analysis of the implications for function. J Mol Biol 1984; 177:531–556.
2. Loebermann H, Lottspeich F, Bode W, Huber R. Interaction of human alpha-1-proteinase inhibitor with chymotrypsinogen A and crystallization of a proteolytically modified alpha-1-proteinase inhibitor. Hoppe-Seyler's A Physiol Chem 1982; 363: 1377–1388.
3. Engh RA, Loebermann H, Schneider M, Wiegand G, Huber R, Laurell C-B. The S-variant of human alpha-1-antitrypsin, structure and implication for function and mutations. Protein Eng 1989; 2:407–415.
4. Huber R, Carrell R. Implications of the three-dimensional structure of alpha-1-antitrypsin for structure and function of serpins. Biochemistry 1989; 28:8951–8966.
5. Wright HT, Qian HX, Huber R. Crystal structure of plakalbumin, a proteolytically nicked form of ovalbumin: Its relationship to the structure of cleaved alpha-1-antitrypsin. J Mol Biol 1990; 213:513–528.
6. Stein PE, Leslie AGW, Finch JT, Turnell WG, McLaughlin PJ, Carrell RW. Crystal structure of ovalbumin as a model for the reactive centre of serpins. Nature 1990; 347:99–102.
7. Mottonen J, Strand A, Symersky J, Sweet RM, Danley DE, Geoghegan KF, Gerard RD, Goldsmith EJ. Structural basis of latency in plasminogen activator inhibitor-1. Nature 1992; 355:270–273.
8. Wei A, Rubin H, Cooperman BS, Christianson DW. Crystal structure of an uncleaved serpin reveals the conformation of an inhibitory reactive loop. Nature Struct Biol 1994; 1:251–258.
9. Schreuder HA, de Boer B, Dijkema R, Mulders J, Theunissen HJM, Grootenhuis PDJ, Hol WGJ. The intact and cleaved human antithrombin III complex as a model for serpin-proteinase interactions. Nature Struct Biol 1994; 1:48–54.
10. Carrell RW, Stein PE, Fermi G, Wardell MR. Biological implications of a 3 Angstrom structure of dimeric antithrombin. Structure 1994; 2:257–270.
11. Schulze AJ, Huber R, Bode W, Engh RA. Structural aspects of serpin inhibition. FEBS Lett 1994; 344:117–124.
12. Engh RA, Schulze AJ, Huber R, Bode W. Serpin structures. Behring Inst Mitt 1993; 93:41–62.
13. Mega T, Luja E, Yoshida A. Studies on the oligosaccharide chains of human alpha-1-proteinase inhibitor. J Biol Chem 1980; 255:4057–4061.
14. Travis J, Salveson G. Plasma proteinase inhibitors. Annu Rev Biochem 1983; 52: 655–709.
15. Bernstein FC, Koetzle TF, Williams GJB, Meyer EF Jr., Price MD, Rogers JR, Kennard O, Shimanouchi T, Tasumi M. The Protein Data Bank: A computer based archival file for macromolecular structures. J Mol Biol 1977; 112:535–542.
16. Abola EE, Bernstein FC, Bryant SH, Koetzle TF, Weng J. In: Allen FH, Berghoff G, Sievers R, eds. Crystallographic Databases: Information Content, Software Systems,

Scientific Applications. Data Commission of the International Union of Crystallography. Bonn, 1987:107–132.
17. Wu Y, Foreman RC. The molecular genetics of alpha-1 antitrypsin deficiency. BioEssays 1991; 13:163–169.
18. Crystal RG. Alpha-1-antitrypsin deficiency, emphysema, and liver disease. J Clin Invest 1990; 85:1343–1352.
19. Stein PE, Carrell PW. What do dysfunctional serpins tell us about molecular mobility and disease? Nature Struct Biol 1995; 2:96–113.
20. Schechter I, Berger A. On the size of active site in proteases. I. Papain. Biochem Biophys Res Comm 1967; 27:157.
21. Bode W, Huber R. Natural protein proteinase inhibitors and their interaction with proteinases. Eur J Biochem 1992; 204:433–451.
22. Laskowski M Jr., Kato I. Protein inhibitors of proteinases. Annu Rev Biochem 1980; 49:593–626.
23. Owen MC, Brennan SO, Lewis JH, Carrell RW. Mutation of antitrypsin to antithrombin: Antitrypsin Pittsburgh (358 Met-Arg), a fatal bleeding disorder. N Engl J Med 1983; 309:694–698.
24. Owen MC, Carrell RW. Alpha-1-antitrypsin: molecular abnormality of S variant. Br Med J 1976; 1:130.
25. Carrell RW, Jeppsson J-O, Laurell C-B, Brennan SO, Owen MC, Vaughan L, Boswell DR. Structure and variation of human alpha-1-antitrypsin. Nature 1982; 298: 329–334.
26. Jeppsson J-O. Amino-acid substitution Glu→Lys in alpha-1-antitrypsin. FEBS Lett 1976; 65:195.
27. Brantly ML, Courtney M, Crystal RG. Repair of the secretion defect in the Z form of alpha-1-antitrypsin by addition of a second mutation. Science 1988; 242:1700–1702.
28. Ogushi F, Fells GA, Hubbard RC, Straus SD, Crystal RG. Z-type alpha-1-antitrypsin is less competent than M1-type alpha-1-antitrypsin as an inhibitor of neutrophil elastase. J Clin Invest 1987; 80:1366–1374.
29. Curiel DT, Vogelmeier C, Hubbard RC, Stier LE, Crystal RG. Molecular basis of alpha-1-antitrypsin deficiency and emphysema associated with the alpha-1-antitrypsin M (mineral springs) allele. Mol Cell Biol 1990; 10:47–56.
30. Kalsheker N. Alpha-1-antitrypsin: Structure, function and molecular biology of the gene. Bioscience Rep 1989; 9:129–138.
31. Kress LF, Kurecki T, Shung Kai Chan, Laskowski M Jr. Characterization of the inactive fragment resulting from limited proteolysis of human alpha-1-proteinase inhibitor. J Biol Chem 1979; 254:5317–5320.
32. Nisbet AD, Sacundry RH, Moir AFG, Fothergill JE. The complete amino acid sequence of hen ovalbumin. Eur J Biochem 1981; 115:335–345.
33. Papamokos E, Weber E, Bode W, Huber R, Empie MW, Kato I, Laskowski M Jr. Crystallographic refinement of Japanese quail ovomucoid, a Kazal-type inhibitor, and model building studies of complexes with serine proteases. J Mol Biol 1982; 158:515–537.
34. Bode W, Papamokos E, Musil D. The high resolution x-ray crystal structure of the

complex formed between subtilisin carlsberg and eglin c, an elastase inhibitor from the leech hirudo medicinalis. Eur J Biochem 1987; 166:673–692.
35. Carrell RW, Owen MC. Plakalbumin, alpha-1-antitrypsin, antithrombin and the mechanism of inflammation. Nature 1985; 317:730–732.
36. Baumann U, Huber R, Bode W, Grosse D, Lesjak M, Laurell C-B. Crystal structure of cleaved alpha-1-antichymotrypsin at 2.7 Angstrom resolution and its comparison with other serpins. J Mol Biol 1991; 218:595–606.
37. Baumann U, Bode W, Huber R, Travis J, Potempa J. Crystal structure of cleaved equine leukocyte elastase inhibitor determined at 1.95 Angstrom resolution. J Mol Biol 1992; 226:1207–1218.
38. Hunt LT, Dayhoff MO. A surprising new protein superfamily containing ovalbumin, antithrombin III and alpha-1-proteinase inhibitor. Biochem Biophys Res Commun 1980; 95:864–871.
39. Stein P, Tewkesbury DA, Carrell RW. Ovalbumin and angiotensinogen lack serpin S-R conformational change. Biochem J 1989; 262:661–663.
40. Gettins P. Absence of large scale conformational change upon limited proteolysis of ovalbumin, the prototypic serpin. J Biol Chem 1989; 264:3781–3785.
41. Miller M, Weinstein JN, Wlodawer A. Preliminary X-ray analysis of single crystals of ovalbumin and plakalbumin. J Biol Chem 1983; 258:5864–5866.
42. Garnier J, Osguthorpe DJ, Robson B. Analysis of the accuracy and implications of simple methods for predicting the secondary structure of globular proteins. J Mol Biol 1978; 120:92–120.
43. Heckman CM, Loskutoff DJ. Endothelial cells produce a latent inhibitor of plasminogen activators that can be activated by denaturation. J Biol Chem 1985; 260: 11581–11587.
44. Carrell RW, Evans D, Stein PE. Mobile reactive centre of serpins and the control of thrombosis. Nature 1991; 353:576–578.
45. Engh RA, Wright HT, Huber R. Modelling the intact form of the alpha-1-proteinase inhibitor. Protein Eng 1990; 3:469–477.
46. Stein PE, Chothia C. Serpin tertiary structure transformation. J Mol Biol 1991; 221:615–621.
47. Bode W, Wei A-Z, Huber R, Meyer E, Travis J, Neumann S. X-ray crystal structure of the complex of human leucocyte elastase (PMN elastase) and the third domain of the turkey ovomucoid inhibitor. EMBO J 1986; 5:2453–2458.
48. Bode W, Mayr I, Baumann U, Huber R, Stone SR, Hofsteenge J. The refined 1.9 Angstrom crystal structure of human alpha-thrombin: Interaction with D-Phe-Pro-Arg chloromethylketone and significance of the Tyr-Pro-Pro-Trp insertion segment. EMBO J 1989; 8:3467–3475.
49. Schulze AJ, Baumann U, Knof S, Jaeger E, Huber R, Laurell CB. Structural transition of alpha-1-antitrypsin by a peptide sequentially similar to b-strand s4A. Eur J Biochem 1990; 194:51–56.
50. Schulze AJ, Huber R, Degryse E, Speck D, Bischoff R. Inhibitory activity and conformational changes in alpha-1-proteinase inhibitor variants. Eur J Biochem 1991; 202:1147–1155.
51. Skriver K, Wikoff WR, Patston PA, Tausk F, Schapira M, Kaplan AP, Bock SC. Sub-

strate properties of C1 inhibitor Ma (alanine 434→glutamic acid). J Biol Chem 1991; 266:9216–9221.
52. Mast AE, Enghild JJ, Salvesen G. Conformation of the reactive site loop of alpha-1-proteinase inhibitor probed by limited proteolysis. Biochemistry 1992; 31:2720–2728.
53. Schulze AJ, Frohnert PW, Engh RA, Huber R. Evidence for the extent of insertion of the active site loop of intact alpha-1-proteinase inhibitor in beta-sheet A. Biochemistry 1992; 31:7560–7565.
54. Potempa J, Shieh BH, Travis J. Alpha-2-antiplasmin: A serpin with two separate but overlapping reactive sites. Science 1988; 241:699–700.
55. Priestle JP. Ribbon: A stereo cartoon drawing program for proteins. J Appl Crystallogr 1988; 21:572–576.

# 7

# The Three-Dimensional Structure of Human Neutrophil Elastase

**WOLFRAM BODE**

Max Planck-Institut für Biochemie
Martinsried, Germany

## I. Introduction

The involvement of human neutrophil elastase (HNE) in various severe pathophysiological disorders has raised interest in searching for appropriate protein inhibitors and in designing potent synthetic inhibitors (reviewed in Refs. 1 and 2). The crystal structure of HNE complexes with inhibitors is important to understanding the inhibitor interaction with HNE and to rationalize the design of better inhibitors.

HNE is a typical vertebrate serine proteinase containing a conserved triad of catalytic residues including Ser195, His57, and Asp102 (the chymotrypsinogen numbering of HNE based on its topological equivalence with chymotrypsin(ogen) and trypsin will be used throughout this chapter; see Fig. 1 and Refs. 3 and 4). Its peptide sequence was established by a combination of peptide sequencing (5) and crystallographic electron-density interpretation (6). The mature HNE consists of a single chain comprising 218 to 220 amino acid residues (3,5,6) and four cross-connecting disulfide bridges. Analysis of the cDNA sequence of HNE (7,8) revealed an additional 20-amino-acid extension at the carboxy terminus, which is probably removed during posttranslational trimming and packaging in the lysosomal granules. Medullasin, an inflammatory serine proteinase derived from bone marrow cells, is similar to HNE but apparently has maintained the carboxy-terminal extension (9,10).

## II. Crystal Structures of HNE

Native HNE produces small crystals that are unsuitable for analysis (E. F. Meyer and W. Bode, unpublished results; 11). However, several HNE-inhibitor complexes have produced useful crystals, and their crystal structures have been determined and crystallographically refined at high resolution: 1) two closely related HNE complexes (4,6) formed with the third protein domain of the ovomucoid inhibitors from turkey (OMTKY3) (12,13) and from Indian peafowl (OMIPF3) (14), 2) one HNE complex (15) formed with a human secretory trypsin inhibitor-like elastase inhibitor (HSTI4a) (16), and 3) two quite similar HNE complexes containing covalently bound small peptidyl methyl moieties (3,17).

The crystallographic and refinement data that characterize these structures are presented in Table 1. The first four of these structures are determined with crystals, which contain HNE samples obtained by pooling the three peaks eluting in the final carboxymethyl cellulose chromatography step (18); the structure of OMTKY3-HNE crystals made with the sialic acid–rich HNE fraction 1 alone (kindly provided by W. Watorek and J. Travis) does not significantly differ from those made from pooled HNE (Bode, unpublished results). The HNE3-MSAAPA

**Table 1** Crystal Structures of Human Neutrophil Elastase

| Structure | Abbreviation | Resolution (Å) | *R*-value[a] | Ref. |
|---|---|---|---|---|
| 1. HNE (pooled)-turkey ovomucoid inhibitor third domain | HNEp-OMTKY3 | 1.8 | 0.166 | 6 |
| 2. HNEp-Indian peafowl ovomucoid inhibitor third domain | HNEp-OMIPF3 | 2.2 | 0.165 | 4 |
| 3. HNEp-human pancreatic secretory inhibitor (K18Y, I19E, D21R, P32A) mutant | HNEp-HSTI4a | 2.5 | 0.172 | 15 |
| 4. HNEp-Met-O-Succinyl AlaAlaProVal-methyl | HNEp-MSAAPV | 2.3 | 0.145 | 3 |
| 5. HNE (60% E4)-MS AlaAlaProAla-methyl | HNE3-MSAAPA | 1.84 | 0.164 | 17 |

[a]The crystallographic *R*-value measures the agreement between the observed and the calculated structure factor amplitudes; lower values indicate better agreement.

crystals (no. 5 in Table 1; Ref. 11) were prepared with HNE samples containing about 60% of HNE fraction 3, which is the least glycosylated and contains the smallest amount of negatively charged sialic acid.

The first and still most accurate of these HNE structures is that of the HNE-OMTKY3 complex (see Fig. 2) (4,6). In this complex, the protein inhibitor interacts in a "canonical" manner with the cognate HNE, i.e., with the conformation and interactions presumably also adopted by a "good" peptide substrate when bound in a productive enzyme-substrate complex (see Refs. 19 and 20). Thus, this HNE-OMTKY3 complex not only gives an accurate picture of the HNE structure itself, but also directly reflects the specific molecular interactions between HNE and bound substrates on both sides of the scissile peptide bond (throughout this chapter I use the nomenclature of Schechter and Berger (21), in which the peptide substrate amino acid residues at the N- and the C-terminal sides of the scissile peptide bond are denoted P1, P2, P3, etc., and P1′, P2′, P3′, respectively, and the corresponding subsites of the cognate enzyme S1, S2, S3, etc., and S1′, S2′, S3′, etc.). The following description of HNE is therefore based mainly on the HNE-OMTKY3 structure. The discussion of the structural and binding properties of HNE and a comparison with the related porcine pancreatic elastase (PPE) have been presented elsewhere (22).

## III. Overall Structure

As with the other vertebrate serine proteinases (see Ref. 23), the polypeptide chain of HNE is organized mainly as two topologically similar cylindrical domains (6). The domains interact with each other through various hydrophobic interactions and hydrogen bonds and by three covalent linkages, namely by an intermediate crossing-over segment (around residue Ala125; see Figs. 1 and 2) and by the amino- and the carboxy-terminal strands. In each domain, most of the polypeptide chain is folded in long loops that form extended β-pleated sheets. Each of these sheets is composed of six antiparallel chain segments, which are heavily twisted and so define two closed barrel-like surfaces (see the six "upper" and six "lower" hydrogen bond–connected antiparallel peptide strands in Fig. 1 and the barrels in Fig. 2).

In HNE there are three short pieces of $3_{10}$-helix (Ala55 to Ala60, Asn63 to Val64, Pro230 to Val235), but only the long carboxy-terminal segment (Phe234 to Glu243) is organized in a regular α-helix (see Figs. 1 and 2). Most of the catalytic residues—especially those of the active-site triad Ser195, His57, and Asp102 (see Fig. 4)—are localized in the crevice formed between both domains. Across the crevice is the cleft-like substrate binding site, which includes parts of each domain. The HNE polypeptide chain is covalently cross-connected by four disulfide bridges, which all have equivalent counterparts in the other serine pro-

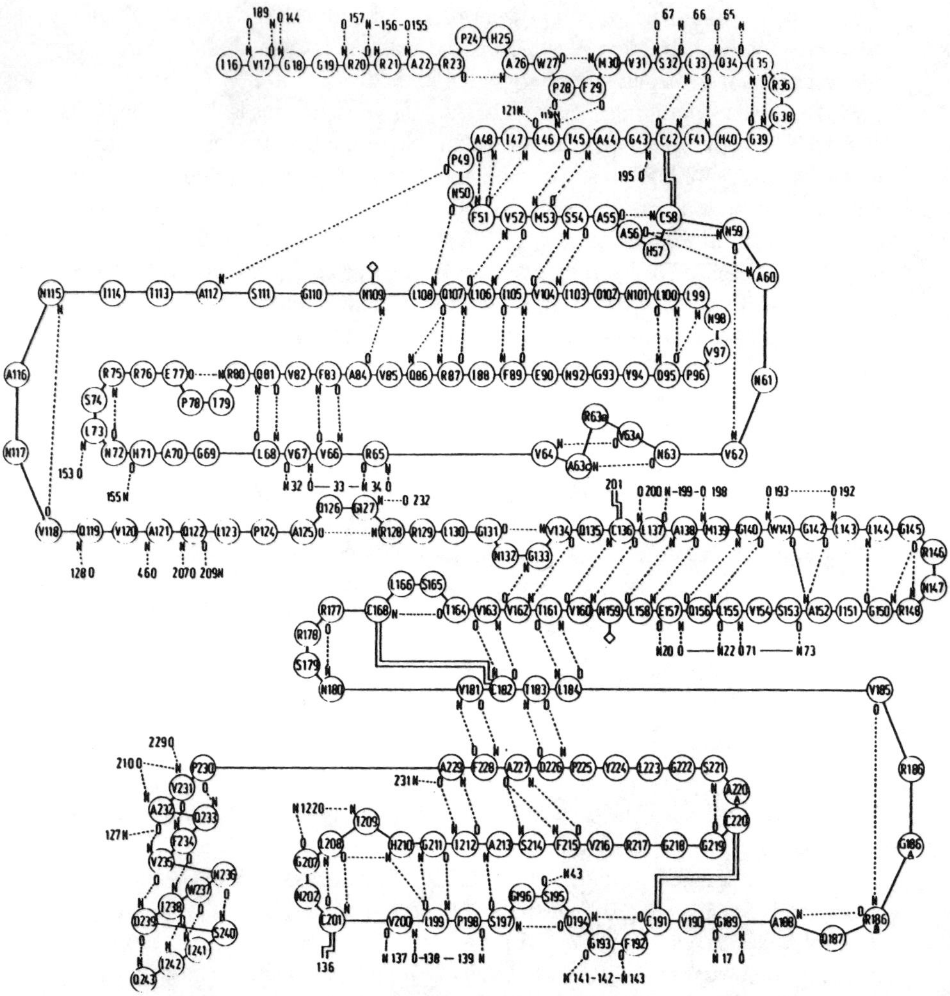

**Figure 1** Secondary structure of HNE. The HNE polypeptide chain extends from Ile16 (top) to Gln243 (bottom). The amino acid residues are designated using the one-letter code. The sequence numbering of HNE is derived from the topological equivalence with chymotrypsin(ogen)/trypsin (3,6). The four disulfide bridges of HNE are indicated by double connections. All inter-main-chain hydrogen bonds, shown by dashed lines, are selected according to criteria (with $E < -0.7$ kcal/Mol) established by Kabsch and Sander (61). (From Ref. 4.)

teinases. Cys42–Cys58 links the second and third strands of barrel 1, whereas Cys136–Cys201 and Cys168–Cys182 cross-connect strands 1 with 4 and 2 with 3 in the carboxy-terminal barrel (see Fig. 1); Cys191–Cys220, surface-located in the carboxy-terminal domain, frames one side of the specificity pocket (see Fig. 4).

As usual, the interior of both barrels is filled with the side chains of hydrophobic residues, whereas the interface between both barrel structures is more polar. Twenty-five fixed solvent molecules of HNE can be assigned as internal water molecules; most of them have equivalent counterparts in the other serine proteinases. About 90 hydrophobic residues of HNE, which represent more than 40% of its total residues, are accessible to bulk water molecules. This high percentage of hydrophobic surface residues is certainly the main reason for the "sticky" character of HNE.

## IV. The Amino-Terminal Domain

As in all other activatable trypsin-like serine proteinases, the amino-terminal residue of the HNE polypeptide chain, Ile16, is completely buried in the carboxy-terminal domain, with its ammonium group forming an internal salt bridge with the side chain carboxylate group of Asp194. This salt bridge is essential for maintenance of the active-enzyme conformation (for more details, see Refs. 23–25). The chain reaches the molecular surface at Gly18–Gly19 (Gly19 is strongly conserved and allows for a disorder–order transition upon activation; see Refs. 25–27), runs along the carboxy-terminal domain surface toward the amino-terminal domain (the right-hand domain in Fig. 2), and enters the barrel proper at Pro28. Noteworthy in this amino-terminal HNE domain are:

1. The 1½-turn $3_{10}$-helix between Ala55 and Ala60, which also provides the active-site residue His57 imidazole side chain
2. The particularly exposed loop 59–63, which is reminiscent of but much smaller than the "60-insertion loop" in thrombin (see Ref. 28)
3. A unique 1½-turn $3_{10}$-helix (five residues) from Asn63 to Val64 (see Fig. 1)
4. The first glycosylation site at Asn109 (see below).

The Ala70–Arg80 loop of HNE is spatially similar to the "calcium-binding loop" in trypsin (29), PPE (30), and chymotrypsin. In these enzymes, the carboxylate groups of two (or three) glutamic acid residues (in trypsin and PPE: Glu70 and Glu80) act as ligands for the central calcium ion, which stabilizes the whole molecule but does not affect the catalytic activity. In HNE, however, Glu80 is replaced by Arg80 (see Fig. 4), whose terminal guanidino group occupies the site at which calcium is found in PPE and trypsin. Thus, HNE carries its own stabilizing cation and does not depend on calcium for stability.

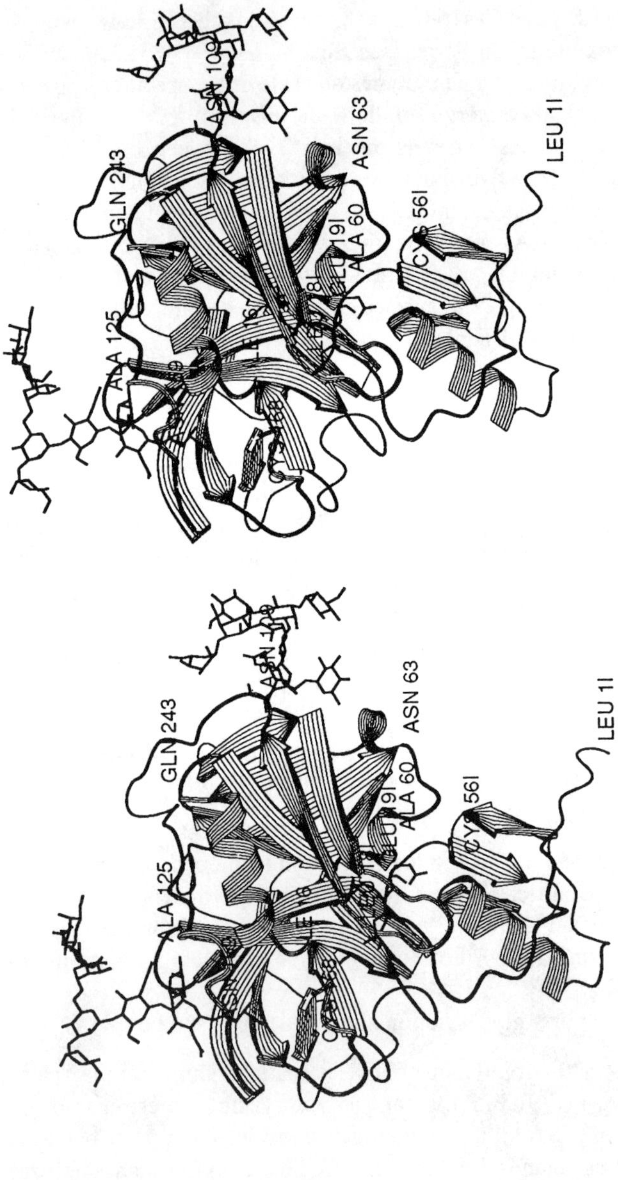


**Figure 2**

## V. The Carboxy-Terminal Domain

Around Ala125 (see Fig. 2), the HNE polypeptide chain crosses over to the carboxy-terminal domain to enter the barrel at Gly133. Noteworthy in this domain are:

1. The Trp141–Gly142 segment (a highly conserved aromate-glycine pair important to mediate refolding of the "activation domain" during activation; see Refs. 23 and 25)
2. The considerable flexibility around Arg146–Asn147 in the exposed (and in other serine proteinases easily autodigestible) "autolysis loop" (see Figs. 4 and 5)
3. The second glycosylation site at Asn159 (see below)
4. An unusually short "methionine loop" (see below)
5. The quite hydrophobic specificity pocket (S1 subsite; see Figs. 4 and 5 and below)
6. A completely buried Asp226 (see below)

Gln243 is the last residue of the HNE chain, which can be traced in the electron-density maps. Its side chain and carboxylate group are completely defined; in the HNE-OMTKY3 crystals there is, however, free space for at least another two carboxy-terminal residues (Arg, Ser).

The largest structural difference between HNE and PPE or trypsin is observed in the so-called "methionine loop" (named for the strong conservation of Met180 in most other serine proteinases), which in HNE is much smaller and has a very different conformation. The topologically equivalent residue 180 in HNE is Asn180, whose carboxamide group is hydrogen-bonded to the neighboring—and also novel—Arg177 side chain (notably, the equivalent residue in the cellular

---

**Figure 2** Stereo ribbon plot of the crystalized complex formed between HNE (top) and OMTKY3 (bottom) (β-strands, helices, and turns are represented by twisted arrows, helical ribbons, and ropes). In this view, the substrate-binding region of HNE points downward. The two sugar chains of HNE, attached to Asn109 (right) and Asn159 (top, back) (shown in full size with a shape expected in analogy to the $C_H2$ domain of the IgG1 (63) for a complex carbohydrate chain), point away from the substrate-binding region. Two times six antiparallel strands form the amino-terminal barrel (right side) and the carboxy-terminal barrel (left side). The prominent carboxy-terminal helix of HNE runs in front of the enzyme molecule.

The OMTKY3 polypeptide chain runs from Leu1I to Cys56I. The inhibitor, with a scaffold consisting of an α-helical segment and a three-stranded β-sheet, nestles with its exposed binding loop toward the substrate-binding site of HNE. Five residues amino-terminal (to the left) and three residues carboxy-terminal of the reactive inhibitor site (scissile peptide bond between P1 residue Leu18I and the P1′ residue Glu19I) are in direct contact with HNE residues. (From Ref. 62, modified by A. Karshikoff.)

serine proteinases rat mast cell protease II (31) and cathepsin G (32) and in most of the granzymes (see Ref. 33) is likewise not a methionine but a glutamine).

## VI. The Active Site

The active-site residues (Ser195, His57, Asp102) have positions in HNE similar to those they occupy in the other vertebrate serine proteinases (see Fig. 4):

1. The completely buried carboxylate group of Asp102 is optimally surrounded by four hydrogen-bond donors (Ser214 Oγ, Ala45 N, His57 N, and Nδ1 of the imidazole ring of His57) that help to stabilize its negative charge.
2. The Nε2 atom of His57 is close enough to the reactive Ser195 Oγ to make a hydrogen bond with its hydroxyl group.
3. The increased nucleophilicity of this surface hydroxyl group promotes (in a productive hydrolytic process) the attack on the carbonyl carbon of the scissile peptide bond of a bound peptide substrate, leading to the tetrahedral intermediate state (for the reaction mechanism of serine proteinases, see, e.g., Refs. 23 and 34–36).

The exact arrangement of the active-site residues is, however, very much influenced by the complex state of the enzyme under study. In all crystal structures of nonliganded serine proteinases determined so far, the Ser195 Oγ–His57 Nε2 hydrogen bond is of normal-to-long length but always has bad geometry. Its conformation is clearly influenced by a fixed solvent molecule (an anion at low pH values but a water molecule at high ones; see Ref. 23) placed close to both polar groups. Upon the approach and binding of a peptide substrate or a protein inhibitor, however, the active-site residues become buried and shielded from the bulk water; consequently, the Ser195 Oγ–His57 Nε2 hydrogen bond becomes stereochemically optimal, facilitating a proton transfer from Ser195 Oγ via His57 Nε2 to the amide nitrogen of the leaving group. The state observed in the HNE-OMTKY3 complexes is almost that expected for a Michaelis-encounter complex; Ser195 Oγ is placed above the carbonyl carbon of the scissile peptide bond of the inhibitor, but is only about 2.7 Å (in sub–van der Waals distance) from it.

In both HNE complexes formed with the peptidyl chloromethylketones (structures 4 and 5 in Table 1), the Ser195 Oγ has moved slightly farther toward the carbonyl group of the P1-residue and forms a covalent bond; the resulting tetrahedral hemiketal structure is thus a stable analog of the putative transient tetrahedral intermediate in real enzyme-substrate complexes.

## VII. Charge Properties

HNE owes its high basicity to the presence of 19 arginines, which considerably outweigh its only eight acidic residues. Two aspartic acid residues and one glutamic acid are involved in buried hydrogen-bonded salt bridges (Asp194 ... Ile16, Asp102 ... His57, Glu77 ... Arg80); another glutamic acid residue (Glu157) forms a surface-located salt bridge (with Arg20). Asp226 is completely buried "beneath" the specificity pocket (see Fig. 4). There is no positively charged residue in the immediate environment that could compensate the (putative) negative charge of the Asp226 carboxyl group; this latter group is hydrogen-bonded with three internal water molecules, which might serve to delocalize its negative charge. Preliminary electrostatic calculations (A. Karshikov and W. Bode) show that the carboxyl group experiences an overall slightly positive electrostatic potential (resulting mainly from the surface-located Arg217), which would stabilize its anionic state and thus would give rise to a slightly decreased pK value compared with intrinsic pK values of model aspartates. The negative charges of three further acidic residues of HNE are likewise uncompensated; these residues (Glu90, Asp95, and Asp239) are situated on the molecular surface in a large surface patch (on the "front" and "top" of HNE in Fig. 2), which completely lacks any basic residue.

All the arginine residues, with the exception of Arg80 in the "calcium-binding loop" (see above), are arranged on the surface of the enzyme. They are not randomly distributed but arranged in a horseshoe-like manner around the active site (running from the "left-hand side" of HNE around its "back" to the "right-hand side" in Fig. 2); several are arranged in pairs (Arg128 and Arg129, Arg177 and Arg178, Arg75 and Arg76, Arg20 and Arg21) and/or form clusters of two to three arginine residues (e.g., Arg75, Arg76, and Arg80; Arg20, Arg21, and Arg23; Arg146 and Arg148; Arg186 and Arg186B; Arg128, Arg129, and Arg178). It is noteworthy that the HNE surface area, which is topologically equivalent to the putative, strongly basic "heparin-binding site" in thrombin (which stretches along the carboxy-terminal helix, i.e., on the "front side" in Fig. 2), lacks any arginine residue; thus, the interaction with heparin shown to affect the HNE properties toward some protein inhibitors (37) probably occurs at different sites.

The arginine surface pattern explains the preferred binding of HNE to linear sulfated polysaccharides and to the negatively charged proteoglycan matrix of the storage granules. Together with other cationic secretory enzymes such as cathepsin G, the rat mast cell proteases I and II, and the cytolytic T-lymphocytic granzymes, HNE might be condensed at these granular matrices as a means of controlling their autodestructive potential (see Ref. 17). The inhibitory effect of glucosaminoglycans (38,39) and of heparin (37,40) on the digestion of synthetic substrates by HNE is less easily explained but might be due to interaction with Arg217 (of all arginine residues localized closest to the active site), through either sterical hindrance or conformational changes (see Refs. 3 and 41).

## VIII. The Glycosylation Sites

Two of HNE's three asparagine residues that are part of glycosylation consensus segments (Asn109–Gly110–Ser111 and Asn159–Val160–Thr161) are linked to varying degrees with carbohydrate chains (see Figs. 2 and 3), giving rise to the three (or four) HNE isoforms (E1, E2, and E3) of almost identical enzymatic activity (18). Both sugar chains extend away from the substrate-binding site and protrude out into solution (Fig. 2); consequently, they should not interfere with the binding of smaller protein substrates or inhibitors, but could become entangled with the extended elastin network. However, the carbohydrate chains affect crystallization. The original HNE-OMTKY3 crystals (no. 1, Table 1) made with "pooled" HNE fractions appear in the presence of 0.5 M sodium citrate, pH8; in contrast, OMTKY3 complexes made with HNE fractions 1 or 3 crystallize from 0.1 M and 1.0 M citrate, respectively. The latter crystals have been analyzed (Bode, Watorek, and Travis); their carbohydrates do not, however, seem to be better defined than those from the original crystals.

The sugar chains are (in structures 1, 2, and 3 of Table 1) defined by proper electron density out to the third sugar and by lower density out to the (branching) fourth, indicating a rigid relationship to the polypeptide backbone in the crystalline complexes (Fig. 3). At both attachment sites, the N-acetyl-glucosamine sugar (2-acetamido-2-deoxy-β-D-glucopyranose) β-N-glycosidically attached to Asn109 and Asn159 is α-1.6-linked to a "side chain" α-L-fucopyranose, and further β-1.4-linked to another N-acetyl-glycosamine, which in turn is connected to a branching mannose (see Fig. 2). The first and the second N-acetyl-glycosamine rings are arranged approximately along a $2_1$-screw axis and form an almost flat ribbon-like glycan structure. Hydrogen bonds between the O3 hydroxyl group of the first sugar and the O5 ring oxygen and the O6 side-chain hydroxyl of the second ring seem to confer stabilization to this arrangement.

The surface buried in the protein–sugar interface is about 400 $Å^2$, i.e., not much smaller than the intermolecular surface buried between HNE and OMTKY3 (600 $Å^2$). The overwhelming majority of noncovalent interactions (see Fig. 3) are made through the "side-chain" fucose (26 and 19 atom–atom contacts below 4.0 Å at the first and second attachment sites) and the covalently linked N-acetyl-glycosamine (16 and 19 such contacts, of which 14 and 17 are, however, made with the respective asparagine residue). Each fucose ring nestles (each with different sides) into flat grooves of surrounding protein loops (see Fig. 3). The protein surfaces around the two sugar-attachment sites of HNE look very different. The only common feature is the semicircular arrangement of arginine residues (Arg75, Arg76, Arg80, Arg36, Arg65, Arg63B, and Arg87 around Asn109 and Arg128, Arg129, Arg178, Arg186, Arg186B, Arg20, Arg21, and Arg23 around Asn159).

This pattern might provide a recognition site for a modifying enzyme (phosphotransferase, see Ref. 42) presumed to be responsible for sorting the lysosomal enzymes from the other secretory proteins and for targeting to the proper destination. Both asparagines are integrated in more or less extended polypeptide strands, with slight kinks at the asparagines. In contrast, Asn72—which is part of a third, but never glycosylated sugar consensus sequence of HNE (Asn72-Leu73-Ser74)—is the first residue of a tight 1-4 turn in the "calcium-

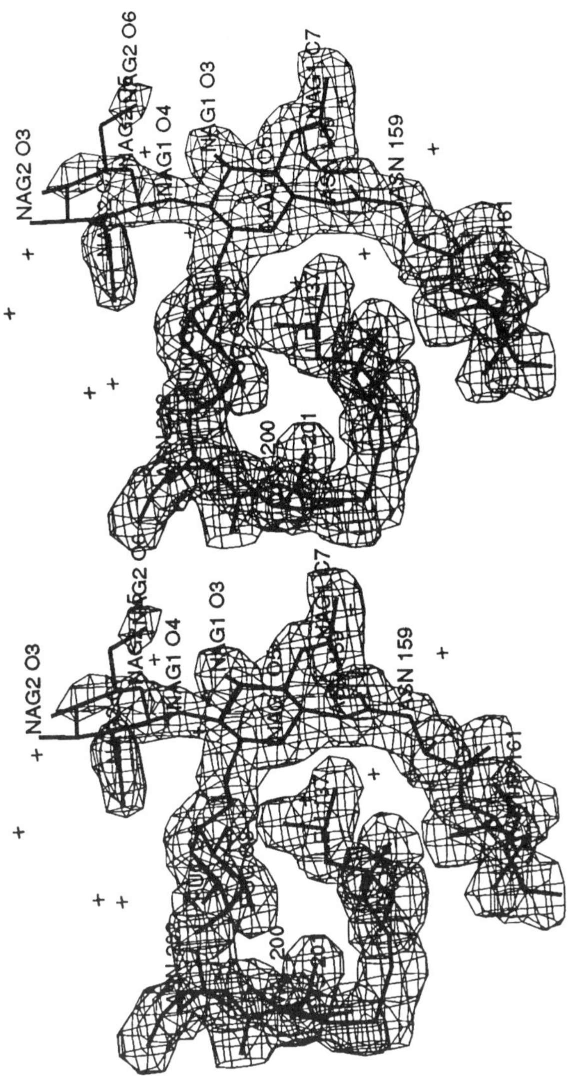


**Figure 3** Stereo plot showing the first three sugars attached to Asn159 and the surrounding polypeptide chains (Asn159–Thr161, Cys136–Leu137, Val200–Asn202, and Cys136–Cys201) of HNE, superimposed with the experimental electron density as observed in the final HNE-OMTKY3 complex. The contour level is at 0.9 σ.

binding loop" (see above). Any attached carbohydrate would lead to overcrowding at this site; however, the first glycosylation step occurs cotranslationally in the nascent chain, so that other (sequential) signals, which determine the actual glycosylation site, must be involved.

## IX. The Substrate-Binding Site

### A. Overall Interaction with Inhibitors/Substrates

The ovomucoid third domain from turkey (OMTKY3) binds to a variety of serine proteinases such as chymotrypsin, PPE, subtilisin, and HNE (see Refs. 12, 13, 43, and 44). Besides the x-ray crystal structures of its HNE complexes (4,6), molecular complexes with the *Streptomyces griseus* proteinase B (45) and with chymotrypsin (46) have been elucidated. OMTKY3 forms a tight complex with HNE characterized by a $K_{assoc}$ of $6.2 \times 10^9\ M^{-1}$ (13,44). This inhibitor, like other Kazal-type inhibitors (47), consists of a molecular scaffold made up of an α-helical segment and a three-stranded β-pleated sheet, from which an extended proteinase-binding loop of a unique "canonical" conformation centered on the reactive-site scissile peptide bond Leu18I–Glu19I (see Refs. 19 and 20) projects toward the cognate enzyme (6,46,48,49).

The substrate-binding site of HNE makes direct contact with eight residues of the "primary binding segment" (P5-Pro14I to P3′-Arg21I) and with an additional three to five residues (Gly32I, Asn33I, and Asn36I) of a "secondary binding segment" of OMTKY3 (see Fig. 4). The majority of the intermolecular contacts (94 of 106 atom–atom contacts with 4 Å) involve the primary binding loop, which mimics a bound substrate. Seven hydrogen bonds are formed between the peptide backbones of the inhibitor segment and HNE (Fig. 5). The P3, P2, and P1 residues of the inhibitor form an antiparallel β-sheet structure with the peptide backbone of Ser214–Val216 of HNE, an interaction that is typical for the binding of peptides to serine proteinases. The carbonyl group of Leu18I is located in the oxyanion hole (Gly193 N, Ser 195 N), and the P2′ residue makes antiparallel β-sheet-like hydrogen bonds with the backbone of Phe41.

The inhibitor peptide chains of both chloromethyl ketone inhibitors in complex with HNE (see Table 1) are bound in a conformation that is similar to the corresponding P4 to P1 residues of OMTKY3. The terminal MeO-Suc group (formally the P5 group) is not rigidly fixed, but runs antiparallel to the backbone residues 216–218. In solution, it could be placed close to Arg217, and a negatively charged succinyl group on an inhibitor could interact with the guanidino group of Arg217.

### B. Interactions Through the Specificity Pocket

One-third of the total contacts between HNE and OMTKY3 are formed between the P1 residue Leu18I of OMTKY3 and the S1-specificity pocket of HNE (see Figs. 4 and 5). The leucine side chain is anchored in the energetically most favorable ($g^+$-t) conformation and fills the pocket almost completely. The opening of this pocket is formed by the flat sides of the peptide backbones of segments 214–216 and 191–192 and is constricted toward its bottom by residues Val190, Phe192, Ala213, Val216, and Phe228 and by the disulfide bridge Cys191–Cys220. The S1 pocket is hemispheric, and is rather hydrophobic in character (see Fig. 5). Thus, it is well adapted to accommodate medium-sized aliphatic side chains such as leucine, isoleucine, or methionine. There is no specific anchoring point in the S1 pocket (such as Asp189 in trypsin) so the aliphatic P1 side chain is not fixed in a distinct orientation and can revolve like a ball-and-socket joint. Accommodation of larger side chains such as phenylalanine would require a considerable expansion of the pocket, and, as a consequence, substrates with phenylalanine are not normally cleaved by HNE behind this residue.

In the structure of the valyl chloromethylketone–HNE complex (3), binding of the β-branched bulky side chain of the P1 valyl residue is accommodated with a slight tilting of its main chain. Simultaneously, the S1 pocket of HNE shrinks slightly and adapts to the reduced size of the smaller side chain.

Among ovomucoid inhibitors (43), HNE slightly prefers leucine over valine at P1; this is in contrast to Kunitz-type protein inhibitors with antielastase specificity, in which valine seems to make the inhibitors bind slightly strongly (50). With synthetic peptide substrates, a P1 norvaline seems to be favored over a valine, which in turn fits better than leucine (51,52).

The P1 residue of the natural plasma inhibitor of HNE, i.e., α1-antitrypsin, is Met358. Modeling experiments show that a methionine residue at P1 should fit easily with a typical bent-side-chain conformation into the S1 pocket of HNE. The extra oxygen of a methionine sulfoxide should, however, create severe sterical hindrance with the S1 pocket. This provides a structural basis for the dramatic decrease in binding affinity of α1-antitrypsin oxidized upon smoking (53–55).

Close to the bottom of the S1 pocket of HNE, the acidic residue Asp226 is somewhat shielded from the exterior of the pocket by Val216 and Val190 (see above and Fig. 4). The valyl side chains are in van der Waals contact with each other; penetration of a basic P1 side chain to form a salt link with Asp226 seems possible only after considerable widening. It is therefore remarkable that the natural basic pancreatic trypsin inhibitor (with a Lys15I-P1 residue) has been found to inhibit HNE with an association constant of $10^6$ $M^{-1}$ (56).

### C. Interactions at Other Subsites

According to the number of intermolecular contacts made with HNE, the P2′ (Tyr20I) and the P2 residue (Thr17I) of OMTKY3 rank next behind the P1 residue, followed by P3 and P1′ (22). HNE subsite S2—complementary to Thr17I and lined by Phe215, Leu99, and the flat side of the imidazole ring of His57—is bowl-shaped and quite hydrophobic (see Fig. 5), but it is similar to that found in all other mammalian serine proteinases. A bound substrate is forced to adopt a kinked polyproline II–like conformation. Medium-sized hydrophobic side chains, including proline, are preferred here.

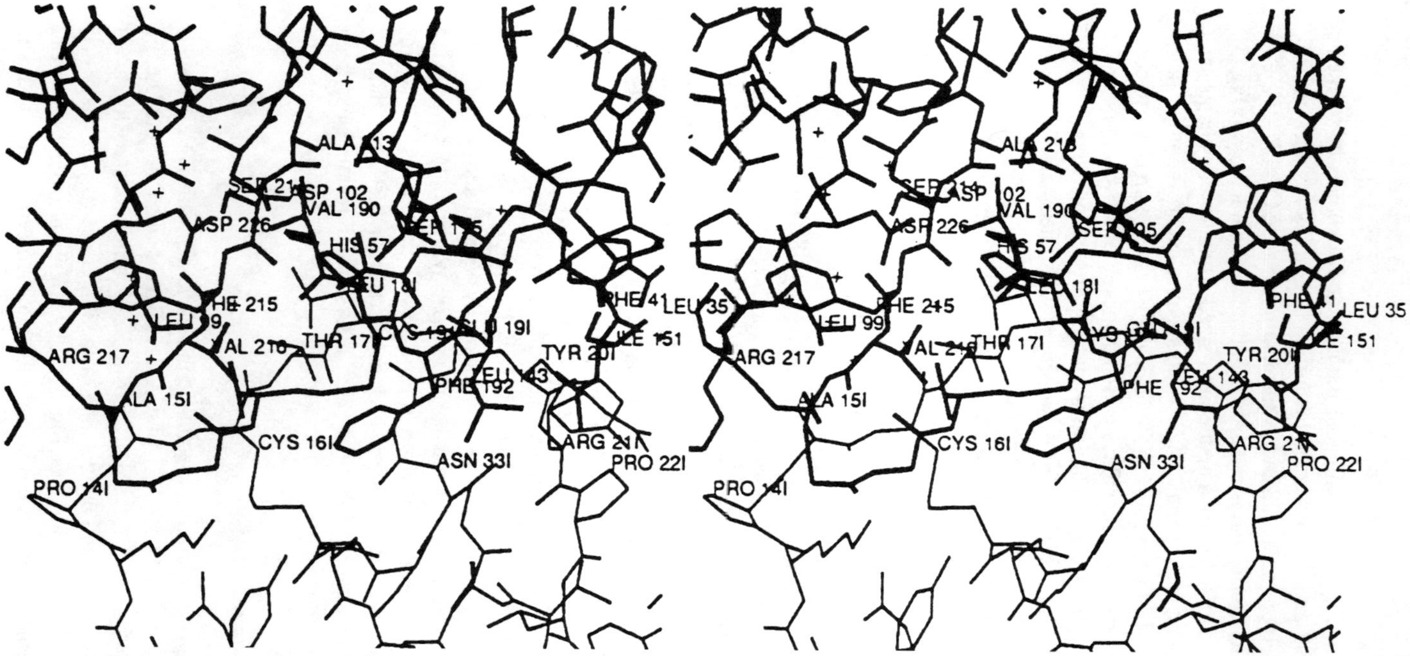


**Figure 4** Stereo plot of the HNE–OMTKY3 interface. The view is similar to that of Fig. 2; HNE residues (top) are shown with bold connections, OMTKY3 residues (bottom) with thin connections and prefixed with *I*. The substrate-binding site of HNE points downward; the specificity pocket, occupied by the P1 residue Leu18I of the inhibitor, opens toward the back. Its entrance frame is formed by peptide segments Ala213–Cys220, Cys191–Ser195, and Cys191–Cys220. Behind this pocket, even farther inside the HNE molecule, is the internal Asp226, with its carboxylate side chain surrounded by several internal solvent (water) molecules (crosses). The side chains of the active site residues Ser195, His57, and Asp102 (center) are arranged to allow good hydrogen-bond interactions.

The inhibitor-binding loop nestles from Pro14I (P5) via Leu18I (P1) and Glu19I (P1′) to Arg21I (P3′) against the HNE-binding site; Ser195 Oγ of HNE is close to the carbonyl carbon of the scissile bond (Leu18I–Glu19I), but remains at a sub–van der Waals distance of 2.7 Å.

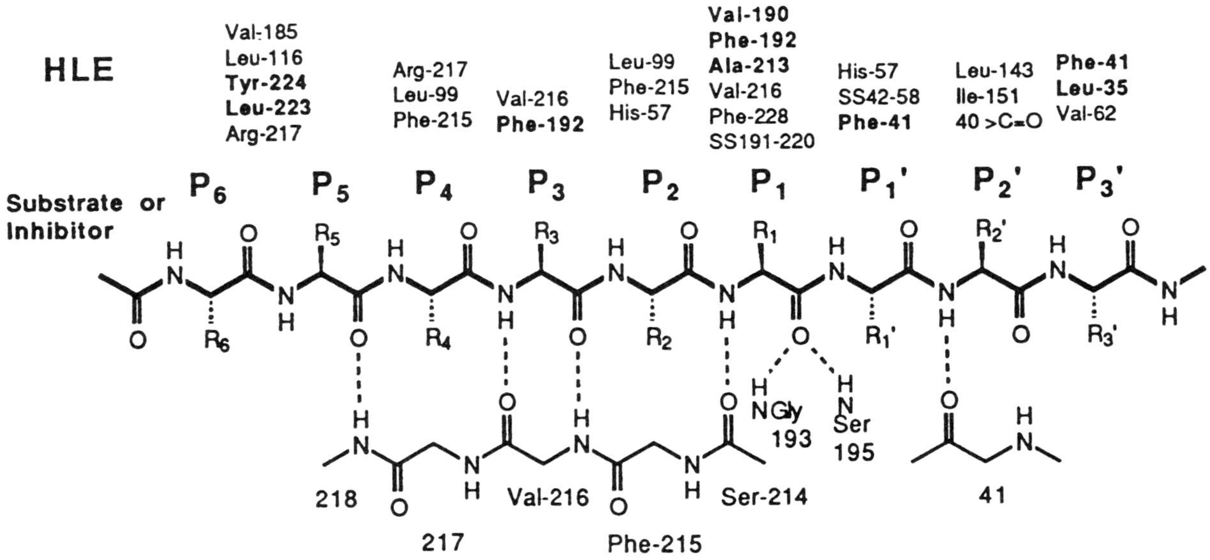


**Figure 5** Schematic representation of the main- and side-chain interactions between the primary binding segment of OMTKY3 or a peptide substrate with HNE. Significant amino acid residues that might particularly influence the specificity of HNE are shown in bold letters. The carbonyl group of the scissile peptide bond (P1–P1′) is shown interacting with the oxyanion hole. (Adapted from Ref. 22.)

The P3 residue Cys16I is in contact with HNE only through main-chain atoms; more elongated side chains would, however, interact with hydrophobic surfaces of HNE, mainly with Phe192 and Val216 (see Fig. 4). In common with similar interactions seen in other serine proteinase complexes with peptides, the P3–S3 contact is characterized by two intermolecular hydrogen bonds made with the backbone amide nitrogen and the carbonyl group of Val216 (see Fig. 5). This interaction must somehow communicate with the catalytic triad in the active site (57), possibly via the S1 subsite (22).

The side chain of Ala15I (P4) is placed along the side chains of HNE residues Phe215 and Arg217. Substrates with aromatic groups or long hydrophobic chains carrying a distal positive charge in P4 are more reactive than the corresponding alanine substrates. These substrates resemble desmosine, the charged, hydrophobic, cross-linking amino acid residue of elastin (22,58). Position and conformation of the P5 residue Pro14I of OMTKY3 are clearly dictated by intramolecular constraints in the ovomucoid inhibitor itself; longer P5 side chains of flexible, bound substrates could, however, interact with Arg217. It has been suggested that the guanidinium groups of this arginine residue, as well as that of the adjacent Arg177, act as anchoring points for some small hydrophobic HNE inhibitors containing an anionic group (see Refs. 3, 22, 41, and 59), because they are (with 14 Å) closest to the reactive Ser195 Oγ. In fact, close to both guanidinium groups is a shallow hydrophobic surface depression (above Leu166 and Leu223), which results mainly from the unique shortening of the "methionine loop" of HNE, and which could accommodate hydrophobic appendices of such inhibitors.

The S1′ subsite of HNE consists of a relatively hydrophobic depression lined by Cys42–Cys58 and Phe41. It can accommodate every amino acid residue except large hydrophobic residues such as tryptophan (for catalytic reasons, proline would lead to slow cleavage). Tyr20I, the P2′ residue of OMTKY3, nestles into a shallow hydrophobic surface depression (see Fig. 4). OMIPF3 (14), which differs from OMTKY3 only in the occurrence of Tyr instead of His at position 20I, binds almost two orders of magnitude more weakly to HNE than does OMTKY3 (Laskowski, private communication). In the crystal structure of HNE-OMIPF3 (4), the imidazole ring of His20I is similarly sandwiched between the S2 subsite of HNE and the neighboring inhibitor residue Pro22I; thus, the affinity differences measured for the closely related ovomucoid derivatives might be due to restrictions in mobility in the histidine variant imposed during complex formation.

Arg21I (P3′) nestles with its (primarily hydrophobic) side chain and the flat side of its guanidino group against the quite hydrophobic surface of the S3′ subsite of HNE. This shallow subsite is formed mainly by the side chains of Phe41, Leu35, and Val63, and probably represents the hydrophobic subsite that binds peptide inhibitors with long carboxy-terminal aliphatic chains (60).

Three residues (Gly32I, Asn33I, and Asn36I) of the "secondary binding segment" of OMTKY3 are in direct contact with HNE, all of them through purely hydrophobic interactions with Phe192. The number and closeness of these "secondary contacts" are not very important (due to the relatively "open" binding cleft of HNE compared, e.g., with thrombin; see Ref. 28) and will clearly vary for different inhibitors.

In α1AT–HNE complexes, the geometry of the inhibitor loop–proteinase interaction might, at first approximation, be similar to that observed for the proteinase complexes with small protein inhibitors (see Chapter 6). Due to the much larger size of the inhibitor scaffold of α1AT, however, the "secondary contacts" with the rim residues of the HNE-binding cleft might become more important.

## Acknowledgment

The help of Dr. Richard Engh, who reviewed this chapter in manuscript, is greatly acknowledged.

## References

1. Trainor A. Synthetic inhibitors of human neutrophil elastase. Trends Pharmacol Sci 1987; 8:303–307.
2. Travis J, Fritz H. Potential problems in designing elastase inhibitors for therapy. Am Rev Respir Dis 1991; 143:1412–1415.
3. Wei A, Mayr I, Bode W. The refined 2.3 Å crystal structure of human leukocyte elastase in a complex with a valine chloromethyl ketone inhibitor. FEBS Lett 1988; 234:367–373.
4. Bode W, Stubbs M, Laskowski M. (1992). Unpublished results.
5. Sinha S, Watorek W, Karr S, Giles J, Bode W, Travis J. Primary structure of human neutrophil elastase. Proc Natl Acad Sci USA 1987; 84:2228–2232.
6. Bode W, Wei A, Huber R, Meyer E, Travis J, Neumann S. X-ray crystal structure of the complex of human leucocyte elastase (PMN, elastase) and the third domain of the turkey ovomucoid. EMBO J 1986; 5:2453–2458.
7. Farley D, Salvesen G, Travis J. Molecular cloning of human neutrophil elastase. Biol Chem Hoppe-Seyler 1988; 369 (suppl):3–7.
8. Takahashi H, Nukiwa T, Basset T, Crystal RG. Myelomonocytic cell lineage expression of the neutrophil elastase gene. J Biol Chem 1988; 263:2543–2547.
9. Okano K, Aoki Y, Sakurai T, Kajitani M, Kanai S, Shimazu H, Natuto M. Molecular cloning of complementary DNA for human medulasin: an inflammatory serine proteinase in bone marrow cells. J Biochem 1987; 102:13–16.
10. Aoki Y, Hase T. The primary structure and elastinolytic activity of medulasin (a serine protease of bone marrow). Biochim Biophys Res Commun 1991; 178:501–506.
11. Williams HR, Lin T-Y, Navia MA, Springer JP, McKeever BM, Hoogsteen K, Dorn

CP. Crystallization of human neutrophil elastase. J Biol Chem 1987; 262:17178–17181.
12. Ardelt W, Laskowski M. Turkey ovomucoid third domain inhibits eight different serine proteinases of varied specificity at the same Leu18-Glu19 reactive site. Biochemistry 1986; 24:5313–5320.
13. Park SJ. Ph.D. Thesis. Purdue University, 1985.
14. Laskowski M, Apostel I, Ardelt W, Cook J, Giletto A, Kelly CA, Lu W, Park SJ, Qasim MA, Whatley HE, Wieczorek A, Wym R. Amino acid sequences of ovomucoid third domain from 25 additional species of birds. J Prot Chem 1990; 9: 715–725.
15. Epp O, Hörlein HD, Wei AZ, Kiefer E, Bode W. Unpublished results.
16. Collins J, Szardening M, Maywald F, Blöcker H, Frank R, Hecht H-J, Vasel B, Schomburg D, Fink E, Fritz H. Human leukocyte elastase inhibitors: designed variants of human pancreatic secretory trypsin inhibitor (hPSTI). Biol Chem Hoppe-Seyler 1990; 371 (suppl).
17. Navia M, McKeever BM, Springer JP, Lin T-Y, Williams HR, Fluder EM, Dorn CP, Hoogsten K. Structure of human neutrophil elastase in complex with a peptide chloromethylketone inhibitor at 1.84 Å resolution. Proc Natl Acad Sci USA 1989; 86:7–11.
18. Baugh RJ, Travis J. Human leukocyte granule elastase: rapid isolation and characterisation. Biochemistry 1976; 15:836–841.
19. Bode W, Huber R. Ligand binding: proteinase–protein inhibitor interactions. Curr Opin Struc Biol 1991; 1:45–52.
20. Bode W, Huber R. Natural protein proteinase inhibitors and their interaction with proteinases. Eur J Biochem 1992; 204:433–451.
21. Berger A, Schechter I. On the size of the active site in proteases. I. Papain. Biochem Biophys Res Commun 1967; 27(2):157–162.
22. Bode W, Meyer J, Powers J. Human leukocyte and porcine pancreatic elastase: X-ray crystal structures, mechanism, substrate specificity, and mechanism-based inhibitors. Biochemistry 1989; 28:1951–1963.
23. Bode W, Huber R. Crystal structures of pancreatic serine endopeptidases. In: Desnuelle P, Sjostrom H, Noren O, eds. Molecular and Cellular Basis of Digestion. Amsterdam: Elsevier, 1986:214–234.
24. Bode W. The transition of bovine trypsinogen to a trypsin-like state upon strong ligand binding. II. The binding of the pancreatic trypsin inhibitor and of isoleucine-valine and of sequentially related peptides to trypsinogen and to p-guanidinobenzoate-trypsinogen. J Mol Biol 1979; 127:357–374.
25. Huber R, Bode W. Structural basis of the activation and action of trypsin. Accounts Chem Res 1978; 11:114–122.
26. Bode W, Fehlhammer H, Huber R. Crystal structure of bovine trypsinogen at 1.8 Å resolution. I. Data collection, application of patterson search techniques and preliminary structural interpretation. J Mol Biol 1976; 106:325–335.
27. Fehlhammer H, Bode W, Huber R. Crystal structure of bovine trypsinogen at 1.8 Å resolution. II. Crystallographic refinement, refined crystal structure and comparison with bovine trypsin. J Mol Biol 1977; 111:415–438.

28. Bode W, Mayr I, Baumann U, Huber R, Stone S, Hofsteenge J. The refined 1.9 Å crystal structure of human alpha-thrombin: interaction with D-Phe-Pro-Arg chloromethylketone and significance of the Tyr-Pro-Pro-Trp insertion segment. EMBO J 1989; 8:3467–3475.
29. Bode W, Schwager P. The refined crystal structure of bovine alpha-trypsin at 1.8 Å resolution. II. Crystallographic refinement, calcium binding site, benzamidine binding site and active site at pH 7.0. J Mol Biol 1975; 98:693–717.
30. Meyer EF, Cole G, Radhakrishnan R, Epp O. Structure of native porcine pancreatic elastase at 1.65 Å resolution. Acta Crystallogr 1988; B44:26–38.
31. Woodbury RG, Katunuma N, Kobayashi K, Titani K, Neurath H. Covalent structure of a group specific protease from rat small intestine. Biochemistry 1978; 17:811–819.
32. Salvesen G, Farley D, Shuman J, Przbyla A, Reiley C, Travis J. Molecular cloning of cathepsin G: Structural similarity to mast cell and cytotoxic lymphocyte proteinases. Biochemistry 1987; 26:2289–2293.
33. Jenne DE, Tschopp J. Granzymes: A family of serine proteinases in granules of cytolytic T lymphocytes. Curr Topics Microbiol Immunol 1988; 140:33–47.
34. Kraut J. Serine proteases: structure and mechanism of catalysis. Annu Rev Biochem 1977; 46:331–358.
35. Kossiakoff AA. Catalytic properties of trypsin. In: Jurnak FA, McPherson A, eds. Biological Macromolecules. New York: John Wiley, 1987:369–412.
36. Dutler H, Bizzozero SA. Mechanism of serine protease reaction: Stereoelectronic, structural, and kinetic considerations a guidelines to deduce reaction paths. Accounts Chem Res 1989; 22:322–327.
37. Frommherz KJ, Faller B, Bieth JG. Heparin strongly decreases the rate of inhibition of neutrophil elastase by α1-proteinase inhibitor. J Biol Chem 1991; 266:15356–15362.
38. Baici A, Salgam P, Fehr K, Böni A. Inhibition of human elastase from polymorphonuclear leukocytes by a glycosaminoglycan polysulfate (Orteparon). Biochem Pharmacol 1980; 29:1723–1727.
39. Rao NV, Wehner NG, Marshall BC, Gray WR, Gray BH, Hoidal JR. Characterization of proteinase-3 (PR-3), a neutrophil serine proteinase. J Biol Chem 1991; 266:9540–9548.
40. Redini F, Tixier J-M, Petiton M, Choay J, Robert L, Hornebeck W. Inhibition of leukocyte elastase by heparin and its derivatives. Biochem J 1988; 252:515–519.
41. Ying Q-L, Rinehart AR, Simon SR, Cheronis JC. Inhibition of human leukocyte elastase by ursolic acid. Biochem J 1991; 277:521–526.
42. Kornfeld S. Trafficking of lysosomal enzymes. FASEB J 1987; 1:462–468.
43. Laskowski M Jr., Kato I, Ardelt W, Cook J, Denton A, Empie MW, Kohr WJ, Park SJ, Parks K, Schatzley BL, Schoenberger OL, Tashiro M, Vichot G, Whatley HE, Wieczorek A, Wieczorek M. Ovomucoid third domains from 100 avian species: Isolation, sequences, and hypervariability of enzyme-inhibitor contact residues. Biochemistry 1987; 26:202–221.
44. Laskowski M, Park SJ, Tashiro M, Wynn R. Design of highly specific inhibitors of serine proteinases. In: Protein Recognition of Immobilized Ligands. New York: Alan R Liss, 1989:149–168.
45. Read RJ, Fujinaga M, Sielecki AR, James MNG. Structure of the complex of

streptomyces grisens protease B and the third domain of the turkey ovomucoid inhibitor at 1.8 Å resolution. Biochemistry 1983; 22:4420–4433.
46. Fujinaga M, James MNG. Rat submaxillary gland serine protease, tonin: Structure solution and refinement at 1.8 Å resolution. J Mol Biol 1987; 195:373–396.
47. Laskowski JM, Kato I. Protein inhibitors of proteinases. Annu Rev Biochem 1980; 49:593–626.
48. Papamokos E, Weber E, Bode W, Huber R, Empie M, Kato I, Laskowski M. Crystallographic refinement of Japanese quail ovomucoid, a Kazal-type inhibitor, and model building studies of complexes with serine proteases. J Mol Biol 1982; 158:515–537.
49. Bode W, Epp O, Huber R, Laskowski J, Ardelt W. The crystal and molecular structure of the third domain of silver pheasant ovomucoid (OMSVP3). Eur J Biochem 1985; 147:387–395.
50. Tschesche H, Beckmann J, Mehlich A, Schnabel E, Truscheit E, Wenzel H. Semisynthetic engineering of proteinase inhibitor homologues. Biochim Biophys Acta 1987; 913:97–101.
51. Zimmermann M, Ashe BM. Substrate specificity of the elastase and the chymotrypsin-like enzyme of the human granulocyte. Biochim Biophys Acta 1977; 480:241–245.
52. Harper JW, Cook RR, Roberts CJ, McLaughlin BJ, Powers JC. Active site mapping of the serine proteases human leukocyte elastase, cathepsin G, porcine pancreatic elastase, rat mast cell proteases I and II, bovine chymotrypsin Aa, and *Staphylococcus aureus* protease V-8 using tripeptide thiobenzylester substrates. Biochemistry 1984; 23:2995–3002.
53. Janoff A. Elastases and emphysema: Current assessment of the protease-antiprotease hypotheses. Am Rev Respir Dis 1985; 132:417–433.
54. Matheson NR, Janoff A, Travis J. Mol Cell Biochem 1982; 45:65–71.
55. Beatty K, Matheson N, Travis J. Kinetic and chemical evidence for the inability of oxidized alpha-1-proteinase inhibitor to protect lung elastin from elastolytic degradation. Hoppe-Seyler's Z Physiol Chem 1984; 365:731–736.
56. Lestienne P, Bieth JG. The inhibition of human leukocyte elastase by basic pancreatic trypsin inhibitor. Arch Biochem Biophys 1978; 190:358–360.
57. Stein RL, Strimpler AM, Hori H, Powers JC. Catalysis by human leukocyte elastase: mechanistic insights into specificity requirements. Biochemistry 1987; 26:1301–1305.
58. Yasutake A, Powers JC. Reactivity of human leukocyte elastase and porcine pancreatic elastase toward peptide 4-nitroanilides containing model desmosine residues: Evidence that human leukocyte elastase is selective for cross-linked regions of elastin. Biochemistry 1981; 20:3675–3679.
59. Tyagi SC, Simon SR. Inhibitors directed to binding domains in neutrophil elastase. Biochemistry 1990; 29:9970–9977.
60. Lentini A, Farchione F, Bernai B, Kreula-Ongarjnukool N, Tovivich P. Synthetic inhibitors of human leukocyte elastase. Part 3: Peptides with alkyl groups at the N- or C-terminus. Biol Chem Hoppe-Seyler 1987; 368:369–378.
61. Kabsch W, Sander C. Dictionary of protein secondary structure: Pattern, recognition of hydrogen-bonded and geometrical features. Biopolymers 1989; 22:2577–2637.

62. Priestle JP. RIBBON: A stereo cartoon drawing program for proteins. J Appl Cryst 1988; 21:572–576.
63. Deisenhofer J. Crystallographic refinement and atomic models of a human Fc-fragment and its complex with fragment B of protein A from *Staphylococcus aureus* at 2.9 and 2.8 Å resolution. Biochemistry 1981; 20:2361–2370.

# 8

# Kinetics of Neutrophil Elastase Inhibition In Vivo

**JOSEPH G. BIETH**

Louis Pasteur University
INSERM U 392
Strasbourg, France

## I. Introduction

One important physiological function of protein proteinase inhibitors is to prevent proteolysis operated by accidentally liberated proteinases. For instance, alpha 1–proteinase inhibitor (α1PI) and mucus proteinase inhibitor (MPI) (also called secretory leukoproteinase inhibitor) are thought to protect the lung tissue against the degrading action of neutrophil elastase (NE) (1). Protein proteinase inhibitors usually exhibit a good proteinase class specificity; e.g., serine proteinase inhibitors do not inhibit cysteine or mettalloproteinases and vice versa. They are, however, poorly specific on an all-or-none basis. For instance, α1PI inhibits trypsin-like, chymotrypsin-like, and elastase-like serine proteinases in vitro (2). Because of this lack of specificity it is difficult to infer the physiological function of inhibitors from simple in vitro inhibition assays. Measurement of the kinetic constants characterizing the proteinase-inhibitor interaction and of the in vivo concentration of the inhibitor helps, however, to predict the proteolysis-preventing function of an inhibitor. This chapter outlines the in vivo inhibition concept (3,4) and illustrates the theory with the NE/α1PI and the NE/MPI systems.

## II. The Delay Time of Inhibition

The delay time of inhibition, d(t), is the time required for almost full inhibition of a proteinase in vivo. Let I be an irreversible inhibitor that inhibits a proteinase E with a second-order association rate constant $k_{ass}$:

$$E + I \xrightarrow{k_{ass}} EI \qquad \text{(Scheme I)}$$

If the in vivo inhibitor concentration $[I_O]$ is at least 10-fold higher than the in vivo proteinase concentration $[E_O]$, the inhibition will be a pseudo-first-order reaction:

$$E \xrightarrow{k_{ass}[I_o]} EI \qquad \text{(Scheme II)}$$

with a half-life of:

$$t_{1/2} = \frac{0.693}{k_{ass}[I_O]} \qquad (1)$$

After seven half-lives, i.e., after d(t), the association will be 99.2% complete. Hence:

$$d(t) \approx \frac{5}{k_{ass}[I_O]} \qquad (2)$$

Now let I be a reversible inhibitor that reacts with E according to scheme III:

$$E + I \underset{k_{diss}}{\overset{k_{ass}}{\rightleftharpoons}} EI \qquad \text{(Scheme III)}$$

where $k_{diss}$ is the dissociation rate constant of the complex. Assuming again that $[I_O] \geqslant 10\,[E_O]$ one gets:

$$E \underset{k_{diss}}{\overset{k_{ass}[I_o]}{\rightleftharpoons}} EI \qquad \text{(Scheme IV)}$$

Since the delay time of inhibition corresponds to 99.2% inhibition, it can be calculated only for those reversible inhibitors that yield at least 99.2% inhibition at equilibrium, i.e., that yield pseudo-irreversible inhibition. This condition is fulfilled if $[I_O]$, the in vivo inhibitor concentration, is much greater than $K_i$, the equilibrium dissociation constant of the complex. It has been shown that for $[I_O] \geqslant 10^3\,K_i$, there is 99.9% or more inhibition at equilibrium (4). From $K_i = k_{diss}/k_{ass}$, one gets $k_{ass}\,[I_O] \geqslant 10^3\,k_{diss}$; i.e., the pseudo-first-order rate constant of complex formation is more than $10^3$-fold larger than the first-order rate constant of complex dissociation (see Scheme IV). This further illustrates the pseudo-irreversible inhibition behavior of a reversible inhibitor.

In summary, the delay time of inhibition d(t) is a tentative but convenient way to quantitate the in vivo potency of an irreversible or a pseudo-irreversible proteinase inhibitor: the lower d(t), the more efficient the inhibition in vivo. The delay time depends on two interchangeable factors: $[I_O]$, the in vivo inhibitor concentration, and $k_{ass}$, the rate constant of proteinase inhibition. Thus, a poor inhibitor (low $k_{ass}$) may have a good in vivo potency if its in vivo concentration is very high and vice versa.

## III. Proteolysis in the Presence of a Proteinase Inhibitor

If a proteinase (E) is released in vivo, it is usually faced with inhibitor (I) and substrate (S). Since both of these ligands are proteins, the inhibition is likely to be competitive; i.e., E binds either S or I, as shown in the following scheme:

$$\begin{array}{ccccc} E + S & \rightleftharpoons & ES & \longrightarrow & E + P \\ + & & & & \\ I & & & & \\ \downarrow k_{ass} & & & & \\ EI & & & & \end{array} \qquad \text{(Scheme V)}$$

Scheme V is valid not only for irreversible inhibitors but also for those reversible inhibitors which exhibit a pseudo-irreversible behavior in vivo, i.e., the inhibitors for which $(I_O) \geqslant 10^3\ K_i$.

Scheme V clearly indicates that there will ineluctably be some substrate breakdown during the delay time of inhibition. The concentration of product [P] increases exponentially with time and reaches a plateau once the bulk of E has transformed into EI (see Figs. 1–3). The concentration of product at the end of the inhibition process, $[P_\infty]$, is given by:

$$[P_\infty] = \frac{k_{cat}[E_O][S_O]}{K_m} \cdot \frac{1}{k_{ass}[I_O]} \tag{3}$$

or by:

$$[P_\infty] = \frac{k_{cat}(E_O)(S_O)}{K_m} \cdot \frac{d(t)}{5} \tag{4}$$

These equations (4) clearly show that the proteolysis-preventing function of a proteinase inhibitor does not depend only on d(t) but also on the efficiency of the proteinase–substrate interaction. As the latter is difficult to estimate, one can only attempt to guess how "small" d(t) should be to have "minute $[P_\infty]$ values" (4). Calculations based on Eqn. 4 with extreme values of $[E_O]$ and $k_{cat}/K_m$ suggest that the highest limit of d(t) compatible with significant prevention of proteolysis is about 1 sec if $[E_O]$ and $k_{cat}/K_m$ are unknown. For instance, if $[E_O]$ is as high as 1 μM and $k_{cat}/K_m$ as large as $10^5$ $M^{-1}$ $sec^{-1}$, no more than 2% substrate will be hydrolyzed if d(t) = 1 sec.

It must be added, however, that an inhibitor with a d(t) as large as $10^3$ sec may nevertheless play a significant proteolysis-preventing function if $k_{cat}$ $[E_O]/K_m$ = $10^{-4}$ sec, e.g., if $[E_O]$ = 1 μM and $k_{cat}/K_m = 10^2$ $M^{-1}$ $sec^{-1}$ or if $[E_O]$ = 1nM and $k_{cat}/K_m = 10^5$ $M^{-1}$ $sec^{-1}$.

In conclusion, if d(t) $\leqslant$ 1 sec, the inhibitor is likely to play an efficient proteolysis-preventing function in vivo.

## IV. Kinetics of NE Inhibition In Vivo

This section attempts to delineate the in vivo inhibitory potential of α1PI and MPI, the physiological NE inhibitors present in the lung. The former is an irreversible inhibitor with a $k_{ass}$ of $9.6 \times 10^6$ $M^{-1}$ $sec^{-1}$ (5) while the latter inhibits NE reversibly with $k_{ass} = 6 \times 10^6$ $M^{-1}$ $sec^{-1}$, $k_{diss} = 2 \times 10^{-3}$ $sec^{-1}$ and $K_i = 3.3 \times 10^{-10}$ M (6).

### A. Inhibition by α1PI

Ogushi et al. (5,7) reported the absolute concentrations of α1PI in the epithelial lining fluids of M1M1, SS, and ZZ subjects, measured the $k_{ass}$ for the inhibition of NE by the three isolated proteins, and calculated d(t) in each case. Table 1 lists their data, together with those obtained for oxidized α1PI (8) Both M1M1 and SS subjects who do not spontaneously develop emphysema have a delay time of inhibition of less than 1 sec. In contrast, the subjects with the ZZ phenotype who are at high risk for emphysema have a d(t) greater than 1 sec. It is remarkable that the 1-second limit proposed in 1984 on pure theoretical grounds (4) was entirely confirmed in 1987 on the NE/α1PI/emphysema system.

Activated neutrophils secrete proteinases and oxidants. The very large d(t) found for oxidized α1PI indicates that NE-mediated proteolysis may occur in an almost unimpaired way in the pericellular space.

Theoretical progress curves have been drawn to further illustrate the compared abilities of M1M1, SS, and ZZ subjects to stop NE-mediated proteolysis in their lower respiratory tract. The curves shown in Fig. 1 have been calculated using the following relationships (9):

$$[P] = \frac{v_Z}{k}(1 - e^{-kt}) \tag{5}$$

**Table 1** Delay Time of Inhibition (d(t)) of NE in the Epithelial Lining Fluids of α1PI-Sufficient and -Deficient Subjects (5,7)

| Phenotype | Concentration (μM) | $k_{ass}$ ($M^{-1}$ $sec^{-1}$) | d(t) (sec) |
|---|---|---|---|
| M1M1 | 4.6 | $9.6 \times 10^6$ | 0.12 |
| SS | 1.2 | $7.1 \times 10^6$ | 0.60 |
| ZZ | 0.46 | $4.6 \times 10^6$ | 2.40 |
| Oxidized α1PI | 4.6 | $7.0 \times 10^3$ [a] | 155.00[b] |

[a]Data from Padrines et al. (8).
[b]For the sake of illustration, calculations have been made assuming that α1PI is fully oxidized in the lower respiratory tract. We are aware that the totality of lung α1PI cannot be oxidized. The present calculation is nevertheless informative since one can imagine that in the vicinity of activated neutrophils a high burden of oxidants may oxidize the totality of the inhibitor present locally. As a result, the local d(t) will be 155 sec and NE-induced lung damage may occur at this site.

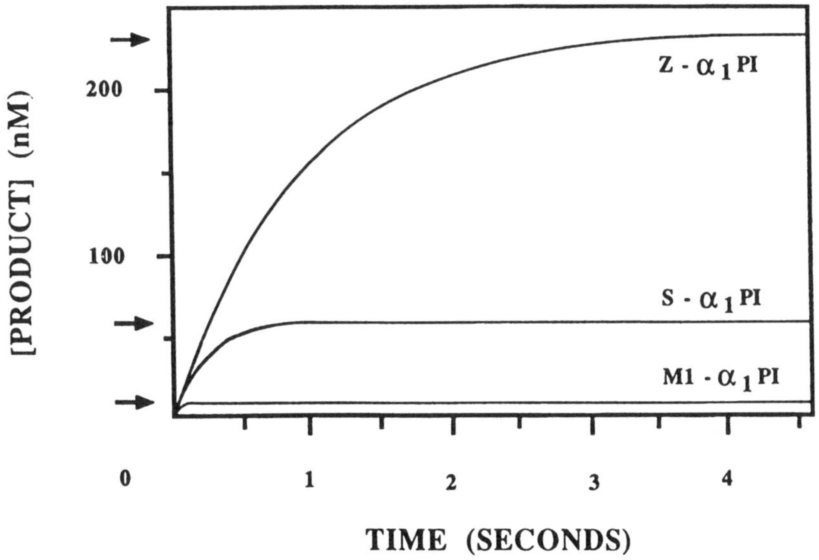


**Figure 1** Theoretical progress curves mimicking the kinetics of NE inhibition by α1PI in the lower respiratory tract of M1M1, SS, and ZZ individuals (M1-α1PI, S-α1PI, Z-α1PI). The curves were calculated using Eqns. 5–7, the $[I_O]$ and $k_{ass}$ values listed in Table 1 and $[E_O] = 50$ nM, $[S_O] = 0.1$ mM $k_{cat} = 10 sec^{-1}$, and $K_m = 0.1$ mM. The arrows indicate $[P_\infty]$.

where $v_Z$ is the velocity in the absence of inhibitor:

$$v_Z = \frac{k_{cat}[E_O]}{\left(1 + \frac{K_m}{[S_O]}\right)} \tag{6}$$

and k is a pseudo-first-order rate constant given by:

$$k = \frac{k_{ass}[I_O]}{\left(1 + \frac{[S_O]}{K_m}\right)} \tag{7}$$

The $k_{ass}$ and $[I_O]$ values used to calculate the three curves are from Table 1. The other concentrations and constants were chosen arbitrarily (see legend to Fig. 1). The curves illustrate the obvious relationship between the delay time of inhibition and the amount of substrate hydrolyzed during this delay time: the lower d(t), the lower $[P_\infty]$. Figure 1 also illustrates the great susceptibility of ZZ subjects to proteolysis; if an equivalent amount of NE is released in the lower respiratory tract of a ZZ and M1M1 subject, it will hydrolyze about 20-fold more substrate in the former individual than in the latter before being irreversibly inhibited.

### B. Inhibition by MPI

The concentration of MPI in the upper respiratory tract is about 5 μM (10). Its absolute concentration in the lower respiratory tract has not been determined directly but may be calculated from the molar ratio of MPI to α1PI (0.15; Ref. 11) and the absolute concentration of α1PI (4.6 μM; Ref. 5). This yields a concentration of about 0.7 μM. If these two in vivo concentrations $[I_O]$ are compared to $K_i$, one gets $[I_O]/K_i = 1.5 \times 10^4$ and $2 \times 10^3$ in the upper and lower respiratory tract, respectively. MPI-mediated inhibition of NE is therefore pseudo-irreversible in the lung so that the delay time of inhibition concept applies to this reversibility-associating system: d(t) = 0.16 and 1.2 sec in the upper and lower respiratory tracts, respectively.

Theoretical progress curves have again been computed to illustrate the inhibitory potential of MPI in vivo. These curves were constructed using equations characteristic of reversible inhibition (9):

$$[P] = v_S \cdot t + \frac{v_Z - v_S}{k}(1 - e^{-kt}) \tag{8}$$

$$k = \frac{k_{ass}[I_O]}{\left(1 + \frac{[S_O]}{K_m}\right)} + k_{diss} \tag{9}$$

where $v_S$ is the steady-state velocity of the reaction ($v_S$ = 0 for irreversible inhibitors).

Figure 2 compares the in vivo potency of MPI in the upper and lower respiratory tracts. The progress curves were calculated using $k_{ass}$, $k_{diss}$, and the two $[I_O]$ values given above. All other parameters were the same as in Fig. 1. The shapes of the two curves calculated using Eqns. 8 and 9, characteristic of reversible inhibitors, closely resemble those calculated with the irreversible inhibitor α1PI. This further illustrates the pseudo-irreversible character of this reversible-inhibition process ($v_S \approx 0$). $[P_\infty]$ is only about sevenfold lower in the upper respiratory tract than in the lower respiratory tract. MPI, which is usually thought to play an antielastase function in airways only, must therefore also be viewed as a physiological antielastase of the lower respiratory tract. Although its $[P_\infty]$ in the alveolar epithelial lining is about 11-fold higher than that of α1PI from M1M1 subjects (compare Figs. 1 and 2), it may compete with α1PI for the binding of NE.

Figure 3 compares the in vivo potency of MPI and α1PI in ZZ subjects: $[P_\infty]$ is about twice as high for α1PI than for MPI. This indicates that MPI is the major

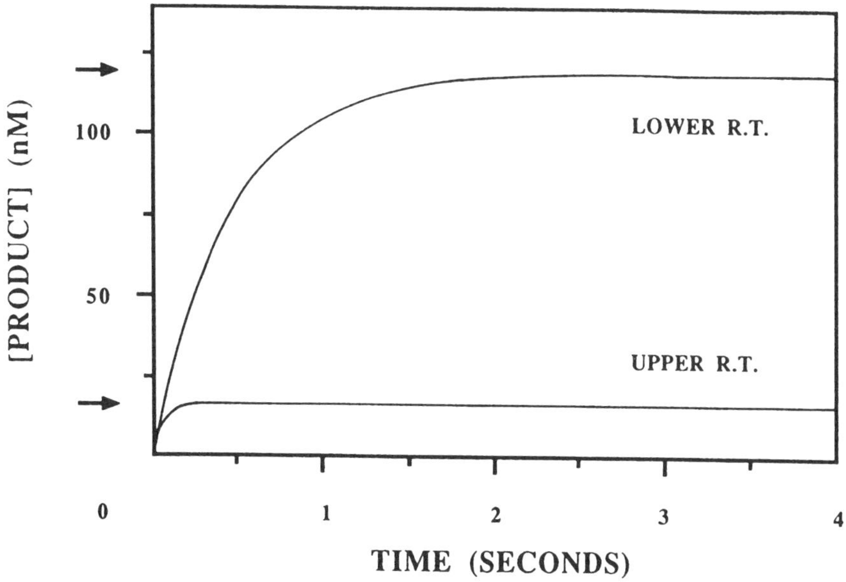


**Figure 2** Theoretical progress curves mimicking the kinetics of NE inhibition by MPI in the lower respiratory tract (LOWER R.T.) and the upper respiratory tract (UPPER R.T.). The curves were calculated using Eqns. 6, 8, and 9; $k_{ass} = 6 \times 10^6\ M^{-1}\ sec^{-1}$, $k_{diss} = 2 \times 10^{-3}\ sec^{-1}$; and $[I_O]$ = 0.7 and 5 μM in the lower and upper respiratory tracts, respectively. All other constants and concentrations were the same as in Fig. 1. The arrows indicate $[P_\infty]$.

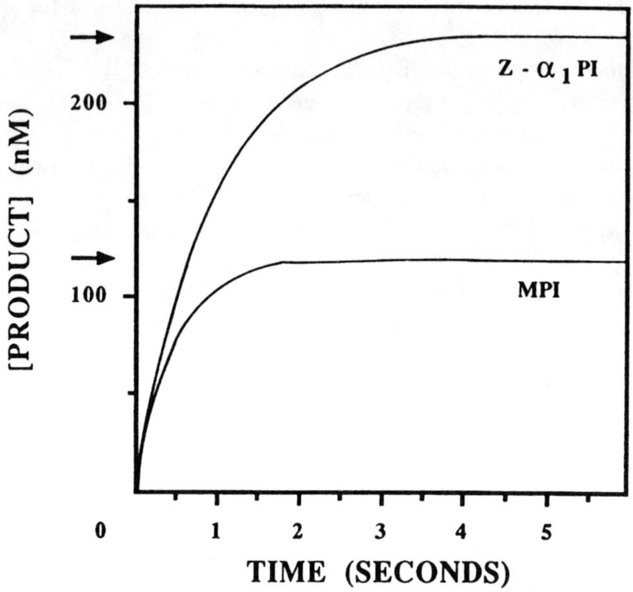


**Figure 3** Theoretical progress curves mimicking the kinetics of NE inhibition by α1PI and MPI in the lower respiratory tract of ZZ subjects. The curves were constructed as shown in the legends to fig. 1 (Z-α1PI) and Fig. 2 (MPI). The arrows indicate [P∞].

NE inhibitor in the lower respiratory tract of ZZ individuals. This observation has not previously been made. It might help explain the resistance to emphysema of a significant number of ZZ individuals.

## V. Predicting the Therapeutic Concentration of a Drug

If the kinetic parameters characterizing an antielastase drug are known, its therapeutic concentration may be tentatively predicted (12). If the drug is an irreversible NE inhibitor characterized by $k_{ass}$, its concentration may be calculated using Eqn. 2 with d(t) = 1 sec. If the NE inhibitor is reversible, its concentration should at least be $10^3$ $K_i$ to make it behave in a pseudo-irreversible fashion. It must next be checked whether this concentration leads to d(t) $\leqslant$ 1 sec.

## VI. Discussion

The present report lays much emphasis on $[P_\infty]$, the in vivo concentration of substrate broken down at the end of the inhibition process. A good inhibitor should make $[P_\infty]$ as low as possible. The inhibitor's efficiency, d(t), is, however, not the sole factor that determines $[P_\infty]$. Equation 4 shows, for instance, that $[P_\infty]$ is proportional to $[E_O]$, e.g., to the concentration of NE released by neutrophils. Since smokers have more lung neutrophils than nonsmokers, they may have significantly more NE-mediated proteolysis than nonsmokers. This might, at least in part, explain why some α1PI-sufficient smokers develop emphysema despite the low d(t) value of their α1PI/NE system. Furthermore, $[P_\infty]$ is proportional to $[S_O]$. This suggests that if neutrophils degranulate in an area where the concentration of extracellular matrix substrates is high, there will be more substrate broken down than in an area of low substrate concentration.

In conclusion, it should be kept in mind that in vivo inhibition is probably always competitive, so some substrate will ineluctably be broken down during the inhibition process. It is extremely difficult, if not impossible, to evaluate the magnitude of $[P_\infty]$. The only measurable parameter is d(t). Inspection of the $[P_\infty]$ values shown in Figs. 1–3 indicates that it can safely be restated that a d(t) close to or less than 1 second predicts an extremely low $[P_\infty]$ value unless $[E_O]$ becomes close to or higher than $[I_O]$. There is no need to add that elastolysis at the cell matrix interface and resistance of elastin-bound NE to α1PI (1) are phenomena that fully escape the above theory.

## Acknowledgment

The author thanks Dr. Faller for computational assistance.

## References

1. Bieth JG. Elastases: catalytic and biological properties. In: Mecham RP, ed. Regulation of Matrix Accumulation. New York: Academic Press, 1986:217–320.
2. Beatty K, Bieth JG, Travis J. Kinetics of association of serine proteinases with native and oxidized $\alpha_1$-proteinase inhibitor and with $\alpha_1$-antichymotrypsin. J Biol Chem 1980; 255:3931–3934.
3. Bieth JG. Pathophysiological interpretation of kinetic constants of protease inhibitors. Bull Eur Physiopathol Respir 1980; (16 (suppl):183–195.
4. Bieth JG. *In vivo* significance of kinetic constants of protein proteinase inhibitors. Biochem Med. 1984; 32:387–397.
5. Ogushi F, Fells GA, Hubbard RC, Straus SD, Crystal RG. Z-type α1-antitrypsin is less competent than M1-type α1-antitrypsin as an inhibitor of neutrophil elastase. J Clin Invest 1987; 80:1366–1374.
6. Boudier C, Bieth JG. Mucus proteinase inhibitor: a fast-acting inhibitor of leucocyte elastase. Biochim Biophys Acta 1989; 995:36–41.
7. Ogushi F, Hubbard RC, Fells GA, Casolaro MA, Curiel DT, Brantly ML, Crystal RG. Evaluation of the S-type of alpha-$_1$-antitrypsin as an *in vivo* and *in vitro* inhibitor of neutrophil elastase. Am Rev Respir Dis 1988; 137:364–370.

8. Padrines M, Schneider-Pozzer M, Bieth JG. Inhibition of neutrophil elastase by $\alpha_1$-proteinase inhibitor oxidized by activated neutrophils. Am Rev Respir Dis 1989; 139:783–790.
9. Morrisson JF, Walsh CT. The behavior and significance of slow-binding enzyme inhibitors. Adv Enzymol Relat Areas Mol Biol 1988; 61:201–301.
10. Kramps JA, Franken C, Dijkman JH. ELISA for quantitative measurement of low-molecular weight bronchial protease inhibitor in human sputum. Am Rev Respir Dis 1984; 129:959–963.
11. Gast A, Dietemann-Molard A. Pelletier A, Pauli G, Bieth JG. The antielastase screen of the lower respiratory tract of alpha$_1$-proteinase inhibitor-sufficient patients with emphysema or pneumothorax. Am Rev Respir Dis 1990; 141:880–883.
12. Bieth JG. The use of inhibition kinetics to delineate the physiological functions of proteinase inhibitors and to predict the potency of antiproteinase drugs. In: Mittman C, Taylor JC, eds. Pulmonary Emphysema and Proteolysis. Vol. II. New York: Academic Press, 1987:93–100.

# 9

# Alpha 1–Antitrypsin Gene Expression in Neutrophils and Other Cells

**ROLAND M. du BOIS**

Royal Brompton Hospital and
National Heart and Lung Institute
London, England

## I. Introduction

Neutrophil polymorphonuclear leukocytes (neutrophils) play a critical role in host defense. A decrease in numbers of neutrophils—which may occur as a consequence of bone marrow suppression due to haematological or lymphoproliferative malignancy and iatrogenic causes, including immunosuppressant drug therapy—results in life-threatening susceptibility to infection. Two major neutrophil microbicidal mechanisms combat microbial infection: the generation of potent oxygen-derived radicals following the triggering of a complex of membrane-associated enzymes and degradation by proteolytic and other neutrophil granule enzymes, including the potent serine protease neutrophil elastase (NE). (For reviews, see Refs. 1–3.)

These protective mechanisms may, however, be responsible for host injury; during phagocytosis, and likely during neutrophil migration through tissue, granule contents leak from the cell into the local milieu (3–6). In the context that 70–100 billion neutrophils are released from the bone marrow each day (7) and end their lifespans within tissue, including lung (2), it is surprising that host injury does not inevitably occur continuously during neutrophil migration unless tight autocrine or paracrine controls exist. Indeed, when neutrophils are attracted into sites of chronic inflammation, such as the lung in idiopathic pulmonary fibrosis as a result of local immune effector mechanisms, there is now clear evidence that neutrophils contribute to further host injury due to the unfettered effects of oxygen radical generation and degranulation in response to activating factors in the local milieu that overwhelm local controls (1,8–10). This chapter explores the concept that the neutrophil may minimize microenvironmental host damage to other cells and tissue matrix due to NE release during neutrophil chemotaxis by synthesizing and secreting alpha 1-antitrypsin ($\alpha$1AT), the natural and most potent inhibitor of NE.

## II. Neutrophil Ontogeny

### A. Neutrophil Origin and Fate

Neutrophils develop from progenitor cells within the bone marrow, and 60% of all bone marrow cells are of neutrophil lineage. Neutrophil production and release from bone marrow are enhanced by proinflammatory cytokines, such as the colony-stimulating factors GCSF and GMCSF; IL-1; TNF$\alpha$; and glucocorticoids (2). On the average, neutrophils remain in the circulating pool for approximately 10 hours before migrating to tissue where, under normal conditions, apoptosis occurs after 2–3 days (11). It is estimated that 55% of all circulating neutrophils are marginated, particularly in the lung, which removes 20% of the $4 \times 10^8$ neutrophils passing through the pulmonary vasculature each second, returning an equal number into the pulmonary veins (12). This huge neutrophil "load" is thus available for lung defenses but is also capable of exerting massive local damage when neutrophils are activated, as seen in adult respiratory distress syndrome.

### B. Neutrophil Granules

The most striking defining feature of neutrophils is the presence of large numbers of intracytoplasmic granules. Ultrastructurally, these granules can be differentiated into primary azurophilic granules, which are relatively electron-lucent, and the denser secondary granules. Primary granules develop almost exclusively during the promyelocyte phase of differentiation, in contrast to the secondary granules, which first appear during the myelocytic stage of neutrophil development (13). Each subset of granules contains a distinct repertoire of enzymes that include NE and myeloperoxidase within primary granules and lactoferrin in secondary granules (3).

### C. Neutrophil Granule Protein Synthesis

The morphological, developmental, and functional differentiation of neutrophils is consistent with immunohistochemical and molecular biological studies that have demonstrated that granule protein gene expression occurs in an ordered fashion; primary granule protein synthesis occurs in promyelocytes, whereas secondary granule proteins such as lactoferrin and collagenase are synthesized during later stages of bone marrow differentiation. Studies of gene-transcription products in bone marrow cells and mature neutrophils have shown (14):

1. mRNA for granule proteins is present in bone marrow cells but not mature neutrophils.
2. Using in situ hybridization, mRNA for the primary granule proteins, NE, and myeloperoxidase are found almost exclusively in promyelocytes, whereas secondary granule protein transcription products such as lactoferrin mRNA are present only in myelocytes and metamyelocytes.
3. Minor differences in expression of myeloperoxidase and elastase are seen at the mRNA level, which suggests that granule protein gene expression is not coordinately controlled in a precise fashion, even for proteins stored within the same compartment (Fig. 1).

Taken together, these observations clearly demonstrate that mature neutrophils are not capable of new granule protein synthesis, and that any modulation of neutrophil protease–antiprotease balance will depend on control of local levels and function of antiptrotease.

## III. Neutrophil Protease, Oxidant, and Antiprotease Interactions

### A. Neutrophil Oxidants

Activated neutrophils generate oxygen-derived products and release their granule contents (for reviews, see Refs. 1 and 3). Surface-membrane triggering of neutrophils activates the membrane-based NADPH–oxidase system, resulting in the generation of superoxide, which dismutes to hydrogen peroxide. Both of these oxidant species can react in vitro, in the presence of an Fe-containing catalyst, to generate $OH^-$ radicals that are more powerful oxidants than either $O_2^{\dot{-}}$ or $H_2O_2$ alone, although it remains unclear whether the neutrophil generates $OH^-$ radicals in vivo. However, neutrophil myeloperoxidase can catalyse the production of hypohalous acids from the halides $C1^-$, Br, $I^-$, and $H_2O_2$. Of these, hypochlorous acid appears to be a most highly reactive compound that interacts with critical cell and tissue substrates, resulting in cell damage and death. Hypochlorous acid oxidation of the active sites of $\alpha 1AT$ can also modulate the function of $\alpha 1AT$ which increases the susceptibility of host tissue to neutrophil elastase damage.

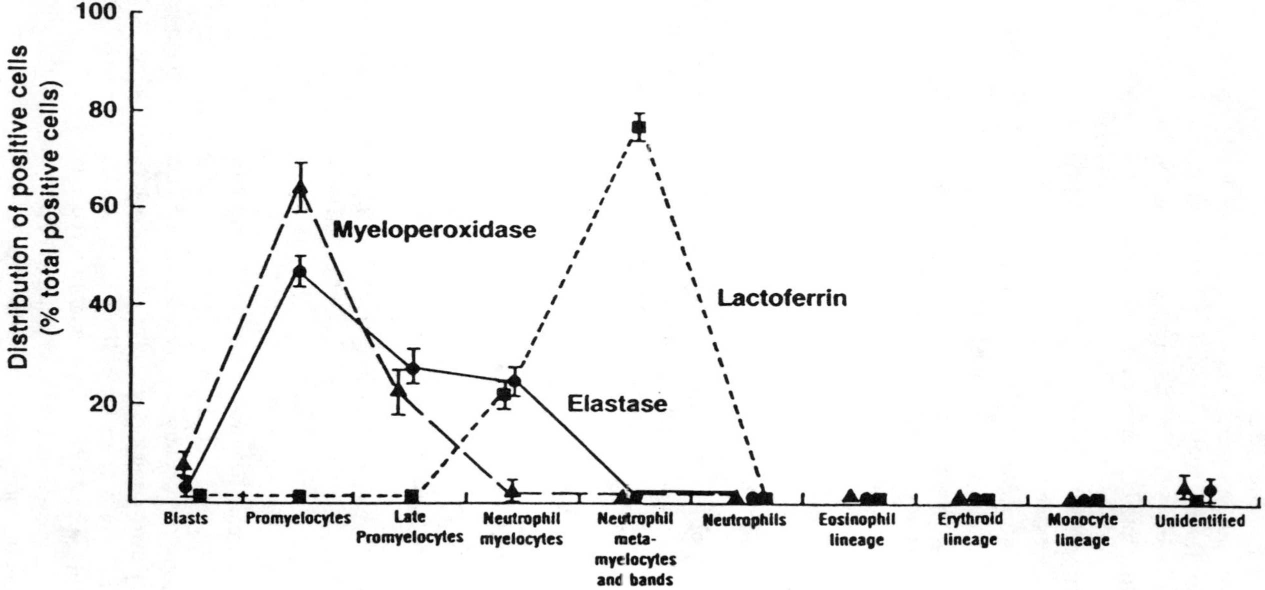


**Figure 1** Distribution of bone marrow cells expressing mRNA trnscripts for the neutrophil elastase (●), myeloperoxidase (▲), and lactoferrin (■) genes. After hybridization with each probe, the number of positive cells in each stage was determined and expressed as a percentage of the total number of cells positive for each gene. (From Ref. 14.)

### B. Neutrophil Elastase

Neutrophil elastase, a 220-residue single-chain glycoprotein, is a potent neutrophil primary granule enzyme capable of destroying a wide range of substrates. These include all major forms of collagen, proteolglycans, laminin, fibronectin, components of the complement and coagulation cascades, and intact cells, including *Escherichia coli* cell walls (15,16). Furthemore, NE has the capability of functioning at neutral pH, i.e., the pH of normal body fluids. Its natural and most potents inhibitor is α1AT.

A triggered neutrophil, by releasing NE and generating oxidants is, therefore, capable of producing a zone of cell and connective tissue damage around itself. Local proteolytic damage is enhanced by oxidative inactivation of the $Met^{358}$ residue within the $Met^{358}$–$Ser^{359}$ active inhibitory site of the α1AT molecule (17,18). This may explain damage to lung tissue evoked in such diseases as emphysema in which excess neutrophils are observed. In these situations, characterized by massive NE and other protease release, it appears that circulating α1AT cannot inhibit NE-induced injury. This is seen most graphically in PiZZ α1AT deficiency, in which α1AT levels are lower than normal and α1AT avidity for NE reduced.

## IV. Neutrophil Diapedesis: The Role of NE

In contrast to the large amounts of NE released following cell-surface-membrane triggering, it is also likely that more controlled release of smaller quantities of granule enzymes, including NE, plays an important role in providing a route for neutrophils migrating through tissue during normal non-inflammatory states. To traverse vascular and epithelial basement membranes during the process of diapedesis, neutrophils must detach from endothelial cell-adhesion molecules, breach the endothelial and epithelial basement membrane barriers, and traverse the connective-tissue matrix. The vast array of neutrophil granule enzymes such as NE are almost certainly involved in this normal neutrophil function (1,3,4–6). In the context that normal homeostatic mechanisms result in neither the autodestruction of neutrophils nor host-tissue damage, connective-tissue breakdown to allow cell traffic must be tightly controlled. Circulating antiprotease levels ought to provide adequate protection in this regard, but, during the migratory process, the neutrophil membrane is closely applied to basement membrane or connective tissue-matrix protein (Fig. 2) sites, where large molecules such as serum- or monocyte-derived α1AT will not diffuse. Within these highly defined and isolated microcompartments, it is possible that release of small amounts of NE is balanced by local anti-NE inhibition. In this regard, the local controlled release by the neutrophil of antiproteases such as α1AT in concert with NE liberation would prevent the unopposed effects of NE producing damage rather than facilitating

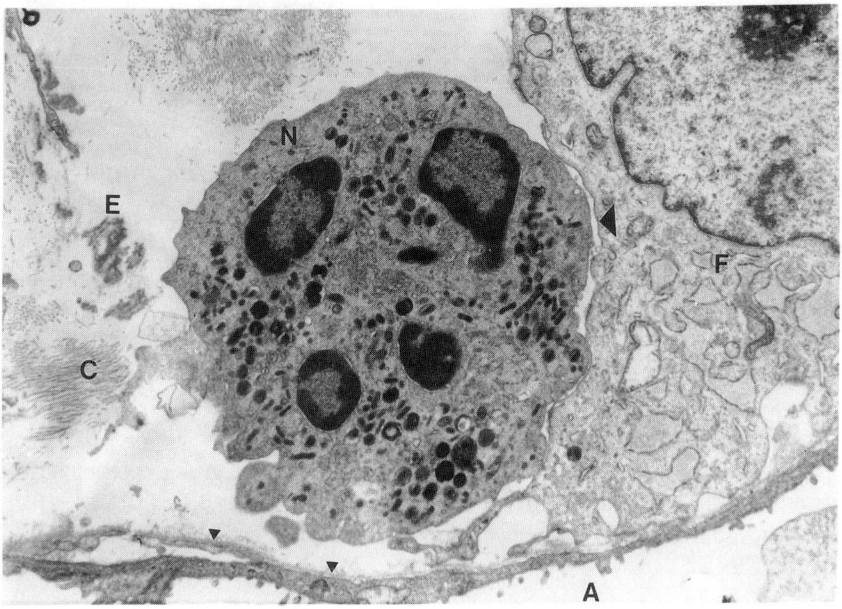


**Figure 2** Compartmentalization of the neutrophil within the lung interstitium—transmission electron micrograph of a section of lung from a patient with acute lung injury. Note the intimate relationship between the neutrophil (N), fibroblast (F), epithelial basement membrane (▼), and the connective tissue matrix proteins, collagen (C) and elastin (E), where little serum protein is likely to diffuse. A = airspace. ×11,000. (Courtesy of A. Dewar, National Heart and Lung Institute, London.)

diapedesis. Several studies have suggested that mature neutrophils may upregulate the expression of a number of genes that influence local inflammation (19–25). More recently, it has been shown that mature neutrophils contain, synthesize, and secrete α1AT (26–28).

## V. De Novo Neutrophil Gene Transcription and Protein Synthesis and Secretion

### A. Mature Neutrophil Gene Expression

Because mature neutrophils are terminally differentiated and do not have the capacity to resynthesize their major protein products, the granule proteins, they have come to be regarded as being incapable of de novo gene transcription, protein synthesis, and secretion. In recent years, it has been shown that appropriately primed and activated neutrophils are capable of expressing a number of genes, including heat-shock proteins, the heavy chain of cytochrome b245, the heavy-chain subunit of cytochrome b558, cfos, the complement receptor CR1, the α-chain of the complement receptor CR3, the Fc receptor, major histocompatibility complex class I proteins, and actin (19–24). More recently, neutrophils after stimulation with LPS or after adherence have been found to contain mRNA for IL-8, a potent neutrophil chemotactic factor and member of the novel chemokine supergene family, indicating that autocrine control mechanisms are likely to play a role in neutrophil recruitment to sites of inflammation (25). These studies provide compelling evidence that mature neutrophils can be activated to synthesize a variety of nongranule proteins and are thus capable of influencing cell function within the local milieu.

### B. Neutrophil α1AT Gene Expression

With the background of the neutrophil's capacity of up-regulating a number of genes, recent studies have been performed to elucidate the potential role of the neutrophil in local NE modulation. It has now been demonstrated that neutrophils are capable, to some extent, of modulating NE activity by synthesizing and secreting α1AT (26–28). Mature neutrophils contain α1AT, express the α1AT gene, synthesize α1AT, and store α1AT in "packages" that are then released, following cell activation, into the extracellular milieu.

### C. α1AT In Neutrophils

Immunohistochemical evaluation of human peripheral blood neutrophils has demonstrated that the majority of cells contain α1AT within the cytoplasm in a granular pattern (26). Studies using polyclonal α1AT antibodies and two-layer immunofluorescence with fluorescence cytometry quantitation have shown that neutrophils contain, cell for cell, more α1AT than autologous blood monocytes; this is confirmed by studies using $^{35}$S-methionine biosynthesis labeling of neutrophil protein synthesis (27).

Ultrastructural studies have confirmed that neutrophils contain α1AT and that this is contained within neutrophil granules (28). Using double ultrastructural labeling with monoclonal or polyclonal antibodies against NE, α1AT, or lactoferrin together with gold-labeled second-layer antibodies, α1AT was seen to be present within granules that are ultrastructurally indistinguishable from primary granules and that are quite distinct from granules containing lactoferrin. Strikingly, α1AT was found to be present in the same primary granules that contained NE; i.e., α1AT and NE colocalized within the same intracytoplasmic compartment but did not appear to be present as complexes. NE was observed mainly in the periphery of the primary granules whereas α1AT was not localized to any particular primary granule site (Fig. 3). However, biosynthetic labeling experiments in

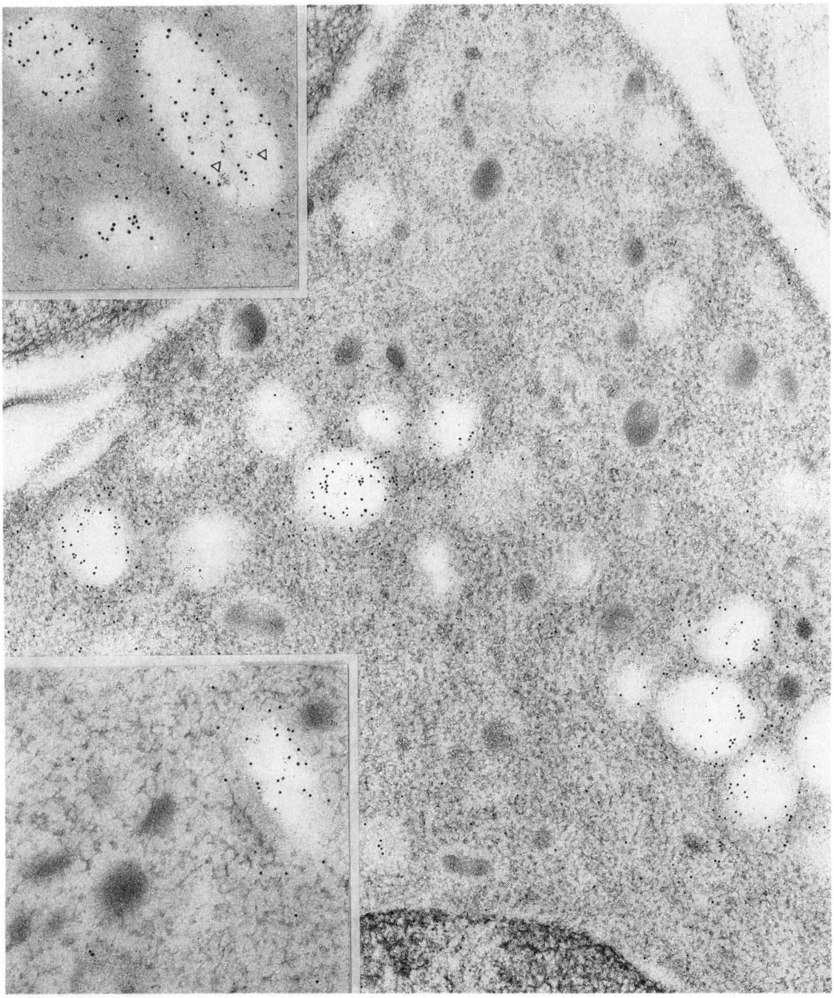

**Figure 3** Immunogold labeling of neutrophil α1AT and neutrophil elastase—transmission electron micrograph of a neutrophil demonstrating large, pale primary granules and denser secondary granules. Polyclonal rabbit anti-α1AT was labeled with small gold particles and the neutrophil elastase monoclonal antibody NP 57 was labeled with large gold particles. The primary granules are colabeled with particles of both sizes, indicating that they contain both elastase and α1AT. Secondary granules are unlabeled (×24,000). (Inset, top) enlargement of three primary granules, two of which show double labeling. The large particles corresponding to elastase tend to be aligned along the periphery of the granule. (×34,500.) (Inset, bottom) the absence of labeling in secondary granules (×34,500). (From Ref. 28.)

conjunction with subcellular fractionation would be needed to confirm that no complexes are formed within the primary granules.

### D. α1AT mRNA in Neutrophils

Mature human peripheral blood neutrophils contain mRNA transcripts for α1AT (26,29). Total RNA extraction from purified blood neutrophils, together with Northern analysis using $^{32}P$-labeled cDNA α1AT probes and in situ hybridization using $^{35}S$-labeled sense and antisense cRNA α1AT probes, has provided clear evidence that 1.8 kb α1AT mRNA transcripts are present within neutrophils (Fig. 4). Although neutrophils yield much less RNA than monocytes or Jurkat T cells (neutrophils, 1 $\mu g/10^7$ cells; monocytes, 10 $\mu g/10^7$ cells; Jurkat T cells, 7 $\mu g/10^7$ cells), the ratio for specific α1AT mRNA transcripts is higher in neutrophils than in monocytes, although the total copy number of mRNA transcripts is lower in neutrophils than in autologous blood monocytes.

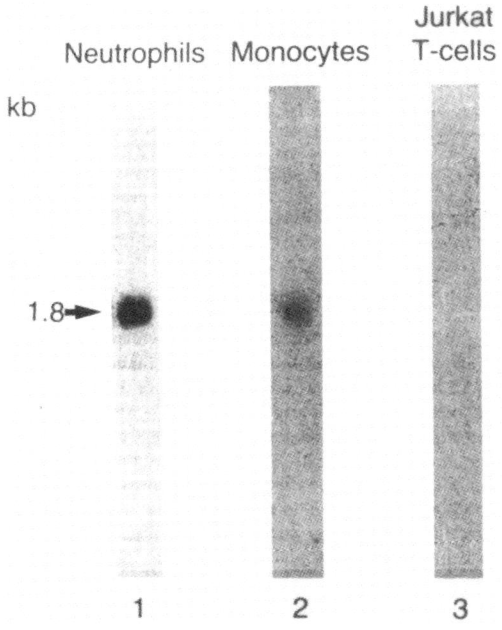


**Figure 4** Identification of α1AT mRNA transcripts in human blood neutrophils—Northern analyses evaluated with a $^{32}P$-labeled α1AT cDNA probe. Lane 1, total cellular RNA (5 μg) from blood neutrophils; lane 2, total cellular RNA (5 μg) from blood monocytes; lane 3, total cellular RNA (5 μg) from Jurkat T-cell line. The 1.8 kDa α1AT mRNA transcript is indicated. (From Ref. 26.)

### E. Synthesis and Secretion of α1AT

In addition to containing α1AT mRNA transcripts, it has been demonstrated that mature neutrophils can synthesize and secrete α1AT de novo in resting (i.e., unstimulated) culture experiments: α1AT secreted by neutrophils has the expected molecular mass of 52 kDa. To put into context the contribution of neutrophil α1AT to total α1AT production, neutrophils synthesize and secrete 40- to 80-fold less α1AT than autologous blood monocytes, and several orders of magnitude less than is secreted by the liver (26,29–31).

In addition to low-grade release of α1AT by unstimulated cells, neutrophils are capable of storing α1AT in a prepackaged form that is available for release minutes after surface stimulation (27). In this regard, stimulated neutrophils contain 60% less α1AT than resting cells, demonstrated by flow-cytometry quantitation of decrease in fluorescence intensity of cells stained with anti-α1AT antibody and FITC-labeled second antibody, and confirmed by biosynthetic experiments using $^{35}$S-methionine, immunoprecipitation, and fluorography. At least some of the newly released α1AT is capable of forming complexes with NE, as shown by the presence of 80 kDa α1AT-NE complexes following immunoprecipitation and fluorography of culture supernatants from neutrophil cultures following neutrophil triggering with fMLP, a powerful stimulus of neutrophil degranulation.

## VI. Functional Role of Neutrophil α1AT

### A. Neutrophil α1AT–NE Balance

In the context that neutrophil α1AT comprises a very small fraction of total α1AT synthesis in humans and that major cell-surface triggering results in the release of amounts of NE that overwhelm the neutrophil's packaged α1AT, it is unlikely that neutrophil α1AT plays a significant role in protecting the host from granule leakage of NE in an inflammatory milieu. However, even after surface triggering with fMLP, which activates oxygen radical production (resulting in local α1AT oxidation, rendering it 2000-fold less efficient than native α1AT at NE inhibition), some neutrophil α1AT is still capable of interacting with its own NE, producing 80 kDa α1AT–NE complexes. This suggests that local leakage of small amounts of granule contents by nonactivated cells may be combatted by the neutrophil's own α1AT. Therefore, a more likely role for neutrophil α1AT is to prevent autocrine or local host damage as the neutrophil performs its homeostatic policing role, migrating from the vascular bed to tissues where apoptosis and removal of apoptotic remnants occur. In this situation, finely controlled degranulation of proteases—particularly NE but also other serine proteases such as proteinase 3—and gelatinase would allow the neutrophil to progress through the normal connective-tissue matrix in a fashion that would not distort the fundamental structural integrity of this matrix, provided it was neutralized rapidly by local α1AT.

### B. α1AT Production by Other Cells

Support for the hypothesis that cells other than liver hepatocytes, monocytes, and macrophages may synthesize α1AT comes from observations of α1AT within other cells, notably human gastrointestinal epithelium and epithelial cell lines and cells of pancreatic and parotid glandular origin—sites where the unopposed effects of proteases are likely to produce stripping of cells from the basement membrane and tissue injury (32). In this regard, α1AT has been observed by immunohistochemistry to be present in gastric mucosal cells, small goblet cells from the small intestine, and pancreatic ducts in humans. Experiments using transgenic mice into which the human α1AT gene had been inserted have supported the concept of de novo synthesis of α1AT in these sites rather than that of exogenous protein being incorporated into cells. First, ultrastructural analysis using gold-labeled α1AT antibodies has localized the α1AT to the rough endoplasmic reticulum, the site of active protein synthesis. Second, the presence of α1AT mRNA transcripts within total RNA extracts of these tissues has been demonstrated by $S_1$ nuclease protection assay (32). These observations are concordant with studies using Northern analysis of total RNA extracted from jejunal mucosa and from the human epithelial cell line Caco2 that demonstrate the presence of α1AT mRNA transcripts (33).

A priori, these observations have supported the concept that a number of cells, including neutrophils, have developed mechanisms for survival within their local microenvironment during resting conditions. Where self-damage through protease degradation may occur, it seem developmentally highly appropriate for such cells as neutrophils to have an intrinsic means of controlling their own local milieu. In this regard, the capacity for neutrophils to synthesize, store within primary granules, and secrete small amounts of α1AT suggests that host tissue may be protected from local release of low concentrations of NE by an autocrine self-protection mechanism. This most likely occurs within the tight microcompartments produced by the close apposition of neutrophils to other cells and connective-tissue-matrix proteins. The colocalization of NE and α1AT within the same primary granule may also allow α1AT to interact within phagolysosomes to inhibit intracellular NE from damaging neutrophils from within.

## References

1. Hogg JC. Neutrophil traffic. In: Crystal RG, West JB, eds. The Lung: Scientific Foundations. New York: Raven Press, 1991:565–579.

2. Abramson L, Malech HL, Gallin JI. Neutrophils. In: Crystal RG, West JB, eds. The Lung: Scientific Foundations. New York: Raven Press, 1991:553–563.
3. Weiss SJ. Tissue destruction by neutrophils. N Engl J Med 1989; 320:365–376.
4. Weissman G, Smolen JE, Korchak HM. Release of inflammatory mediators from stimulated neutrophils. N Engl J Med 1980; 303:27–34.
5. Harlan JM, Schwartz BR, Reidy MA, Schwartz SM, Ochs HD, Harker LA. Activated neutrophils disrupt endothelial monolayer integrity by an oxygen radical-independent mechanism. Lab Invest 1985; 52:141–150.
6. Smedley LA, Tonnesen MG, Sandhouse RA, Haslett C, Guthrie LA, Johnston RB Jr, Henson PM, Worthen GS. Neutrophil-mediated injury to endothelial cells: enhancement by endotoxin and essential role of neutrophil elastase. J Clin Invest 1986; 77:1233–1243.
7. Dancey JT, Deubelbeiss KA, Harker LA, Finch CA. Neutrophil kinetics in man. J Clin Invest 1976; 58:705–715.
8. Cantin AM, North SL, Fells GA, Hubbard RC, Crystal RG. Oxidant mediated epithelial cell injury in idiopathic pulmonary fibrosis. J Clin Invest 1987; 79:1665–1675.
9. Gadek JE, Kellman JA, Fells GA, Weinberger SE, Horwitz AL, Reynolds HY, Fulmer JD, Crystal RG. Collagenase in the lower respiratory tract of patients with idiopathic pulmonary fibrosis. N Engl J Med 1979; 301:737–742.
10. Hallgren R, Bjermer L, Lundgren R, Venge P. The eosinophil component of the alveolitis in idiopathic pulmonary fibrosis: Signs of eosinophil activation in the lung are related to impaired lung function. Am Rev Respir Dis 1989; 139:373–377.
11. Golde DW. Neutrophil kinetics: production, distribution and fate of neutrophils. In: Williams WJ, Beutler E, eds. Haematology. New York: McGraw-Hill 1983:759–765.
12. Muir AL, Cruz M, Martin BA, Thommasen HV, Belzberg A, Hogg JC. Leukocyte kinetics in the human lung: role of exercise and catecholamines. J Appl Physiol 1984; 57:711–719.
13. Bainton DF, Ullyot JL, Farquhar MG. The development of neutrophilic polymorphonuclear leukocytes in human bone marrow: origin and content of azurophil and specific granules. J Exp Med 1971; 134:907–934.
14. Fouret P, du Bois RM, Bernaudin J-F, Takahashi H, Ferrans VJ, Crystal RG. Expression of the neutrophil elastase gene during human bone marrow cell differentiation. J Exp Med 1989; 169:833–845.
15. Bieth JG. Elastases: catalytic and biological properties. In: Mecham R, ed. Regulation of Matrix Accumulation. New York: Academic Press, 1986:217–320.
16. Janoff FA. Eloastase in tissue injury. Annu Rev Med 1985; 36:207–216.
17. Hubbard RC, Ogushi F, Fells GA, Cantin AM, Jallat S, Courtney M, Crystal RG. Oxidants spontaneously released by alveolar macrophages of cigarette smokers can inactivate the active site of $\alpha 1$-antitrypsin rendering it ineffective as an inhibitor of neutrophil elastase. J Clin Invest 1987; 80:1289–1295.
18. Weiss SJ, Curnutte JT, Regiani S. Neutrophil mediated solublization of the subendothelial matrix: oxidative and non-oxidative mechanisms of proteolysis used by normal and chronic granulomatous disease phagocytes. J Immunol 1986; 136: 636–641.

19. Berton G, Zeni L, Cassatella MA, Rossi F. Gamma interferon is able to enhance the oxidative metabolism of human neutrophils. Biochem Biophys Res Commun 1986; 138:1276–1282.
20. Eid NS, Kravath RE, Lanks KW. Heat-shock protein synthesis by human polymorphonuclear cells. J Exp Med 1987; 165:1448–1452.
21. Jack RM, Fearon DT. Selective synthesis of mRNA and proteins by human peripheral blood neutrophils. J Immunol 1988; 140:4286–4293.
22. Newberger PE, Ezekowitz RAB, Whitney C, Wright J, Orkin SH. Induction of phagocytes cytochrome-b heavy chain gene expression by interferon-gamma. Proc Natl Acad Sci USA 1988; 85:5215–5219.
23. Itami M, Kuroki T, Nose K. Induction of c-fos protooncogene by chemotactic peptide in human peripheral granulocytes. FEBS Lett 1987; 222:289–292.
24. Cassatella MA, Bazzoni F, Flynn RM, Dusi S, Trinchieri G, Rossi F. Molecular bases of interferon-gamma and lipopolysaccharide enhancement of phagocyte respiratory burst capability: Studies on the gene expression of several NADPH oxidase components. J Biol Chem 1990; 265:20241–20246.
25. Strieter RM, Kasahara K, Allen R, Showell HJ, Standiford TJ, Kunkel SL. Human neutrophils exhibit disparate chemotactic factor gene expression. Biol Biophys Res Commun 1990; 173:725–730.
26. du Bois RM, Bernaudin J-F, Paakko P, Hubbard R, Takahashi H, Ferrans V, Crystal RG. Human neutrophils express the α1AT gene and produce α1AT . Blood 1991; 77: 2724–2730.
27. Pääkö P, Bernaudin J-F, Kirby M, Gillissen A, du Bois RM, Ferrans VJ, Crystal RG. Manifestations of the Z mutation of α1-antitrypsin differ among α1-antitrypsin synthesizing cells. Clin Res 1990; 38:266A.
28. Mason DY, Cramer EM, Massé J-M, Crystal R, Bassot J-M, Breton-Gorius J. α1AT is present within the primary granules of human polymorphonuclear leukocytes. Am J Pathol 1991; 139:623–628.
29. Mornex J-F, Chytil-Weir A, Martinet Y, Courtney M, LeCocq J-P, Crystal RG. Expression of the α1AT gene in mononuclear phagocytes of normal and α1AT deficient individuals. J Clin Invest 1986; 77:1952–1961.
30. Crystal RG, Brantly ML, Hubbard RC, Curiel DT, States DJ, Holmes MD. The α1-antitrypsin gene and its mutations: clinical consequences and strategies for therapy. Chest 1989; 95:196–208.
31. Perlmutter DH, Cole FS, Kilbridge P, Rossing TH, Colten HR. Expression of the α1-proteinase inhibitor gene in human monocytes and macrophages. Proc Natl Acad Sci USA 1985; 82:795–799.
32. Carlson JA, Rogers BB, Sifers RN, Hawkins HK, Finegold MJ, Woo SLC. Multiple tissues express α1AT in trangenic mice and man. J Clin Invest 1988; 82:26–36.
33. Perlmutter DH, Daniels JD, Auerbach HS, De Schryver-Kecskemeti K, Winter HS, Alpers DH. The α1AT gene is expressed in the human intestinal epithelial cell line. J Biol Chem 1989; 264:9485–9490.

# 10

# Alpha 1–Antitrypsin Gene Expression in Hepatocytes

**ALFREDO NICOSIA and PAOLO MONACI**

Istituto di Ricerche
di Biologia Molecolare P. Angeletti
Pomezia, Rome, Italy

## I. Introduction

Alpha 1–antitrypsin (α1AT) is one of the most abundant serine protease inhibitors present in the bloodstream of mammals. As with to many serum proteins, the major site of α1AT synthesis is the liver, from which it is secreted into the plasma (1). In the blood circuit, α1AT exerts its inhibitory action on plasma proteases. Other sites displaying a lower degree of α1AT expression are the kidney, lung, and small intestine, where additional localized action is required (2–4). In the lung, α1AT acts to protect the tissue from hydrolytic destruction by excessive neutrophil elastase (NE) (5–7). The physiological role of α1AT expression in the kidney is still unclear. In contrast, because it is capable of inactivating several pancreatic digestive enzymes, it has been postulated that gastrointestinal α1AT modifies protein digestion when secretion of digestive enzymes is reduced, as in the case of pancreatic insufficiency (4). A severe deficiency of α1AT in serum is associated with chronic liver disease and premature development of pulmonary emphysema (8). α1AT also belongs to a family of proteins called acute-phase reactants because their rate of synthesis is modified in response to inflammation. Its concentration in serum increases three- to four-fold following inflammation or tissue injury (9).

Medical interest in this inhibitory protein is high, and considerable information has been accumulated on its biochemistry and genetics. This has promoted the study of regulation of α1AT gene expression, making it a model system for the understanding of molecular mechanisms governing tissue-specific expression.

Control of α1AT expression acts mainly at the transcription initiation level. Several studies with different experimental approaches have investigated its transcription regulation in humans and mice. Selectivity of transcription is retained by the α1AT promoter when introduced into eukaryotic cells by transfection. Reverse-genetics experiments using cultured hepatoma cells have defined the DNA sequences responsible for efficient and tissue-specific transcription from the mouse and human α1AT promoters. These findings have been confirmed in vivo transgenic mice, in which it has been possible to follow gene expression throughout development and in different tissues. Cell-free systems that reproduce in vitro the selectivity of transcription observed in vivo have allowed the *trans*-acting factors involved in α1AT liver-specific transcription to be identified and characterized. Finally, cloning the genes that code for these regulatory proteins and their structural and functional characterization has expanded our comprehension of the molecular mechanism regulating α1AT mRNA synthesis.

In this chapter we review the current knowledge of the regulation of α1AT gene expression, with particular emphasis on the *cis*-acting elements and the *trans*-acting factors responsible for the tissue specificity of α1AT transcription in hepatocytes.

## II. Regulation of the Human α1AT Gene

### A. Tissue-Specific Expression of the Human α1AT Gene

The amount of human α1AT (hAT) transcripts found in different tissues varies significantly. It is higher in liver and lower in kidney, lung, and small intestine (3,4).

Extrahepatic synthesis of hAT mRNA is partly related to transcription initiation sites that show distinct cell specificity. In hepatocytes, hAT transcription starts in the first exon, and gives rise to a transcript of about 1.6 kilobases (kb), which accounts for most of the hAT mRNA present in the adult liver (10). The same initiation site is used in human intestinal epithelial Caco2 cells, leading to accumulation of the 1.6 kb mRNA species. This transcript significantly increases during differentiation of Caco2 cells from crypt-type to villous-type enterocytes (11). Transcription initiation at the same position is also detected in kidney, lung, and small intestine (3,4).

In macrophages, longer hAT mRNAs of 1.8 and 2 kb are present, as there are three macrophage-specific transcription start sites located about 2 kb upstream of the hepatic one (11,12). Transcripts of the same length are detected in lung (3).

Different sequences are responsible for hAT mRNA synthesis in hepatocytes and in macrophages. The two promoters do not display significant homology and are alternatively used: the hepatocyte promoter is inactive in macrophages, while the macrophage one is silent in hepatocytes (12). However, upon stimulation with the acute-phase mediator interleukin-6 (IL-6), both hepatocytes and enterocytes switch on transcription from the upstream macrophage initiation sites (11).

Transcription from two mutually exclusive promoters is a common way to express the same gene in distantly related cells during ontogenesis (13). Macrophages originating from the embryonal mesoderm and hepatocytes deriving from the endodermal layer have evolved specialized transcriptional apparati in order to prevent ubiquitous expression of tissue-specific genes. Thus, during basal transcription the *trans*-acting factors that recognize the hepatocyte-specific promoter are not present in macrophages and vice versa. Transcription of the hAT gene is achieved in the two cell types by making use of different sets of *cis*-acting elements. This does not necessarily apply to IL-6-induced transcription, since both macrophage and hepatocyte promoters respond to IL-6 induction and contain sequences homologous to the DNA recognition site of the transcription factor IL-6DBP, a major mediator of IL-6-induced response (11,14–16).

Expression of the hAT gene has been extensively studied in vivo in transgenic mice. The human gene is appropriately regulated when introduced into the mouse genome (3,17,18). Transcription activation of the transgene in the mouse liver follows the same kinetics observed in the human embryonic tissue during differentiation, and leads to the accumulation of hAT mRNA levels similar to those synthesized in humans. Physiological amounts of hAT protein are also secreted into the blood of transgenic animals. The distribution and the quantities of both the hepatocyte- and macrophage-specific hAT transcripts in other organs closely reflect the human pattern (3,18). The most striking differences between the expression pattern of the transgene and the normal human pattern are the persistence of high levels of hAT mRNA in adult transgenic mouse small intestine and the lack of mRNA induction in response to inflammation in transgenic mice (3,18).

The correct regulation of the human gene in the mouse context indicates that a common set of *trans*-acting factors that has been conserved between two species is able to recognize homologous *cis*-acting elements present in the promoters of the two genes.

### B. Organization of the Human α1AT Hepatic Promoter

DNA sequences responsible for hepatic-specific hAT transcription have been localized in the 5′ flanking region of the gene by transfection assays using human hepatoma Hep3B and HepG2 cells (10,19,20). A short DNA fragment containing the first 732 base pairs (bp) upstream of the hepatic transcription start site is still able to direct efficient and specific transcription of a chloramphenicol acetyltransferase transgene in mice (21).

The first 557 bp upstream of the cap site stimulate maximal and accurate transcription of a reporter gene in HepG2 cells, but are inactive in nonhepatoma HeLa cells. Detailed characterization of this DNA fragment has allowed the identification of an essential TATA box situated 20 nucleotides upstream of the transcription start site, and three additional regions that contribute to the efficiency and tissue specificity of transcription. These regions have been designated Y (nucleotides −488/−356), X (nucleotides −261/−210), and P (nucleotides −137/−37) (Figure 1; 19). Both X and P elements are required for maximal transcription in hepatoma cells, while removal of the Y block does not affect hAT promoter activity. Thus, the −261/−37 promoter fragment contains all the information sufficient for hAT expression in hepatoma cells. All three hAT regulatory elements can enhance transcription when fused to a truncated SV40 promoter, but the extent and specificity of their activity differ significantly. The X and Y regions are active in HepG2 and HeLa cells (the latter being stronger in both kinds of cells), while the P element has a strong enhancer effect in hepatoma cells but is silent in HeLa cells (19). Even on its own, the P element is still able to stimulate transcription in a hepatic-specific manner, although at a reduced level with respect to longer promoter segments. This minimal hepatic-specific promoter in turn is composed of multiple regulatory sequences. Among these elements, two *cis*-acting signals—A (nucleotides −119/−104) and B (nucleotides −77/−64)—positively modulate transcription activity in HepG2 cells (19).

In vitro transcription experiments with rat nuclear extracts from liver and spleen led to the same conclusions drawn on the ground of the results obtained in the in vivo system. hAT promoter sequences from −137 to −37 represent the minimal DNA fragment capable of directing accurate and efficient transcription in a liver-specific manner (22). Within this minimal tissue-specific promoter, two *cis*-acting elements are required for maximal transcription in vitro using liver extracts. The boundaries of these elements coincide with those of the A and B regions defined by transfection experiments in hepatoma cells (22).

In short, the hAT control region can be viewed as a tripartite structure composed of two distal enhancer sequences, whose activity is not restricted to hepatic cells, and a tissue-specific proximal element. The importance of the Y region has yet to be addressed. It may be a redundant signal that substitutes the downstream X element to prevent loss of promoter activity following a mutational event. Alternatively, the Y block might play an important role in cell types other than hepatocytes. The lack of activity in HeLa cells of a DNA segment containing only the X and P elements indicates that in this promoter context a dominant mechanism restricts the transcription potential of the X element to hepatic cells.

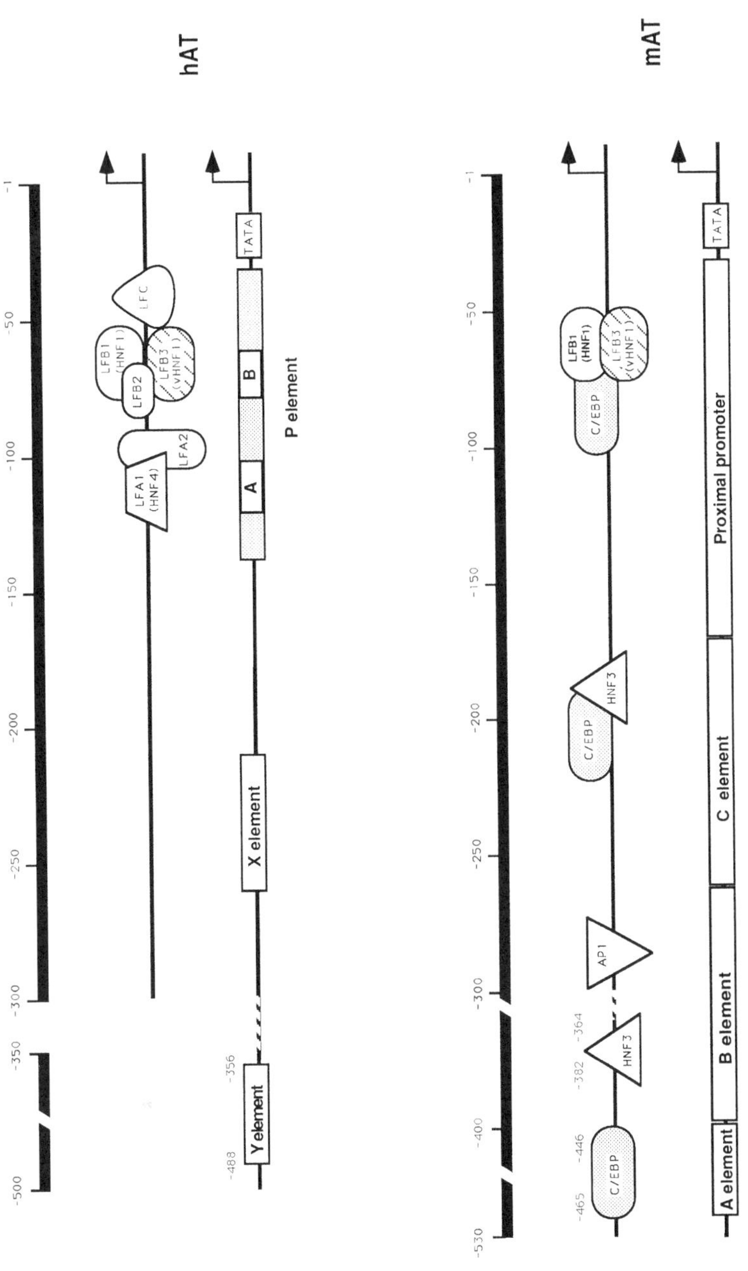


**Figure 1** Schematic representation of the *cis*-elements and *trans*-acting factors binding to the human and *M. domesticus* α1AT promoters.

### C. Nuclear Proteins Interacting with the hAT Minimal Promoter

The current view is that tissue specificity of transcription is due mainly to the interaction of DNA-binding proteins with specific sequences located in the regulatory regions of the genes (23,24). In vitro studies using protein extracts from rat liver nuclei have shown that multiple factors specifically recognize DNA sequences within the hAT minimal promoter. Among these factors, five DNA-binding proteins have been identified and further characterized: LFA-1/HNF-4, LFA-2, LFB-1/HNF-1, LFB-2 and LFC. The sites of interaction of these factors on the hAT promoter are shown in Figure 1. Virtually all DNA sequences between nucleotides −138 and −20 of the hAT promoter appear to be covered by these proteins. The complex interplay of these factors with their cognate sequences results from cooperative interactions or mutually exclusive binding. Stable interaction of LFC depends on the concomitant occupancy of the upstream sites by LFA-1/HNF-4 and LFB-1/HNF-1; in fact, removal of LFA- 1/HNF-4 or LFB-1/HNF-1 protein–DNA interaction by oligonucleotide competition also abolishes LFC binding (22). In contrast, LFA-2 interaction with DNA is enhanced when binding of LFA-1/HNF-4 to the adjacent sequences is prevented. Finally, LFB-1/HNF-1 and LFB-2 bind to DNA in a mutually exclusive fashion. Their recognition sites on the DNA are distinct but overlapping. In rat liver nuclear extracts, LFB-1/HNF-1 is more abundant than LFB-2; however, it would appear that the latter has a higher affinity for DNA than the former, since in vitro footprinting experiments clearly show that LFB-2 binding is dominant over that of LFB-1/HNF-1 (22).

As for the role played by each of these factors, a series of data indicates that LFA-1/HNF-4 and LFB-1/HNF-1 are positive transactivators of the hAT promoter in all experimental systems. There is a good correlation between the sites of interaction of LFA-1/HNF-4 and LFB-1/HNF-1 on the DNA and the A and B *cis*-acting elements essential for hAT promoter activity. Oligonucleotides capable of binding LFA-1/HNF-4 or LFB-1/HNF-1 specifically inhibit hAT promoter activity in competition experiments in vitro. Mutations that abolish LFA-1/HNF-4 or LFB-1/HNF-1 binding to the DNA are detrimental for hAT promoter activity in vitro, in cultured hepatoma cells, and in transgenic mice (19,22,25).

Of the various DNA-binding proteins that interact with the hAT minimal promoter, LFC is revealed as being the most elusive, and its role, if any, in transcription control is at the moment unknown.

LFA-2 is not a positive transcription factor, since its depletion does not affect hAT promoter activity in vitro. In addition, a fine 5′ deletion analysis of the hAT proximal element reveals a negative *cis*-element in correspondence to the LFA-2 binding site (P. Monaci and A. Nicosia, unpublished).

LFB2 does not stimulate transcription from the hAT minimal promoter in vitro either. Considering the relative concentrations of LFB-1 and LFB-2 in liver cells and their affinity for DNA, it is possible that LFB-2 quantitatively controls the level of transcription by displacing LFB-1 from its target sequence. A similar mechanism has been shown to operate in the LAP/LIP pair of DNA-binding proteins (26).

Tissue-specific expression of hAT can be explained by the cell-type specific distribution of the positive transcriptional factors acting on its promoter (see Section VI). However, some evidence suggests that negative control might also play a role in hAT transcription regulation (27; P. Monaci and A. Nicosia, unpublished). Negative *cis*-elements may be involved in the modulation of hAT transcription in liver cells, or they may repress the activity of transcriptional factors in nonhepatic cells to restore the tightness of hAT transcription. At present it is not possible to include all the results in a coherent picture of how the hAT promoter is regulated.

## III. Regulation of the Mouse α1AT Gene

### A. Organization of the Mouse α1AT Promoter

The mouse α1AT gene (mAT) is more strictly liver-specific than the human gene. High levels of mAT protein are found in liver, but not in the majority of other cell types in the animal (28,29). The most significant difference between murine and human genes is the absence of mAT protein in mouse macrophages. Consistent with this finding, no transcriptional start sites other than the hepatocyte-specific one have been detected in mice (J. E. Darnell, personal communication). In addition, the macrophage-specific intron–exon splicing junctions are not conserved in the muring gene (30).

Expression of mAT mainly reflects the gene-transcription rate. Reverse genetics experiments using differentiated cell lines have identified sequences that participate in mAT transcription regulation. About 500 bp of sequences upstream of the transcription start site are sufficient for full hepatocyte-specific expression. No further transcriptional stimulation is afforded by any other DNA segment, either extending up to 2 kb 5′ from the RNA start site or within the long first intron (31).

The 170 bp immediately upstream of the cap site contain sufficient information for hepatoma-specific transcription, but display reduced efficiency compared to the full-length promoter. Within this proximal promoter, binding sites for the liver-enriched transcription factors C/EBP (−85/−62) (31–34) and LFB-1/HNF-1 (−75/−63) have been identified (35). Figure 1 shows a schematic representation of the *trans*-acting factors interacting with the mAT promoter.

The upstream region (from −523 to −168) is required for maximal expression and exhibits hepatoma-specific enhancer function. Dissecting this enhancer region has revealed three separate domains that contribute to its activity: the A element, from −523 to −397; the B element, from −397 to −263; and the C element, from −263 to −168 (Fig. 1; 31). All three elements, which on their own are incapable of activating a heterologous promoter, interact with nuclear proteins. C/EBP, or a related factor, binds to sites within the A and C elements of the enhancer (−465/−446 and −211/−200) (31–33). The B element of the mouse enhancer interacts with a nuclear protein present in many cell types. A GTGACTCA motif, previously reported to be the binding site of the transcription factor AP1 (36), is contained within this element (−292/−282) (32).

Binding of hepatocyte nuclear factor III (HNF-3) has been detected at two sites in the mAT enhancer region (−382/−364 and −199/−181). Deletion of the latter element reduces promoter activity by about 50% (37).

A comparison of the mouse and human α1AT regulatory regions reveals over 80% of identity within the first 140 bp upstream of the transcription start site. Despite this, the human, but not the mouse, proximal promoter is able to direct efficient hepatoma-specific transcription. This difference might be explained by a 4 bp insertion within the mouse sequence, which corresponds to the human A domain. Mutation in this region has been shown to impair promoter activity of the human gene and concomitantly abolish binding activity of the LFA-1/HNF-4 transcription factor (19,22,38). Other short blocks of homology are scattered throughout several hundred nucleotides upstream of the proximal element. In particular, the putative AP1-binding site of the mAT enhancer is almost perfectly conserved in the X element of the hAT enhancer. However, a substantial difference exists between the enhancer elements of two genes. The X and Y elements of the human gene can activate (either together or independently) the expression of a heterologous promoter in both hepatoma and HeLa cells, while the murine enhancer stimulates transcription in a liver-specific fashion (31).

### B. Alternative Strategies for Regulation of α1AT Expression

The study of mAT expression in the wild-derived mouse species *M. caroli* reveals a mode of regulation distinct from that of the *M. domesticus*. In *M. caroli*, the mRNA is expressed not only in the liver but also in the kidney, using the same transcription start site (37). Although the 5′-flanking regions of the genes in the two species show a 93% sequence homology, the activity of *cis*-regulatory elements governing liver-specific expression is strikingly different. The proximal region of the *M. caroli* promoter (i.e., between −120 and −2 relative to the transcriptional start site) is an efficient tissue-specific promoter, while the analogous region of *M. domesticus*—only two nucleotides distinguishing the two species—shows very little activity. In addition, the upstream region between −520 and −199 in *M. domesticus*, but not in *M. caroli*, acts as a liver-specific enhancer of expression.

There appear to be several arrangements for the organization of the regulatory elements that determine the pattern of liver-specific α1AT expression. The human gene is controlled primarily by the proximal region, along with upstream enhancers active in all cell types. In contrast, most of the regulatory information in the *M. domesticus* gene is confined to a strong upstream hepatocyte-specific enhancer, which compensates for the presence of a weak proximal promoter region. Finally, despite the extensive homology shared with the *M. domesticus* species, the regulatory information of *M. caroli* is concentrated in the proximal promoter region. Thus, liver-specific expression of the α1AT gene is maintained by different promoter organizations in the three species, reflecting the accumulation of regulatory mutations since they diverged. Regardless of molecular mechanisms, the three strategies generate distinct, yet equally active, modes of hepatocyte-specific expression.

## IV. Architecture of the α1AT Promoter

A number of recurrent features can be identified as a result of the definition and characterization of the *cis*-elements acting on human and mouse α1AT promoters, as well as the information acquired through the study of promoters of several different liver-specific genes.

As for many RNA polymerase II genes, the *cis*-regulatory signals governing liver-specific gene expression are interspersed throughout several kilobases of 5′- and 3′-noncoding sequence. However, in most cases, the proximal promoter region, e.g., the first 100–200 bp upstream of the transcription start site, contains sufficient information for efficient hepatocyte-specific transcription. Within this region, binding sites for ubiquitous and liver-enriched factors are concomitantly present, suggesting that both kinds of transactivators are required for maximal gene transcription in the hepatocyte (39).

Detailed characterization of the hAT promoter and its liver-specific A and B boxes has led to experiments aimed at understanding the rules governing the organization of the transcriptional signals being made. The A and B elements enhance transcription from a heterologous promoter in a tissue-specific manner (22). Liver-specific promoter elements can thus confer a tissue-specific phenotype on ubiquitously expressed promoters, as if they were independent functional units.

Many *cis*-elements exert their function irrespective of their position and orientation relative to the direction of transcription. For example, the A and B boxes can modulate transcription from a heterologous promoter in either orientation. The B element maintains its function in the original promoter even if the orientation is inverted (22; P. Monaci and A. Nicosia, unpublished). Finally, the orientation and position of the A and B elements vary in different liver genes. The different arrangement of the same regulatory sequences in several liver-specific promoters shows that various regulatory elements have a broad functional compatibility. It appears that a unique architecture of *cis*-elements is not essential for their function, but rather that variable assortments of transcriptional signals can lead to liver-specific expression.

In all the promoters examined, at lease one *cis*-element recognized by C/EBP, LFB-1/HNF-1, HNF- 3, or HNF-4/LFA-1 is always present. Very often, there is a binding site for a liver-enriched transcription factor located close to the TATA box. Whenever a direct correlation has been established between binding and functional data, this tissue-specific proximal element has been shown to limit the rate of promoter activity. The particular function that a liver-specific binding site in such a position could have is the ability to assemble an active transcription complex in the vicinity of the start site. The hAT promoter is a typical case of the central role played by tissue-specific proximal elements. Its activity in transiently transfected hepatoma cells or in liver extracts is largely dependent on the two binding sites for HNF-4/LFA-1 and LFB-1/HNF-1. However, the relative importance of these two elements emerges when their contribution to the promoter activity is analyzed in the context of the entire gene in transgenic mice. In this case, disruption of the HNF-4/LFA-1 *cis*-element has a detrimental effect on promoter activity only in embryonal tissue, while mutation of the more proximal LFB-1/HNF-1-binding site drastically reduces hAT transcription throughout development and in the adult animal (25).

## V. Structure and Tissue Distribution of the Transcription Factors Binding to the α1AT Promoter

Most of the accumulated information on the factors that interact with the α1AT promoter deals with the structure of the DNA-binding domain and the molecular mechanisms of protein–DNA recognition. Protein domains mediating transcription activation have been identified; however, the rules governing transcription stimulation by these factors are largely unknown.

Expression of the *trans*-acting factors described below occurs at transcriptional level. How such control is brought about is still unclear, but it has been established that a cascade of sequential transcriptional events contributes to the realization of the "hepatic program."

### A. LFB-1/HNF-1

The palindromic consensus sequence GTTAATNATTAAC is a well characterized *cis*-element present in the regulatory region of several hepatocyte-specific promoters. Mutations of this sequence severely impair promoter cell-type specific transcriptional activity. At least two related proteins recognize this *cis*-element: LFB-1, (also called HNF-1α) and LFB-3 (also called vHNF-1 or HNF-1β).

LFB-1/HNF-1 and LFB-3 are both transcriptional activators. On the basis of their structural similarity, they are considered related members of the same family of DNA binding proteins.

LFB-1 is composed of two physically separable fragments: the DNA-binding domain, consisting of 281 N-terminal amino acids, and the C-terminus, where sequences responsible for transcriptional enhancement are present (40).

Within the C-terminal half of LFB-1, two distinct protein elements—ADI (from aa547 to aa628) and ADII (from aa281 to aa318)—are required for maximal induction of liver-specific promoter activity in vitro (40). ADI, which is rich in serine and threonine residues, is also necessary for full activity in vivo and activates transcription when fused to a heterologous DNA-binding domain (41). In contrast, ADII, a proline-rich peptide sequence, does not show any activation function in cell-transfection assays (41,42). Another domain that is active only in vivo has been localized between aa440 and aa506, in a protein fragment rich in glutamine residues. This protein region acts as a very powerful activator when fused to the GAL-4 DNA-binding moiety (41,42).

A distinctive feature of LFB-1 is that efficient and specific DNA binding requires three protein domains. Region A (amino acids 1–31) is necessary and sufficient to guide DNA-independent dimerization of the protein through an original type of coiled-coil structure (40,43,44). The B region (amino acids 100–184) is distantly related to the subdomain A of POU proteins (45) and determines dimer geometry and sequence specificity (46). The C region (amino acids 198–281) is a novel type of homeodomain containing 19 extra–amino acids with respect to the canonic homeodomain, and is required for DNA recognition (40,47).

LFB-1 is a liver-enriched *trans*-acting factor that is also present in similar amounts in kidney. Lower levels are found in intestine, stomach, spleen, pancreas, and thymus (48,49).

The LFB-3 DNA-binding moiety shares several regions of significant homology with LFB-1. In particular, the three most conserved amino acid sequences correspond to the A, B, and C domains essential for LFB-1–DNA interaction. In contrast, the glutamine-enriched region is the only C-terminal protein fragment that is conserved between the two factors. As in the case of LFB-1, deletion of this glutamine-enriched stretch abolishes the *trans*-activation properties of LFB-3 (V. De Simone, personal communication).

During mouse development, LFB-3 transcription precedes that of LFB-1, which appears in concomitance with the yolk sac and the embryonal liver. LFB-3 is expressed abundantly in kidney and to a lesser extent in liver and lung (48).

LFB-1 and LFB-3 are expressed in a variety of tissues characterized by the presence of polarized epithelia. This lends support to the idea that both factors are involved in establishing and maintaining the differentiated status of epithelial cells.

Both LFB-1 and LFB-3 bind to DNA as dimers, and already exist in solution in dimeric form prior to DNA binding (40,48). Thanks to the structural similarity between their dimerization domains, LFB-1 and LFB-3 form heterodimers in the cells in which both factors are expressed. In addition, homo- or heterodimeric molecules from rat liver are stabilized by the association of an 11 kDa polypeptide named DCoH. This protein enhances LFB-1 transcriptional activity in cotransfection experiments (50).

### B. C/EBP

The CCAAT/enhancer binding protein (C/EBP) is a heat-stable DNA-binding activity present in rat liver nuclei, capable of selective binding to the CCAAT motif of several viral promoters and to the SV40 core enhancer (51,52). C/EBP also binds to the ATTGCGCAAT palindromic sequence present in the regulatory regions of many liver-specific genes (39).

C/EBP is composed of two physically separable domains: an N-terminal transcription activating domain and a DNA-binding domain, which is located at the C-terminus of the protein (53). Two subregions contribute to the transactivation potential of C/EBP: the first (aa62 to aa89) might fold as an α-helix, while the second (aa150 to aa196) is formed by three redundant elements (54). This second region is characterized by a significant enrichment in prolines and histidines; however, mutant analysis indicates that a specific proline content is not essential for transcription activity (55).

C/EBP binds to DNA as a dimer through a bipartite structure called the basic-zipper (b-Zip) domain. The b-Zip domain is composed of a dimerization domain containing a repeat of five leucines (leucine zipper) and a second region enriched with basic residues. The leucine zipper domain forms a parallel coil of two α-helices in which the conserved leucine residues make side-to-side interactions, in a handshake fashion (53,56). The paired set of basic regions formed by dimeric C/EBP begins DNA contact at a central point and tracks in opposite directions along the major groove, forming a molecular clamp around DNA (57).

Recently, cDNAs encoding for proteins whose DNA-binding domain is highly homologous to the b-Zip of C/EBP have been cloned, leading to the definition of a family of C/EBP-related transcription factors (58–62). These factors differ significantly in the N-terminal region in which sequences responsible for transcription activity are located. Heterodimerization between different members of the C/EBP family gives rise to protein complexes with new transactivating specificity and/or potential (58).

C/EBP is expressed in liver, intestine, and several other tissues characterized by metabolism of high levels of lipids and cholesterol-related compounds, such as gut, white and brown fat, lung, adrenal gland, and placenta (64). High expression of C/EBP in both hepatocytes and adipocytes is limited to terminally differentiated cells (63–65). In the mouse brain, C/EBP transcription is switched on in the adult animal but not in the embryo (66). All these data suggest that C/EBP is involved in maintaining the differentiated state of the cell.

### C. HNF-3

Hepatocyte nuclear factor III (HNF-3) is a DNA-binding protein capable of interacting with sequences located in the regulatory regions of many liver-specific genes (39). Liver nuclear extracts contain three major binding activities for these sites: HNF-3α, HNF-3β, and HNF-3γ. Cloning the relative cDNAs revealed a striking homology in the protein regions responsible for DNA binding (67,68). Within this protein fragment, a cluster of basic amino acids is present (RRQKRFK) that is reminiscent of the basic region of the b-Zip DNA-binding domain. However, in contrast to the b-Zip proteins, HNF-3 binds to the DNA as a monomer, suggesting that its DNA binding motif is of a novel type. Interestingly, the HNF-3 DNA-binding domain is highly homologous to the corresponding region of the *Drosophila forkhead* protein (69).

All three cloned HNF-3 genes are expressed in liver and intestine. HNF-3α and HNF-3β are also transcribed in lung, while HNF-3γ mRNA is also found in testis (68). Therefore, it appears that expression of the HNF-3 family of factors is restricted to cells deriving from the primitive gut. Interestingly, the product of the *forkhead* gene is expressed in those cells of the *Drosophila* embryo from which the anterior and posterior gut structures originate.

### D. HNF-4/LFA-1

Hepatocyte nuclear factor IV (HNF-4) is a DNA-binding protein interacting with the mouse transthyretin and the hAT promoters (70,71). Cloning the rat HNF-4 cDNA revealed that it is a member of the steriod/thyroid hormone receptor superfamily, whose DNA binding domain is of the zinc-finger type (72). Members of this superfamily have been classified according to the amino acids present in the knuckle of the first finger, which is critical for the sequence specificity of DNA recognition (73,74). The HNF-4 sequence in this region (DGCKG) is highly homologous to the corresponding sequence (EGCKG) of the thyroid hormone receptor (TR). The similarity between HNF-4 and TR also extends to the nucleotide sequence of their cognate DNA-binding sites (nine identical residues over 12). Despite these homologies, HNF-4 does not bind to a thyroid-response element (72). The HNF-4 recognition sequence appears to be composed of two short motifs (consensus: TGGAC$^{T}$/c$^{T}$/c and TGGCCC) separated by a variable "spacer" region whose mutation does not affect protein–DNA interaction (75). Consistent with this observation, and similarly to other hormone receptors, HNF-4 binds to DNA as a dimer. Dimerization of steriod/thyroid receptors is mediated by a series of heptad repeats of hydrophobic amino acids (73). HNF-4 also contains

12 heptad repeats in a region essential for DNA binding. No ligand able to interact with HNF-4 has been identified yet.

Transcription factor LFA-1 was identified independently from HNF-4 as an activity binding to the essential A element of the hAT promoter (19,22,38). Cross-competition studies in DNA-binding assays suggested that HNF-4 and LFA-1 are related factors. On the basis of their immunological cross-reactivity it has also been proposed that HNF-4 and LFA-1 are the same protein (72). As with the other transcription factors involved in liver-specific gene control, HNF-4 expression is not restricted to hepatocytes. In fact, significant levels of HNF-4 mRNA are also detected in kidney and intestine (72,76).

## VI. Conclusions

It has been well established that regulation at the transcriptional level accounts for α1AT tissue–specific expression. The simple model involving the existence of one, or a few, hepatocyte-specific transcription factors does not correlate with the tissue distribution of the *trans*-acting factors controlling the α1AT transcription rate. In fact, the proteins identified as binding to several functionally important sites on the hepatic α1AT promoter of both the human and the mouse genes include four factors that, based on DNA-binding and mRNA-detection assays, are highly enriched in liver, but are also found in other tissues (Table 1). None of these proteins appears to act as a "master" positive acting factor, as in the case of the muscle determination factor MyoD (77). A similar situation has been found for other *trans*-acting factors mediating tissue-specific gene expression. The octamer-binding protein Oct-2 is found in cells other than lymphocytes (78); the pituitary *trans*-acting factor Pit- 1 is also expressed in the brain (79); and Eryf-1, a regulator of the erythroid lineage, is also present in megakaryocytes (80).

The picture that emerges is that transcription factors have a wider domain of

**Table 1** Tissue Distribution of the *trans*-Acting Factors Binding to the Human and Mouse AT Promoters

| | Liver | Kidney | Intestine | Lung |
|---|---|---|---|---|
| hAT | +++ | + | + | + |
| mAT (*M. domesticus*) | +++ | − | − | − |
| mAT (*M. caroli*) | +++ | + | − | − |
| LFB-1/HNF-1 | +++ | +++ | + | − |
| LFA-1/HNF-4 | +++ | +++ | +++ | − |
| C/EBP | +++ | − | +++ | + |
| HNF-3α | +++ | − | + | +++ |

expression than the genes they control. Two important conclusions can be drawn from this observation. The first is that variable assortments of a limited number of regulatory proteins can differentially control a large number of tissue-specific genes. Second, such a combinatorial model would allow transcription to occur from the same promoter in different tissues, provided that a sufficient concentration of the right transcription factors is attained in the cells.

Dissecting the promoters of many genes that are specifically or preferentially transcribed in hepatocytes has shown that their activity is dependent largely on interaction with a common set of transactivators (39). Therefore, a network of *trans*-acting factors of limited tissue distribution appears to determine the liver-specific phenotype of these promoters. As shown in Table 1, simultaneous expression of high levels of LFB-1/HNF-1 and HNF-4/LFA-1 determines appropriate transcription of hAT in hepatic cells as well as in kidney and intestine. The more restricted tissue specificity of the murine gene also reflects the pattern of expression of the relevant transcription factors. For the *M. domesticus* gene, whose transcription is dependent primarily on the distal enhancer sequences, these factors are C/EBP and HNF-3, which are concomitantly present at high levels only in liver. In the case of the *M. caroli* gene transcription, whose principal regulatory region corresponds to the proximal promoter element, expression in both liver and kidney correlates with the levels of LFB-1/HNF-1 in these tissues.

Transcription regulation of liver-specific genes probably represents the endpoint of a cascade of transcriptional events that control cell fate during development. Recently, two features of the hepatic transcriptional network have emerged: cross-regulation between liver factors and autoregulation loops. For instance, efficient transcription of the LFB-1/HNF-1 gene depends on HNF-4/LFA-1 (81), while overexpression of LFB-1/HNF-1 down-regulates its own promoter (G. Piaggio, personal communication). In the case of the HNF-3β promoter, positive autoregulation has also been observed (82).

The progress being made in the characterization of *cis*-elements and *trans*-acting factors controlling α1AT transcription will soon provide full knowledge of the molecular mechanisms underlying α1AT expression in the liver as well as in other tissues. This information has practical relevance in relation to the feasibility of using the α1AT promoter in gene therapy.

## Acknowledgment

We wish to thank Janet Clench for proofreading the manuscript.

## References

1. Laurell CB, Jeppsson JO. In: Putnam FW, ed. The Plasma Proteins. New York: Academic Press, 1975:229–264.

2. Perlmutter DH, Kay RM, Cole FS, Rossing TH, Van-Thiel D, Colten HR. The cellular defect in alpha1-proteinase inhibitor (alpha1-PI) deficiency is expressed in human monocytes and in xenopus oocytes injected with human liver mRNA. Proc Natl Acad Sci USA 1985; 82:6918–6921.
3. Kelsey GD, Povey S, Bygrave AE, Lovell-Badge RH. Species- and tissue-specific expression of human alpha1-antitrypsin in transgenic mice. Genes Devel 1987; 1: 161–171.
4. Perlmutter DH, Daniels JD, Auerbach HS, DeSchryver-Kecskemeti K, Winter HS, Alpers DH. The alpha1-antitrypsin gene is expressed in human intestinal epithelial cell line. J Biol Chem 1989; 264:9485–9490.
5. Olsen GN, Harris JO, Castle JR, Waldman RH, Karmgard HJ. Alpha-1-antitrypsin content in the serum, alveolar macrophages, and alveolar lavage fluid of smoking and nonsmoking normal subjects. J Clin Invest 1975; 55:427–430.
6. Gadek JE, Fells GA, Wright DG, Crystal RG. Human neutrophil elastase functions as a type III collagen "collagenase." Biochem Biophys Res Commun 1980; 95:1815–1822.
7. Kidd VJ, Wallace RB, Itakura K, Woo SL. Alpha 1-antitrypsin deficiency detection by direct analysis of the mutation in the gene. Nature 1983; 304:230–234.
8. Gitlin D, Gitlin JD. In: Putnam FW, ed. The Plasma Proteins Vol. 2. New York: Academic Press 1975:334–339.
9. Dickson ER, Alper CA. Changes in serum proteinase inhibitor levels following bone surgery. Clin Chim Acta 1974; 54:381–385.
10. Ciliberto G, Dente L, Cortese R. Cell-specific expression of a transfected human alpha 1-antitrypsin gene. Cell 1985; 41:531–540.
11. Hafeez W, Ciliberto G, Perlmutter DH. Constitutive and modulated expression of the human alpha 1-antitrypsin gene: different transcriptional initiation sites. J Clin Invest 1992; 89:1214–1222.
12. Perlino E, Cortese C, Ciliberto G. The human alpha 1-antitrypsin gene is transcribed from two different promoters in macrophags and hepatocytes. EMBO J 1987; 6: 2767–2771.
13. Schibler U, Sierra F. Alternative promoters in developmental gene expression. Annu Rev Genet 1987; 21:237–257.
14. Oliviero S, Cortese R. The human haptoglobin gene promoter: interleukin-6 responsive elements interact with a DNA binding protein induced by interleukin-6. EMBO 1989; 8:1145–1151.
15. Poli V, Cortese R. Interleukin 6 induces a liver specific nuclear protein that binds to the promoter of acute phase genes. Proc Natl Acad Sci USA 1989; 86:8202–8206.
16. Majello B, Arcone R, Toniatti C, Ciliberto G. Constitutive and IL-6-induced nuclear factors that interact with the human C-reactive protein promoter. EMBO J 1990; 9: 457–465.
17. Sifers RN, Carlson JA, Clift SM, DeMayo FJ, Bullock DW, Woo SLC. Tissue-specific expression of the human alpha 1-antitrypsin gene in trangenic mice. Nucl Acids Res 1987; 15:1459–1475.
18. Rüther U, Tripodi M, Cortese R, Wagner E. The expression of the human alpha-1-antitrypsin gene in transgenic mice. Nucl Acids Res 1987; 15:7519–7529.

19. De Simone V, Ciliberto G, Hardon E, Paonessa G, Palla F, Lundberg L, Cortese R. Cis- and trans-acting elements responsible for the cell-specific expression of the human alpha 1-antitrypsin gene. EMBO J 1987; 6:2759–2766.
20. Shen RF, Li Y, Sifers RN, Wang H, Jardick C, Tsai SY, Woo SLC. Tissue-specific expression of the human alpha 1-antitrypsin gene is controlled by multiple cis-regulatory elements. Nucl Acids Res 1987; 15:8399–8415.
21. Shen RF, Clift SM, DeMayo FJ, Sifers RN, Finegold MJ, Woo SLC. Tissue-specific regulation of the human alpha 1-antitrypsin gene expression in transgenic mice. DNA 1989; 8:111–118.
22. Monaci P, Nicosia A, Cortese R. Two different liver-specific factors stimulate in vitro transcription from the human alpha 1-antitrypsin promoter. EMBO J 1988; 7:2075–2087.
23. Maniatis T, Goodbourn S, Fischer JA. Regulation of inducible and tissue-specific gene expression. Science 1987; 236:1237–1244.
24. Wasylyk B. Transcription elements and factors of RNA polymerase B promoter of higher eukaryotes. CRC Crit Rev Biochem 1988; 23:77–120.
25. Tripodi M, Abbott C, Vivian N, Cortese R, Lovell-Badge R. Disruption of the LF-A1 and LF-B1 binding sites in the human alpha-1-antitrypsin gene has a differential effect during development in transgenic mice. EMBO J 1991; 10:3177–3182.
26. Descombes C, Schibler U. A liver-enriched trancriptional activator protein, LAP, and a trancriptional inhibitory protein, LIP, are translated from the same mRNA. Cell 1991; 67:569–579.
27. De Simone V, Cortese R. Negative regulatory element in the promoter of the human alpha 1-antitrypsin gene. Nucl Acids Res 1989; 17:9407–9415.
28. Derman E, Krauter K, Walling L, Weinberger C, Ray M, Darnell JE. Transcriptional control in the production of liver specific mRNAs. Cell 1981; 23:731–739.
29. Costa RH, Lai E, Darnell JE. Transcriptional control of the mouse prealbumin (transthyretin) gene: both promoter sequences and district enhancers are cell specific. Mol Cell Biol 1986; 6:4697–4708.
30. Krauter KS, Citron BA, Hsu MT, Powell D, Darnell JE. Isolation and characterization of the alpha 1-antitrypsin gene in mice. DNA 1986; 5:29–36.
31. Grayson DR, Costa RH, Xanthopoulos KG, Darnell JE Jr. A cell-specific enhancer of the mouse alpha 1-antitrypsin gene has multiple functional regions and corresponding protein-binding sites. Mol Cell Bio 1988; 8:1055–1066.
32. Grayson DR, Costa RH, Xanthopoulos KG, Darnell JE Jr. One factor recognizes the liver-specific enhancers in alpha 1-antitrypsin and transthyretin genes. Science 1988; 239:786–788.
33. Costa RH, Grayson DR, Xanthopoulos KG, Darnell JE Jr. A liver-specific DNA-binding protein recognizes multiple nucleotide sites in regulatory regions of transthyretin, alpha 1-antitrypsin, albumin, and simian virus 40 genes. Proc Natl Acad Sci USA 1988; 85:3840–3844.
34. Costa RH, Grayson DR, Darnell JE Jr. Multiple hepatocyte-enriched nuclear factors function in the regulation of transthyretin and alpha 1-antitrypsin genes. Mol Cell Biol 1989; 9:1415–1425.
35. Courtois G, Morgan JG, Campbell LA, Fourel G, Crabtree GR. Interaction of a liver-

specific nuclear factor with the fibrinogen and alpha 1-antitrypsin promoters. Science 1987; 238:688–692.

36. Bohmann D, Bos TJ, Admon A, Nishimura T, Vogt PK, Tjian R. Human proto-oncogene c-jun encodes a DNA binding protein with structural and functional properties of transcription factor AP-1. Science 1987; 238:1386–1392.
37. Latimer JJ, Berger FG, Baumann H. Highly conserved upstream regions of the alpha 1-antitrypsin gene in two mouse species govern liver-specific expression by different mechanism. Mol Cell Biol 1990; 10:760–769.
38. Hardon EM, Frain M, Paonessa G, Cortese R. Two distinct factors interact with the promoter regions of several liver-specific genes. EMBO J 1988; 7:1711–1719.
39. Ciliberto G, Colantuoni V, De Francesco R, De Simone V, Monaci P, Nicosia A, Ramji D, Toniatti C, Cortese R. Transcriptional control of gene expression in hepatic cells. In: Karin M. ed. Research in Gene Expression Series. Boston: Birkhauser, 1993: 162–242.
40. Nicosia A, Monaci P, Tomei L, De Francesco R, Nuzzo M, Stunnenberg H, Cortese R. A myosin-like dimerization helix and an extra-large homeodomain are essential elements of the tripartite DNA binding structure of LFB1. Cell 1990; 61:1225–1236.
41. Toniatti C, Monaci P, Nicosia A, Cortese R, Ciliberto G. A bipartite transactivation domain in transcriptional activator LFB1/HNF-1a functions in cells of non-hepatic origin. DNA Cell Biol 1993; 12:199–208.
42. Raney AK, Easton AJ, Milich DR, McLachlan A. Promoter-specific transactivation of hepatitis B virus transcription by a glutamine-and proline-rich domain of hepatocyte nuclear factor 1. J Virol 1991; 65:5774–5781.
43. De Francesco R, Pastore A, Vecchio G, Cortese R. A circular dichroism study on the conformational stability of the dimerization domain of the transcription factor LFB1. Biochemistry 1991; 30:143–147.
44. Pastore A, De Francesco R, Barbato G, Castiglione Morelli MA, Motta A, Cortese R. $^{1}$H-Resonance assignment and secondary structure determination of the dimerization domain of the transcription factor LFB1. Biochemistry 1991; 30:148–153.
45. Herr W, Sturm RA, Clerc RG, Corcoran LM, Baltimore D, Sharp PA, Ingraham HA, Rosenfeld MG, Finney M, Ruvkun G, Horvitz HR. The POU domain: A large conserved region in the mammalian pit-1, oct-1, oct-2 and *Caenorhabditis elegans* unc-86 gene products. Genes Dev 1988; 2:1513–1516.
46. Tomei L, Cortese R, De Francesco R. A POU-A related region dictates DNA binding specificity of LFB1/HNF1 orienting the two XL-homeodomains in the dimer. EMBO J 1992; 11:4119–4129.
47. Scott MP, Tamkun JW, Hartzell GW III. The structure and function of the homeodomain. Biochim Biophys Acta 1989; 989:25–48.
48. De Simone V, De Magistris L, Lazzaro D, Gerstner J, Monaci P, Nicosia A, Cortese R. LFB3, a heterodimer-forming homeoprotein of the LFB1 family, is expressed in specialized epithelia. EMBO J 1991; 10:1435–1443.
49. Baumhueter S, Mendel DB, Conley PB, Kuo CJ, Turk C, Graves MK, Edwards CA, Courtois G, Crabtree GR. HNF-1 shares three sequence motifs with the POU domain proteins and is identical to LF-B1 and APF. Genes Dev 1990; 4:372–379.

50. Mendel DB, Khavari PA, Conley PB, Graves MK, Hansen LP, Admon A, Crabtree GR. Characterization of a cofactor that regulates dimerization of a mammalian homeodomain protein. Science 1991; 254:1762–1767.
51. Graves B, Johnson PF, McKnight SL. Homologous recognition of a promoter domain common to the MSV LTR and the HSV tk gene. Cell 1986; 44:565–576.
52. Johnson PF, Landschulz WH, Graves BJ, McKnight SL. Identification of a rat liver nuclear protein that binds to the enhancer core element of three animal viruses. Genes Dev 1987; 1:133–146.
53. Landschulz WH, Johnson PF, McKnight SL. The DNA binding domain of the rat liver nuclear protein C/EBP is bipartite. Science 1989; 243:1681–1688.
54. Friedman AD, McKnight SL. Identification of two polypeptide segments of CCAAT/enhancer-binding protein required for transcriptional activation of the serum albumin gene. Genes Dev 1990; 4:1416–1426.
55. Pei D, Shih C. Transcriptional activation and repression by cellular DNA-binding protein C/EBP. J Virol 1990; 64:1517–1522.
56. O'Shea EK, Rutkowski R, Stafford WF III, Kim PS. Preferential heterodimer formation by isolated leucine zippers from fos and jun. Science 1989; 245:646–648.
57. Vinson CR, Sigler PB, McKnight SL. Scissors-grip model for DNA recognition by a family of leucine zipper proteins. Science 1989; 246:911–916.
58. Poli V, Mancini FP, Cortese R. IL-6DBP, a nuclear protein involved in interleukin-6 signal transduction, defines a new family of leucine zipper proteins related to C/EBP. Cell 1990; 63:643–653.
59. Akira S, Isshiki H, Sugita T, Tanabe O, Kinoshita S, Nishio Y, Nakajima T, Hirano T, Kishimoto T. A nuclear factor for IL-6 expression (NF-IL6) is a member of a C/EBP family. EMBO J 1990; 9:1897–1906.
60. Mueller CR, Maire P, Schibler U. DBP, a liver-enriched transcriptional activator, is expressed late in ontogeny and its tissue specificity is determined posttranscriptionally. Cell 1990; 61:279–291.
61. Cao Z., Umek RM, McKnight SL. Regulated expression of three C/EBP isoforms during adipose conversion of 3T3-L1 cells. Genes Devel 1991; 5:1538–1552.
62. Kinoshita S, Akira S, Kishimoto T. A member of the C/EBP family, NF-IL6b, forms a heterodimer and transcriptionally synergized with NF-IL6. Proc Natl Acad Sci USA 1992; 89:1473–1476.
63. Birkenmeyer EH, Gwynn B, Howard S, Jerry J, Gordon JI, Landschultz WH, McKnight SL. Tissue-specific expression, developmental regulation, and genetic mapping of the gene encoding CCAAT/enhancer binding protein. Genes Dev 1989; 3: 1146–1156.
64. Friedman AD, Landschultz WH, McKnight SL. CCAAT/enhancer binding protein activates the promoter of the serum albumin gene in cultured hepatoma cells. Genes Dev 1989; 3:1314–1322.
65. Christy RJ, Yang VW, Ntambi JM, Geiman DE, Landschulz WH, Friedman AD, Nakabeppu Y, Kelly TJ, Lane MD. Differentiation-induced gene expression in 3T3-L1 preadipocytes: CCAAT/enhancer binding protein interacts with and activates the promoters of two adipocyte-specific genes. Genes Dev 1989; 3:1323–1335.

66. Kuo, CF, Xanthopoulos, K, Darnell, JE. Fetal and adult localization of C/EBP: evidence for combinatorial action of transcription factors in cell-specific gene expression. Development 1990; 109:374–481.
67. Lai E, Prezioso VR, Smith E, Litvin O, Costa RH, DArnell JE. HNF-3A, a hepatocyte-enriched transcription factor of novel structure, is regulated transcriptionally. Genes Dev 1990; 4:1427–1436.
68. Lai E, Prezioso VR, Tau W, Chen W, Darnell JE. Hepatocyte nuclear factor 3a belongs to a gene family in mammals that is homologous to the Drosophila homeotic gene forkhead. Genes Dev 1991; 5:416–427.
69. Weigel D, Jackle H. Forkhead: a new eukaryotic DNA binding motif? Cell 1990; 63: 455–456.
70. Costa, RH, Grayson, DR, Darnell, JE Jr. Multiple hepatocyte-enriched nuclear factors function in the regulation of transthyretin and alpha 1-antitrypsin genes. Mol. Cell. Biol 1989; 9:1415–1425.
71. Costa RH, Van Dyke TA, Yan C, Kuo F, Darnell JE Jr. Similarities in transthyretin gene expression and differences in transcription factors: liver and yolk sac compared to choroid plexus. Proc Natl Acad Sci USA 1990; 87:6589–6593.
72. Sladek FM, Zhong WM, Lai E, Darnell JE. Liver-enriched transcription factor HNF-4 is a novel member of the steroid hormone receptor superfamily. Genes Dev 1990; 4: 2353–2365.
73. Forman BM, Samuels HH. Interactions among a subfamily of nuclear hormon receptors: the regulatory zipper model. Mol Endocrinol 1990; 4:1293–1301.
74. Harrison SC. A structural taxonomy of DNA-binding domains. Nature 1991; 353:715.
75. Ramji DP, Tadros MH, Hardon EM, Cortese R. The transcription factor LF-A1 interacts with a bipartite recognition sequence in the promoter regions of several liver-specific genes. Nucl Acids Res 1991; 19:1139–1146.
76. Xanthopoulos KG, Prezioso VR, Chen WS, Sladek FM, Cortese R, Darnell JE. The different tissue transcription patterns of genes for HNF-1, C/EBP, HNF-3, and HNF-4, protein factors that goven liver-specific transcription. Proc Natl Acad Sci USA 1991; 88:3807–3811.
77. Weintraub H, Tapscott SJ, Davis RL, Thayer MJ, Adam MA, Lassar AB, Miller AD. Activation of muscle-specific genes in pigment, nerve, fat, liver and fibroblast cell lines by forced expression of MyoD. Proc Natl Acad Sci USA 1989; 86:5434–5438.
78. Cockerill PN, Klinken SP. Octamer-binding proteins in diverse hemopoietic cells. Mol Cell Biol 1990; 10:1293–1296.
79. Sharp ZD, Cao Z. Regulation of cell-type-specific transcription and differentiation of the pituitary. Bioessays 1990; 12:80–85.
80. Romeo PH, Prandini MH, Joulin V, Mignotte V, Prenant M, Veinchenker W, Marguerie G, Uzan G. Megakaryocytic and erythrocytic lineages share specific transcription factors. Nature 1990; 344:447–449.
81. Kuo CJ, Conley PB, Chen L, Sladek FM, Darnell JE, Crabtree GR. A transcriptional hierarchy involved in mammalian cell-type specification. Nature 1992; 355:457–460.
82. Pani L, Xiaobing Q, Clevidence D, Costa RH. The restricted promoter activity of the liver transcription factor HNF3b involves a cell specific factor and positive autoactivation. Mol Cell Biol 1992; 12:552–562.

# 11

# Alpha 1–Antitrypsin Gene Expression in Mononuclear Phagocytes

**GREGG JOSLIN and DAVID H. PERLMUTTER**

Washington University School of Medicine
St. Louis, Missouri

## I. Introduction

Alpha 1–antitrypsin ($\alpha$1AT) is the major physiological inhibitor of neutrophil elastase, an enzyme capable of degrading many constituents of the extracellular matrix. The net concentration of $\alpha$1AT in plasma and tissues is, therefore, thought to be an important determinant of tissue remodeling during homeostasis, tissue injury, and inflammation. Although plasma $\alpha$1AT is derived predominantly from the liver, as shown by changes in allotype after orthotopic liver transplantation, there are also extrahepatic sites of its synthesis (1,2). We have demonstrated expression of the $\alpha$1AT gene in human monocytes, bronchoalveolar and breast-milk macrophages, and enterocytes (3–5). Because monocytes can be relatively easily obtained from human donors, the study of $\alpha$1AT synthesis in these cells has provided further understanding of several aspects of the biology and pathobiology of this protein.

First, monocytes have been used as a model primary cell culture system in which the cellular basis for inherited $\alpha$1AT deficiencies could be determined. This has been especially important for homozygous PiZZ $\alpha$1AT deficiency, the most common genetic cause of pulmonary emphysema in adults and chronic liver injury in infants. Studies of monocytes from PiZZ individuals showed that the abnormal α1AT molecule was selectively retained within the intracellular portion of the secretory pathway and that this abnormality could, at least in large part, explain the 85–90% reduction in plasma concentrations of α1AT in these individuals (4,6). Second, monocytes have been used as a model cell culture system in which putative regulating factors could be identified. This has also provided information about several aspects of α1AT deficiency. For example, factors that mediate increases in synthesis of α1AT have the potential of mediating increases in intracellular accumulation of the abnormally folded α1AT molecule and, therein, to have the potential for hepatotoxic consequences. Finally, studies of α1AT synthesis and its regulation in macrophages—cells that constitute the first line of host defense at epithelia—have been used to provide further understanding of the role of α1AT in the host response to tissue injury and inflammation.

In this chapter we review current literature on the expression and regulation of the α1AT gene in mononuclear phagocytes in normal and deficient individuals. A novel mechanism for regulation of α1AT gene expression involving the recognition of α1AT–elastase complexes by a specific cell-surface receptor is discussed in detail.

## II. Synthesis

Human monocytes synthesize α1AT as 48 and 52 kDa underglycosylated precursor polypeptides and convert these precursors into the mature 55 kDa polypeptide for secretion with a half-time of 40–50 minutes (3). The kinetics of synthesis and secretion of α1AT by monocytes are similar to those of human hepatoma HepG2 cells. The α1AT secreted by monocytes is functionally active, as evidenced by the presence of complexes with neutrophil elastase in the extracellular medium. This is thought to result from the concomitant spontaneous release of the small amount of preformed neutrophil elastase found in freshly isolated monocytes.

Biosynthesis of α1AT by monocytes is greatest during the first 24 hours in culture and progressively declines over the next 10 days (3). This reduction in α1AT biosynthesis in vitro involves a pretranslational mechanism, as α1AT mRNA levels also decline over 10 days in culture. The decrease in expression of α1AT cannot be explained by a change in viability or total metabolic activity because total RNA content, steady-state levels of specific mRNAs, total protein synthesis, and synthesis of other specific secretory proteins increase during the same interval. Furthermore, it cannot be explained by the differentiation of monocytes into macrophage-like cells, because there is also a decrease in α1AT gene expression in bronchoalveolar and breast-milk macrophages during the same time interval in culture.

These observations suggested that expression of α1AT in monocytes and macrophages is down-regulated by a factor elaborated in tissue culture or by removal from an in vivo up-regulating factor. We examined the latter possibility first and found that addition of exogenous elastase to primary cultures of blood monocytes prevented the decrease in α1AT synthesis during the first week in culture (7). The results then suggested that expression of α1AT decreases in cell culture because the cells have been removed from elastase present in vivo or because there is exhaustion of the small stores of preformed neutrophil elastase present in freshly isolated monocytes and spontaneously released into the extracellular medium. In fact, in the presence of crude lymphokine supernatants or endotoxin, synthesis of α1AT can be "reinduced" in monocytes after 10 days in culture, a time point by which there is ordinarily negligible synthesis of α1AT and no further release of neutrophil elastase, and the α1AT is secreted as a completely active native molecule (8). Thus, in cultured monocytes and macrophages, there is a concomitant progressive decline in the spontaneous release of preformed neutrophil elastase stores, in the concentration of α1AT–elastase complexes in the extracellular medium and in α1AT gene expression. In studies discussed below, we have identified a mechanism for this decline in α1AT gene expression.

There are at least four transcriptional initiation sites in the 5′ flanking region of the human α1AT gene (9–11) (Fig. 1). Three of these (−2110, −2073, and −1892) are called *macrophage-specific* because these initiation sites are used only for constitutive α1AT gene expression in cells of mononuclear phagocyte origin. The downstream transcriptional initiation site (+1) is termed *hepatocyte-specific* because it is used by hepatocytes for constitutive α1AT gene expression. This downstream transcriptional initiation site is also used for constitutive α1AT gene expression by cells of enterocytic origin, whether crypt-like or having undergone differentiation to villous-like enterocytes (11). It is not yet known whether an alternative upstream translational initiation site at −354 is used in mononuclear phagocytes. This translational initiation site is followed by a short open-reading frame and a termination codon. Furthermore, this translational codon is encoded within a context that is favorable for initiation of translation according to the Kozak consensus sequence principles (12,13). Other factors, however, such as a surrounding upstream flanking region that is heavily encumbered by secondary structure, probably prevent efficient initiation at this site.

## III. Regulation

α1AT synthesis in mononuclear phagocytes is regulated by several inflammatory mediators (Fig. 2). Introduction of bacterial lipopolysaccharide (LPS) into monocyte cultures results in a five- to 10-fold increase in α1AT synthesis (14,15). This effect is due predominantly to an increase in translational efficiency of the α1AT mRNA. In normal monocytes, the increase in synthesis results in an increase in secretion; however, in monocytes derived from PiZZ patients, LPS induces an

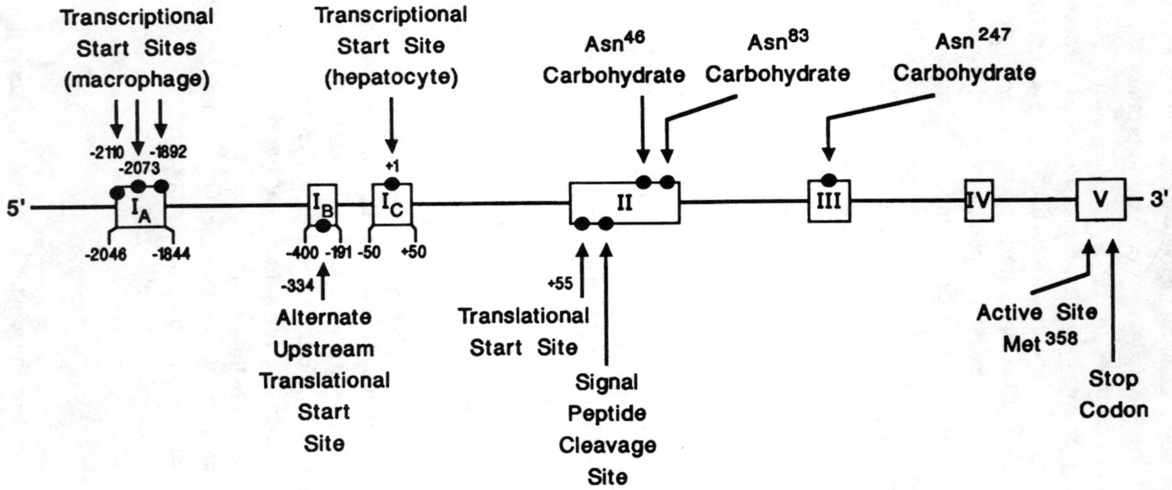


**Figure 1** Map of the human alpha 1–antitrypsin gene—transcriptional and translational initiation sites. (Reproduced with permission from Perlmutter DH, Alpha-1-antitrypsin: structure, function, physiology. In: Makiewicz A, Kushner I, Baumann H, eds. *Molecular Biology, Biochemistry, Clinical Applications*. Miami: CRC Press, 1993:152.)

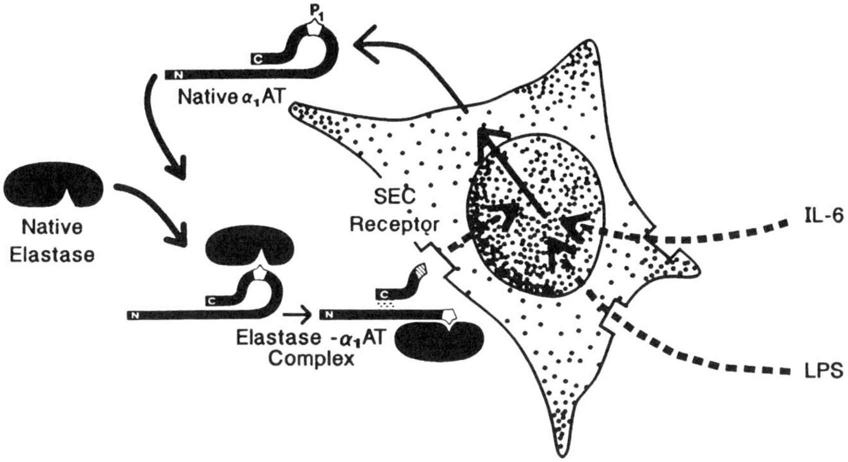


**Figure 2** Physiological factors that regulate α1AT synthesis. (Adapted with permission from Perlmutter DH, Alpha-1-antitrypsin: structure, function, physiology. In: Makiewicz A, Kushner I, Baumann H, eds. *Molecular Biology, Biochemistry, Clinical Applications*. Miami: CRC Press, 1993:156.)

increase in intracellular accumulation concurrent with an increase in α1AT synthesis. LPS does not affect the synthesis of α1AT in human hepatoma HepG2 cells or in human intestinal adenocarcinoma Caco2 or T84 cells. In a recent study employing ribonuclease protection assays and primer extension analysis, the increase in translational efficiency of α1AT mRNA mediated by endotoxin could not be attributed to a change in transcriptional initiation to the downstream "hepatocyte-specific" promoter (11). Endotoxin mediated increases in three α1AT mRNA species, all initiated at the upstream "macrophage-specific" transcriptional initiation sites. By exclusion of this latter mechanism, the translational effect of endotoxin on α1AT gene expression must, therefore, involve a change in specific RNA–protein interactions or a change in specific RNA folding.

Expression of α1AT in mononuclear phagocytes is also regulated by the acute-phase monokine IL-6 (16). When recombinant IL-6 is added to monocyte cultures, there is an increase in α1AT-specific mRNA and in synthesis of α1AT. This autocrine or paracrine pathway is distinct from that of LPS since the effect of IL-6 is blocked by antibody to IL-6 but not by antibody to the lipid A moiety of LPS or by polymyxin B, and the effects of LPS are blocked by antibody to lipid A and polymyxin B but not by antibody to IL-6. Moreover, the effect of IL-6 is almost exclusively at a pretranslational level. IL-6 also mediates an increase in synthesis of α1AT in human hepatoma HepG2 cells (16) and in human intestinal adenocarcinoma Caco2 cells when they have differentiated into villous-like enterocytes (17,18). Thus, IL-6 regulates α1AT synthesis in several cell types. Ribonuclease protection assays have shown that IL-6 not only mediates a modest increase in α1AT mRNA transcripts initiated at the downstream "hepatocyte-specific" transcriptional initiation site in HepG2 and Caco2 cells but also induces α1AT mRNA transcripts initiated at the three upstream "macrophage-specific" transcriptional initiation sites in these cell lines (11). In blood monocytes and tissue macrophages, IL-6 mediates an increase only in transcripts initiated at the upstream transcriptional initiation sites.

It is not yet known whether these effects are mediated by two sequences—similar to the proximal portion of the IL-6 response element and approximately 200 nucleotides upstream from the "hepatocyte" transcriptional initiation site—and/or by one sequence—even more homologous with the IL-6 response element and approximately 200 nucleotides upstream from the most remote "macrophage" transcriptional initiation site. It is also not yet known if these effects involve the IL-6-inducible *trans*-acting DNA-binding protein called IL-6DBP, or LAP (19,20). This *trans*-acting protein is characterized by leucine zipper domains, similar to that of C/EBP, a transcription factor implicated in terminal differentiation. A recent study (21) has shown that use of a downstream translational initiation site within the IL-6DBP/LAP mRNA leads to a shorter protein, which binds to the IL-6 response element with high affinity but cannot activate transcription. It is, in effect, a transcriptional repressor. Relative ratios of the two translational products and their relative affinities for *cis*-acting structural elements upstream of IL-6-responsive genes may therefore determine the magnitude of the effect of IL-6 on those particular genes. Finally, it is not yet known whether the alternative upstream translational initiation site within the IL-6-inducible, longer α1AT mRNA is actually used. There is no evidence that α1AT gene expression is significantly modulated by other acute-phase mediators, including IL-1β, TNF-α, and IFNγ (16,22–24).

Synthesis of α1AT in mononuclear phagocytes is also modulated in the presence of elastase (7). When nanomolar concentrations of elastase are added to monocytes in culture, there is a dose- and time-dependent increase in α1AT mRNA levels and α1AT synthesis. This effect is abrogated by the addition of antisera to elastase or by pretreatment of elastase with the organic protease inhibitor DFP. However, addition of preformed α1AT–elastase complexes results in an increase in α1AT mRNA and α1AT synthesis. These data suggested the existence of a signal-transduction mechanism that was dependent on α1AT, either endogenous or exogenous in origin. We believed that it was important to determine the biochemical basis of this particular signal-transduction mechanism for several reasons: experiments with blood monocytes and bronchoalveolar and breast-milk macrophages provided circumstantial evidence that constitutive expression of α1AT in mononuclear phagocytes was almost completely dependent on the presence of elastase–α1AT complexes in the extracellular fluid; the effect of this signal-transduction mechanism on monocytes from PiZZ individuals was greater intracellular accumulation of the mutant α1AT molecule, a potentially hepatotoxic effect; from a teleological point of view, this mechanism had the characteristics of a system that would be well adapted for control of proteolytic activity of a migrating cell, integrating protease inhibitor production with protease activity and, in turn, protease inhibitor activity.

With these observations in mind, we proposed that this particular regulatory mechanism involved the recognition of α1AT in its complex form by a specific cell-surface receptor, or receptors (25). Several other observations have suggested the presence of a receptor that recognizes α1AT–elastase complexes. First, several lines of evidence suggest that a receptor is responsible for in vivo clearance/catabolism of α1AT–elastase as well as other serpin–enzyme complexes. In experimental animals, clearance of α1AT–protease complexes is more rapid than clearance of native α1AT (26,27). Labeled α1AT–elastase complexes are rapidly distributed to the tissues, predominantly the liver. Clearance of α1AT–elastase complexes is also inhibited by antithrombin III–thrombin, heparin cofactor II–thrombin, and alpha 1–antichymotrypsin–cathepsin G complexes but not by alpha 2–macroglobulin–protease complexes. Second, α1AT–elastase complexes and proteolytically modified α1AT mediate directed migration of neutrophils (28,29).

To test the hypothesis, we used synthetic peptides based on the sequence of the carboxyl-terminal fragment of α1AT as candidate mediators for regulation of α1AT synthesis and as candidate ligands for cell-surface binding. This region was selected because it had been previously implicated in the chemotactic properties of α1AT–elastase (28,29) complexes and because crystal-structure analysis predicted that a domain within this region was exteriorly exposed after formation of a complex (30,31). The results indicated that a synthetic peptide (peptide 105Y) based on amino acids 359–374 of α1AT mediated a selective increase in α1AT synthesis in human monocytes and in HepG2 cells (25). Radioiodinated peptide 105Y bound specifically and saturably to HepG2 cells, defining a single class of receptors with a $K_d$ of ~40 nM at a density of ~$4.5 \times 10^5$ plasma membrane receptor molecules per cell. Binding of $^{125}$I–peptide 105Y was blocked by unlabeled elastase–α1AT complexes and unlabeled peptide 105Y blocked binding of $^{125}$I–α1AT–elastase complexes, $^{125}$I–elastase–α1AT complexes and $^{125}$I–trypsin–α1AT complexes. Antisera to keyhole-limpet hemocyanin-coupled peptide 105Y blocked binding of $^{125}$I–α1AT–elastase complexes and blocked the increase in synthesis of α1AT mediated by α1AT–elastase complexes (D. H. Perlmutter, unpublished). These results provide confirmatory evidence that at least part of the region corresponding to peptide 105Y represented the receptor-binding domain of α1AT–elastase complexes and was capable of transducing a signal to increase synthesis of α1AT.

Next, we examined the significance of the high degree of primary sequence homology within this receptor-binding domain of α1AT and in the corresponding regions of other serpins AT III, alpha 1–antichymotrypsin (α1ACT), and C1 inhibitor (Fig. 3). In competitive binding assays, we found that binding of $^{125}$I peptide 105Y was displaced by AT III–thrombin, α1ACT–cathepsin G, and, to a lesser extent, C1 inhibitor–C1s complexes, but not by the corresponding proteins in their native forms. Moreover, we have recently found that binding of $^{125}$I–elastase–α1AT complexes is displaced by these other serpin–enzyme complexes (32). These data indicated that the receptor that recognizes peptide 105Y and α1AT–elastase complexes also recognizes these other serpin–enzyme complexes, so we have called it the serpin–enzyme complex, or SEC, receptor. These data also showed that the SEC receptor recognizes the serpin only after it has undergone the

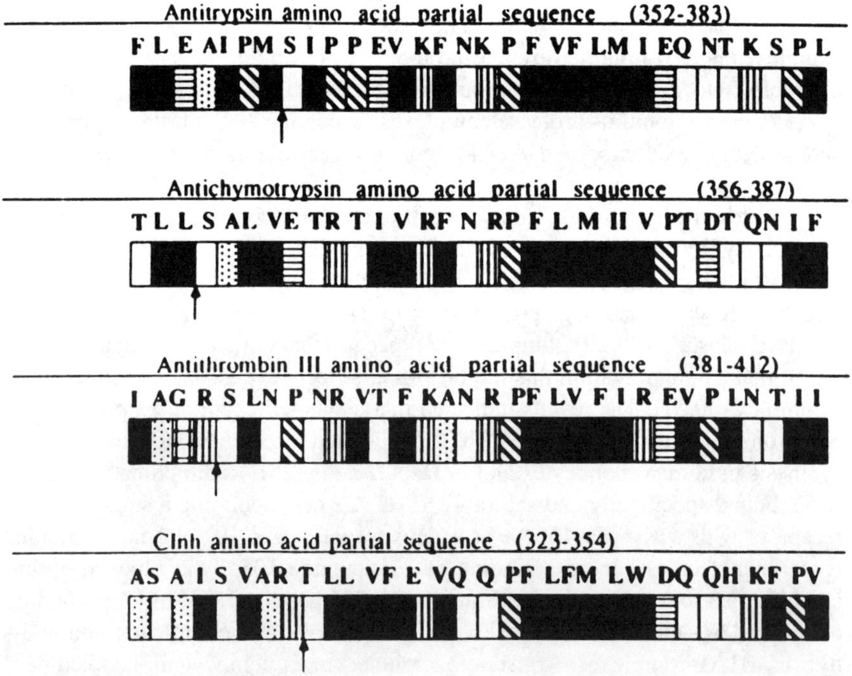


**Figure 3** Functional homology within the carboxyl-terminal fragments of serpins (kindly provided by C. Schasteen, St. Louis, MO). Amino acids with similar functional units are indicated by open bars, solid bars, diagonal hatched bars, vertical hatched bars, horizontal hatched bars or bars with dotted lines. (Reproduced with permission from Perlmutter DH, Alpha-1-antitrypsin: structure, function, physiology. In: Makiewicz A, Kushner I, Baumann H, eds. *Molecular Biology, Biochemistry, Clinical Applications*. Miami: CRC Press, 1993:159.)

structural rearrangement that accompanies formation of a complex with its cognate enzyme. Other experimental results showed that the SEC receptor also recognizes α1AT after it has undergone proteolytic modification at its reactive site by the action of the metalloelastase of *Pseudomonas aeruginosa* (33). Even more recently, we have observed binding to the SEC receptor of α1AT that has undergone proteolytic modification of its reactive site by the collaborative action of oxidizing agents and neutrophil elastase (32). In each case, the SEC receptor recognizes a domain within the carboxyl-terminal fragment of α1AT, which has stayed associated with the rest of the α1AT molecule by tenacious hydrophobic interactions at the extreme carboxyl-terminus and therein carries to the cell-surface receptor-binding site the larger amino-terminal portion of α1AT. The SEC receptor has subsequently been found on a number of cell types, including hepatoma cells, mononuclear phagocytes, neutrophils, human intestinal epithelial cell line Caco2, mouse fibroblast L cells, Cos cells, and PC12 cells, but is not present on Chinese hamster ovary cells or HeLa cells (G. Joslin, R. Fallon, and D. H. Perlmutter, unpublished).

We have also examined the possibility that the SEC receptor is involved in clearance/catabolism of serpin–enzyme complexes in vivo by determining whether it mediated internalization and/or degradation of serpin–enzyme complexes in tissue culture. As mentioned above, α1AT–protease complexes are subjected to rapid in vivo clearance and are catabolized predominantly in the liver. The pathway for clearance/catabolism is shared by other serpin–enzyme complexes, including AT III–thrombin and α1ACT–cathepsin G. Our studies showed that α1AT–elastase and α1AT–trypsin complexes were internalized in hepatoma HepG2 cells by SEC receptor–mediated endocytosis and delivered to an acidic compartment—either late endosome or lysosome—for degradation (34). Thus, these results provide evidence that the characteristics of the SEC receptor in cell culture are similar to those that would be expected for the receptor responsible for in vivo clearance/catabolism of, at least several, serpin–enzyme complexes.

Photoaffinity cross-linking studies have shown that the ligand-binding domain of the SEC receptor is an ~78 kDa single-chain polypeptide (G. Joslin, R. Fallon, and D. H. Perlmutter, unpublished). For these studies the photoreactive reagent NHS-ASA was radioiodinated and then coupled to peptide 105Y. HepG2 cells were incubated for 2 hours at 4°C in the dark with $^{125}$I–ASA–peptide 105Y, in the absence or presence of unlabeled peptide 105Y, and then exposed to UV light. The results demonstrate concentration-dependent labeling of a single ~78 kDa polypeptide. The labeling is completely blocked by unlabeled peptide 105Y.

In more recent studies, we have used synthetic peptides to determine the minimal structural requirements for binding of α1AT–elastase complexes by the SEC receptor. These studies have shown that a pentapeptide domain with the carboxyl-terminal fragment of α1AT (amino acids 370–374, FVFLM) is sufficient for binding to the SEC receptor (35). A synthetic analog of this pentapeptide

(peptide 105C, FVYLI) blocked binding and internalization of [125]I–trypsin–α1AT complexes by HepG2 cells. [125]I-peptide 105C bound specifically and saturably to HepG2 cells, and its binding was blocked by unlabeled trypsin–α1AT or elastase–α1AT complexes. Alterations of the sequence of the pentapeptide introduced into synthetic peptide (mutations, deletions, or scrambling) demonstrated that recognition by the SEC receptor was sequence-specific. The study of synthetic peptides in which each of the five amino acids is individually replaced by alanine indicates that the two amino acids at the carboxyl-terminus of the pentapeptide are most critical for interacting with the SEC receptor. Photoaffinity cross-linking studies have shown that the pentapeptide (peptide 105C) blocks photoaffinity cross-linking of the SEC receptor by [125]I–ASA–peptide 105Y. Tetrapeptides in which the carboxyl- or amino-terminal amino acids of peptide 105C are deleted do not block cross-linking of the SEC receptor (G. Joslin, R. Fallon, and D. H. Perlmutter, unpublished). Synthetic peptapeptides were also capable of mediating an increase in synthesis of α1AT. As might have been predicted from competitive binding of other serpin–enzyme complexes to the SEC receptor, the SEC receptor–binding pentapeptide neodomain of α1AT is highly conserved in the corresponding regions of these other serpins.

The SEC receptor-binding pentapeptide of α1AT was also found to be remarkably similar to sequences in substance P, several other tachykinins, and bombesin (Fig. 4). These peptides have a number of different biological activities. In many cases, these biological activities are mediated by specific cell-surface

| | | | |
|---|---|---|---|
| | 360 | | 380 |
| $\alpha_1$-AT seq | S I P P E V K F N K P | F V F L M | I E Q N T K |
| 105Y | S I P P E V K F N K P | F V Y L I | |
| 105C | | F V Y L I | |
| 105B | V K F N K P | | |
| 105C-S | | I L V F Y | |
| 105C-C | | F V Y L | |
| 105C-N | | V Y L M | |
| SP | R P K P Q Q | F F G L M | NH2 |
| Bb | E Q R L G N Q W A | V G H L M | NH2 |
| | 17 | | 42 |
| β-AM | L V F F A E D V G S N K G A | I I G L M | V G G V V I A |

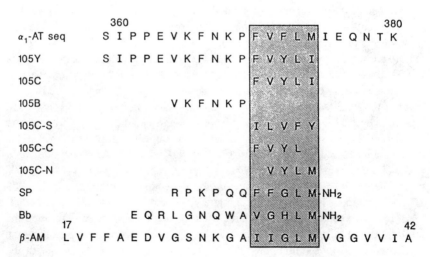

**Figure 4** Map of synthetic peptides used to define the SEC receptor, aligned with tachykinin and amyloid-β peptides.

receptors, including tachykinin receptors NK-1 (substance P receptor), NK-2 (substance K receptor), NK-3 (neurokinin B receptor), and several bombesin receptors (36,37). Because these cell-surface receptors have only recently been described and because there are only a few highly selective, high-affinity receptor antagonists, it has not yet been possible to attribute all the biological activities of these peptides to the known receptors. With these considerations in mind, we examined the possibility that the tachykinins and bombesin bind to the SEC receptor (38). The results indicated that substance P, several other tachykinins, and bombesin compete for binding to, and cross-linking of, the SEC receptor. These other ligands also mediated an increase in synthesis of α1AT in monocytes and HepG2 cells. These results were not surprising in that the two residues within the receptor-binding pentapeptide of α1AT that were most affected by mutations—the carboxyl-terminal leucine and methionine (35) residues—are the ones mostly highly conserved in comparison to the tachykinins and bombesin.

The SEC receptor was found to be distinct from the substance P receptor by several criteria (38). There was no substance P receptor mRNA in HepG2 cells or human liver as assessed by ribonuclease protection assays with human substance P receptor cRNA as probe. The SEC receptor recognized synthetic peptide ligands with carboxyl-terminal carboxy-acid or carboxy-amide moieties with equivalent affinity, whereas the substance P receptor recognized substance P carboxy-amide with affinity several orders of magnitude higher than that for substance P carboxy-acid. The SEC receptor bound its ligands at lower affinity than the substance P receptor. The SEC receptor was much less restricted in the specificity with which it recognized ligands—i.e., ligands for the SEC receptor including peptide 105Y (based on α1AT sequence 359–374), α1AT–protease complexes, and bombesin did not compete for binding of substance P to a stable transfected cell line expressing the substance P receptor. Several of these criteria also make it highly likely that the SEC receptor is distinct from the substance K, neurokinin B, and bombesin receptors. Partial structural characterization of the SEC receptor also suggests that the SEC receptor is distinct from the tachykinin receptors and the bombesin receptors. As mentioned above, the ligand-binding subunit of the SEC receptor in HepG2 cells is a single-chain polypeptide of 78 kDa (38). The SEC receptor has also been purified to homogeneity as an ~78–80 kDa polypeptide from HepG2 cell membranes by ligand-affinity chromatography with α1AT–elastase complexes. Amino-terminal amino acid sequence analysis clearly demonstrates that it is distinct from the tachykinin and bombesin receptors (R. J. Fallon, G. Joslin, and D. H. Perlmutter, unpublished).

A pentapeptide sequence within the amyloid-β peptide is also similar to the SEC receptor–binding pentapeptide of α1AT (Fig. 4). In fact, amyloid-β peptide binds specifically and saturably to the SEC receptor and blocks the binding of $^{125}$I–peptide 105Y and $^{125}$I–elastase–α1AT complexes to the SEC receptor of HepG2 cells (38 and Fig. 5). Recent data have suggested that the amyloid-β

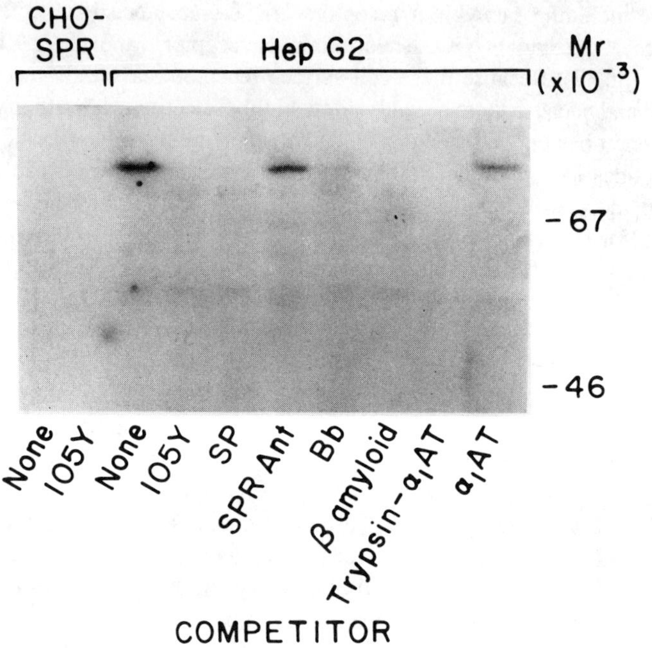


**Figure 5** Competition for cross-linking of the SEC receptor of HepG2 cells. Peptide 105Y was coupled to N-hydroxysuccinimidyl-3-iodo-4-azidosalicylic acid and labeled with $^{125}$I. HepG2 cells or CHO-SPR cells were incubated in the dark for 2 hours at 4°C with the resulting $^{125}$I–ASA–peptide 105Y in subsaturating concentrations (50 nM) in the absence or presence of competitor at 100-fold molar excess. Cells were then photolyzed at 366 nm, homogenized in Laemmli sample buffer, and subjected to SDS-PAGE next to molecular-mass markers as shown at the right margin. CHO-SPR cells are Chinese hamster ovary cells transfected with the substance P receptor cDNA and expressing 531,000 sites/cell with a $K_d$ of ~0.73 nM using $^{125}$I–Y-SP as ligand. (Reproduced with permission from Ref. 38.)

peptide—the major constituent of the cerebral extracellular deposits that characterize the presenile dementia of Alzheimer's disease and Down's syndrome—is neurotrophic/neurotoxic (39). Moreover, its neurotrophic/neurotoxic effects have been attributed to the same domain that would be recognized by the SEC receptor and these effects have been blocked by substance P. This peptide is probably generated by aberrant proteolytic cleavage of a transmembrane precursor protein, the amyloid precursor protein (APP) (reviewed in Refs. 40 and 41). In normal individuals, APP undergoes a complex series of proteolytic processing reactions that may result in cleavage within the amyloid-β peptide as well as an alternative proteolytic pathway in which an intact soluble amyloid-β peptide is generated. Two observations have, to a certain extent, clarified the relationship between the amyloid-β peptide, Alzheimer's disease, and Down's syndrome. First, the locus responsible for familial Alzheimer's disease maps to the gene for the APP on chromosome 21 (42). Second, single amino acid substitutions can be found in the amyloid-β peptide region in these individuals. It has therein been suggested that familial Alzheimer's disease is associated with aberrant proteolytic processing of APP as a result of mutations in the amyloid-β peptide and that Down's syndrome is associated with gene duplication, resulting in excess production of APP, saturation of normal processing pathways, and utilization of the alternative processing pathway (43–45). Thus, the SEC receptor may play an important role in presenile dementia if it is involved in intracellular processing of amyloid-β peptide/APP or in neurotrophic/neurotoxic effects of amyloid-β peptide.

A sequence similar to α1AT 368–374, the receptor-binding region, has also been found in the carboxyl-terminal propeptide of mouse β-glucuronidase (46) and a collagen-binding protein gp46 (47). β-glucuronidase is ordinarily a lysosomal enzyme, but a significant proportion of newly synthesized β-glucuronidase is retained within the endoplasmic reticulum of murine hepatocytes in a serpin-like complex with the esterase-active site of the protein egasyn. Similarly, gp46, a collagen-binding protein found in human fibroblasts, is also retained in the endoplasmic reticulum (47). It is homologous with several different proteins: a rat skeletal myoblast protein, expression of which is modulated by heat shock; the J6 protein from mouse F9 embryonal carcinoma cells, expression of which is modulated by retinoic acid; hsp 47 from chick-embryo fibroblasts. The β-glucuronidase–egasyn complex and collagen–gp46 complex are presumably retained in the endoplasmic reticulum by KDEL-like sequence in egasyn and gp46, respectively, but it will be interesting to determine whether these interact with the SEC receptor and whether these potential interactions shed some light on the mechanism by which the mutant Z α1AT protein is retained in the endoplasmic reticulum in individuals with homozygous PiZZ α1AT deficiency.

We have recently examined the possibility that the SEC receptor mediates the neutrophil chemotactic effects of α1AT–elastase complexes (48). Previous studies have shown that α1AT–elastase complexes and proteolytically modified α1AT are chemotactic for neutrophils and that the carboxyl-terminal fragment of α1AT possessed all of this biological activity (28,29). First, receptor-binding studies with $^{125}$I–peptide 105Y showed that there was a single class of receptors on human neutrophils with $K_d$ (~43 nM) almost identical to that previously reported for HepG2 cells. There were ~13,000–500,000 plasma membrane SEC-receptor molecules on each human neutrophil as compared to ~450,000 plasma membrane receptors on each human hepatoma HepG2 cell. Second, chemotactic studies showed that peptide 105Y and pentapeptide 105C mediated neutrophil chemotaxis with maximal stimulation at $10^{-9}$ to $10^{-8}$ M. The magnitude of the effect was comparable to that of the chemotactic peptide fMLP of $10^{-8}$ M. The specificity of the effect was consistent with its being mediated by SEC receptor as shown by negative control peptides. Most importantly, the neutrophil chemotactic effect of α1AT–elastase complexes was completely blocked by antiserum to keyhole-limpet hemocyanin-coupled peptide 105Y and by anti-SEC receptor antiserum but not by a control antiserum. Other ligands for the SEC receptor, including the amyloid-β peptide, mediated neutrophil chemotaxis. Finally, preincubation of neutrophils with peptide 105Y completely abrogated the chemotactic effect of amyloid-β peptide by inducing homologous desensitization of the SEC receptor. Preincubation with substance P also desensitized the SEC receptor to the neutrophil chemotactic effects of amyloid-β peptide. Thus, the SEC receptor mediated the previously recognized chemotactic effect of α1AT–elastase complexes and the previously unrecognized chemotactic effect of amyloid-β peptide. It is also likely to mediate the recently described chemotactic effect of α1ACT–cathepsin G complexes (27). One might also predict that it mediates any chemotactic effect of HCII–thrombin complexes, although a structurally distinct region in the amino-terminal domain of HCII has been shown to possess neutrophil chemotactic activity (49). Further studies will be necessary to determine whether two regions of HCII can mediate neutrophil chemotactic effects through two distinct receptors. Although it has not been completely excluded, there is no current evidence to suggest that other regions with the α1AT molecule, or within other serpin molecules, contribute to binding to the SEC receptor.

The effect of amyloid-β peptide on neutrophils, which is mediated by the SEC receptor, may also be important in Alzheimer's disease. Microglial cells, which are also of myeloid lineage, are prominent cellular constituents of amyloid deposits. Reactive astrocytes, which are phagocytic in function, are often found surrounding the amyloid deposits. Activation of these inflammatory cells is thought to play a secondary damaging role in the neuropathology of Alzheimer's disease (50).

Taken together, these studies define the cellular biochemistry of an interesting and physiologically relevant network for regulation of α1AT activity and, therein, extracellular proteolytic activity. Formation of covalently stabilized inhibitory complexes with neutrophil elastase, or proteolytic modification by metalloelastases such as that of *Pseudomonas aeruginosa*, induces structural rearrangement of α1AT and, in so doing, exposes a pentapeptide receptor-binding domain in the carboxyl-terminal fragment of α1AT. This domain can, in turn, be recognized by a single class of receptors with a $K_d$ of ~40 nM and a ligand-binding subunit of ~78 kDa. The receptor-binding domain is highly conserved among the serpin family, and several serpin–enzyme complexes can be recognized by the same receptor, the SEC receptor. The receptor-binding domain is also conserved among several tachykinins, bombesin, and the amyloid-β peptide. These other ligands are also recognized by the SEC receptor. Once engaged, the SEC receptor is capable of activating a signal-transduction pathway for increased synthesis of α1AT. Thus, the regulatory effect maintains an excess of inhibitor in the extracellular milieu, an effect that is likely to be important for control of limited proteolytic cascade pathways at sites of inflammation, for orderly initiation of tissue repair, or for prevention of excessive connective-tissue destruction around migrating cells and sprouting cell processes. The SEC receptor is also capable of internalizing its ligands and delivering them to an acidic compartment—either late endosome or lysosome—for degradation. Based on this property and the similarity of its specificity for recognition of ligands to the specificity of pathways for in vivo clearance/catabolism of serpin–enzyme complexes, the SEC receptor probably mediates in vivo clearance/catabolism of certain serpin–enzyme complexes. The SEC receptor also mediates neutrophil chemotactic activities. Identification of amyloid-β peptide as a ligand for the SEC receptor and identification of SEC receptor in cells of neuronal origin (38) raise the possibility that the SEC receptor is involved in the neuropathology of Alzheimer's disease and presenile dementia in Down's syndrome. Finally, the signal-transduction pathway activated by the SEC deficiency works to the disadvantage of individuals with homozygous PiZZ α1AT deficiency, leading to greater intracellular accumulation of the mutant α1AT molecule and, therein, to greater potential for liver injury.

## Acknowledgments

The studies described in this chapter were supported in part by grant HL-37784 from the National Institutes of Health, by an Established Investigator Award from the American Heart Association, by the Monsanto/Washington University Biomedical Program, by the Arthritis Foundation, and by the March of Dimes.

## References

1. Alper CA, Raum, D, Awdeh ZI, Petersen RH, Taylor PD, Starzl TE. Studies of hepatic synthesis in vivo of plasma proteins including orosomucoid, transferrin, alpha-1-antitrypsin, C8 and factor B. Clin Immunol Immunopathol 1990; 16:84–88.
2. Hood JM, Koep L, Peters RF, Schroter GPJ, Well R, Redeker AG, Starzl TE. Liver transplantation for advanced liver disease with alpha-1-antitrypsin deficiency. N Engl J Med 1989; 302:272–276.
3. Perlmutter DH, Cole FS, Kilbridge P, Rossing TH, Colten HR. Expression of alpha-1-proteinase inhibitor gene in human monocytes and macrophages. Proc Natl Acad Sci USA 1985; 82:795–799.
4. Perlmutter DH, Kay RM, Cole FS, Rossing TH, Van Thiel DH, Colten HR. The cellular defect in alpha-1-proteinase inhibitor deficiency is expressed in human monocytes and in xenopus oocytes injected with human liver mRNA. Proc Natl Acad Sci USA 1985; 82:6918–6921.

5. Perlmutter DH, Daniels JD, Auerbach HS, De Schryver-Kecskemeti K, Winter HS, Alpers DA. The alpha-1-antitrypsin gene is expressed in a human intestinal epithelial cell line. J Biol Chem 1989; 264:9485–9490.
6. Mornex J-F, Chytil-Weir A, Martinet Y, Courtney M, LeCocq J-P, Crystal RG. Expression of the alpha-1-antitrypsin gene in mononuclear phagocytes of normal and alpha-1-antitrypsin-deficient individuals. J Clin Invest 1986; 77:1952–1961.
7. Perlmutter DH, Travis J, Punsal PI. Elastase regulates the synthesis of its inhibitor alpha-1-proteinase inhibitor and exaggerates the defect in homozygous PiZZ $\alpha 1$ PI deficiency. J Clin Invest 1988; 81:1774–1780.
8. Takemura S, Rossing TH, Perlmutter DH. A lymphokine regulates expression of alpha-1-proteinase inhibitor in human mononuclear phagocytes. J Clin Invest 1986; 77:1207–1213.
9. Perlino E, Cortese R, Ciliberto G. The human alpha-1-antitrypsin gene is transcribed from two different promoters in macrophages and hepatocytes. EMBO J 1987; 6: 2767–2771.
10. Kelsey GD, Povey S, Bygrave AE, Lovell-Badge RH. Species- and tissue-specific expression of human alpha-1-antitrypsin in transgenic mice. Genes Dev 1987; 1: 161–171.
11. Hafeez W, Ciliberto G, Perlmutter DH. Constitutive and modulated expression of human alpha-1-antitrypsin gene: Different transcriptional initiation sites used in three different cell types. J Clin Invest 1992; 89:1214–1222.
12. Kozak, M. Structural features in eukaryotic mRNAs that modulate the initiation of translation. J Biol Chem 1991; 166:19867–19870.
13. Kozak, M. An analysis of vertebrate mRNA sequence: Intimations of translation control. J Cell Biol 1991; 115:887–903.
14. Barbey-Morel C, Pierce JA, Campbell EJ, Perlmutter DH. Lipopolysaccharide modulates the expression of alpha-1-proteinase inhibitor and other serine proteinase inhibitors in human monocytes and macrophages. J Exp Med 1987; 166:1041–1054.
15. Perlmutter DH, Punsal PI. Distinct and additive effects of elastase and endotoxin on alpha-1-proteinase inhibitor expression in macrophage. J Biol Chem 1988; 263: 16499–16503.
16. Perlmutter DH, May LT, Sehgal PG. Interferon $\beta 2$/interleukin-6 modulates synthesis of alpha-1-antitrypsin in human mononuclear phagocytes and in human hepatoma cells. J Clin Invest 1989; 84:138–144.
17. Molmenti EP, Ziambaras T, Perlmutter DH. Evidence for an acute phase response in human intestinal epithelial cells. J Biol Chem 1993; 268:14116–14124.
18. Molmenti EP, Perlmutter DH, Rubin DC. Cell-specific expression of $\alpha_1$-antitrypsin in human intestinal epithelium. J Clin Invest 1993; 92:2022–2034.
19. Poli V, Mancini FP, Cortese R. IL-6DBP, a nuclear protein involved in interleukin-6 signal transduction, defines a new family of leucine zipper protein related to C/EBP. Cell 1990; 63:643–653.
20. Descombes P, Chojker M, Lichsteiner S, Falvey E, Schibler U. LAP, a novel member of the C/EBP gene family, encodes a liver enriched transcriptional activator protein. Genes Dev 1990; 4:1541–1551.
21. Descombes P, Schibler U. A liver-enriched transcriptional activator protein, LAP,

and a transcriptional inhibitor protein, LIP, are translated from the same mRNA. Cell 1991; 67:569–579.
22. Perlmutter DH, Goldberger G, Dinarello CA, Mizel SB, Colten HR. Regulation of class III major histocompatibility complex gene products by interleukin-1. Science 1986; 232:850–852.
23. Perlmutter DH, Dinarello CA, Punsal PI, Colten HR. Cachectin/tumor necrosis factor regulates hepatic acute-phase expression. J Clin Invest 1986; 78:1349–1354.
24. Perlmutter DH. Cytokines and the hepatic acute phase response. In: Multiple Systems Organ Failure: Hepatic Regulation of Systemic Host Defense. Matuschak GM, ed. New York: Marcel Dekker, 1993.
25. Perlmutter DH, Glover GI, Rivetna M, Schasteen CS, Fallon RJ. Identification of serpin-enzyme complex (SEC) receptor on human hepatoma cells and human monocytes. Proc Natl Acad Sci USA 1990; 87:3753–3757.
26. Mast AE, Enghild JJ, Pizzo SV, Salvesen G. Analysis of plasma elimination kinetics and conformational stabilities of native, proteinase-complexes and reactive site cleaved serpins: comparison of alpha-1-proteinase inhibitor, alpha-1-antichymotrypsin, antithrombin III, alpha-2-antiplasmin, angiotensinogen, and ovalbumin. Biochemistry 1991; 30:1723–1730.
27. Potempa J, Fedek D, Duhn A, Mast A, Travis J. Proteolytic inactivation of alpha-1-antichymotrypsin: site of cleavage and generation of chemotactic activity. J Biol Chem 1991; 266:21482–21487.
28. Banda MJ, Rice AG, Griffin GL, Senior RM. Alpha-1-proteinase inhibitor is a neutrophil chemoattractant after proteolytic inactivation by macrophage elastase. J Biol Chem 1988; 263:4481–4484.
29. Banda MJ, Rice AG, Griffin GL, Senior RM. The inhibitory complex of human alpha-1-proteinase inhibitor and human leukocyte elastase is a neutrophil chemoattractant. J Exp Med 1988; 168:1608–1615.
30. Huber R, Carrell RW. Implication of the three-dimensional structure of alpha-1-antitrypsin for structure and function of serpins. Biochemistry 1990; 28:8951–8966.
31. Loebermann H, Tokuoka R, Deisenhofer J, Huber R. Human alpha-1-proteinase inhibitor: crystal structure analysis of two crystal modifications, molecular model and preliminary analysis of the implications for function. J Mol Biol 1984; 177:531–556.
32. Joslin G, Wittwer A, Adams S, Tollefsen DM, August A, Perlmutter DH. Cross-competition for binding of $\alpha_1$-antitrypsin-elastase complexes to the serpin-enzyme complex receptor by other serpin-enzyme complexes and by proteolytically modified $\alpha_1$AT. J Biol Chem 1993; 268:1886–1893.
33. Barbey-Morel C, Perlmutter DH. Effect of pseudomonas elastase on human mononuclear phagocyte alpha-1-antitrypsin expression. Ped Res 1991; 29:133–140.
34. Perlmutter DH, Joslin G, Nelson P, Schasteen CS, Adams SP, Fallon RJ. Endocytosis and degradation of alpha-1-antitrypsin-protease complexes is mediated by the SEC receptor. J Biol Chem 1990; 265:16713–16716.
35. Joslin G, Fallon RJ, Bullock J, Adams SP, Perlmutter DH. The SEC receptor recognizes a pentapeptide neodomain of alpha-1-antitrypsin-protease complexes. J Biol Chem 1991; 266:11282–11288.
36. Helke CJ, Krause JE, Mantyh PW, Couture R, Bannon MJ. Diversity in mammalian

tachykinin peptidergic neurons: multiple peptides, receptors and regulatory mechanisms. FASEB J 1990; 4:1605–1615.
37. Battey J, Wada E. Two distince receptor subtypes for mammalian bombesin-like peptides. Trends Neurolog Sci 1991; 14:524–528.
38. Joslin G, Krause JE, Hershey AD, Adams SP, Fallon RJ, Perlmutter DH. Amyloid-beta peptide, substance P, and bombesin bind to the serpin-enzyme complex receptor. J Biol Chem 1991; 266:21897–21902.
39. Yankner BA, Duffy LK, Kirschner DA. Neurotrophic and neurotoxic effects of amyloid beta protein: reversal by tachykinin neuropeptides. Science 1990; 250: 279–282.
40. Selkoe DJ. Amyloid-beta protein precursor and the pathogenesis of Alzheimer's disease. Cell 1989; 58:611–612.
41. Katzman R, Saitoh T. Advances in Alzheimer's disease. FASEB J 1991; 5:278–286.
42. St. George-Hyslop PH, Tanzi RE, Polinsky RJ, et al. The genetic defect causing familial Alzheimer's disease maps on chromosome 21. Science 1987; 235:885.
43. Goate A, Chartier-Harlin M-C, Mullan M, et al. Segregation of a missense mutation in the amyloid precursor protein gene with familial Alzheimer's disease. Nature 1991; 349:704–706.
44. Murrell J, Farlow M, Ghetti B, Benson MD. A mutation in the amyloid precursor protein associated with hereditary Alzheimer's disease. Science 1991; 254:97–99.
45. Levy E, Carman MD, Fernandez-Madrid IJ, Power MD, Lieberburg I, van Duinen SG, Bots G, Luyendijk W, Frangione B. Mutation of the Alzheimer's disease amyloid gene in hereditary cerebral hemorrhage, Dutch type. Science 1990; 248:1124–1126.
46. Li H, Takeuchi KH, Manly K, Chapman V, Swank RT. The propeptide of beta-glucuronidase. Further evidence of its involvement in compartmentalization of beta-glucuronidase and sequence similarity with portions of the reactive site region of the serpin superfamily. J Biol Chem 1990; 265:14732–14735.
47. Clarke EP, Cates GA, Ball EH, Sanwal BD. A collagen-binding protein in the endoplasmic reticulum of myoblasts exhibits relationship with serine proteinase inhibitors. J Biol Chem 1991; 266:17230–17235.
48. Joslin G, Griffin GL, August AM, Adams S, Fallon RJ, Senior RM, Perlmutter DH. The serpin-enzyme complex (SEC) receptor mediates the neutrophil chemotactic effect of $\alpha_1$-antitrypsin-elastase complexes and amyloid-$\beta$ peptide. J Clin Invest 1992; 90:1150–1154.
49. Church FC, Pratt CW, Hoffman M. Leukocyte chemoattractant peptides from the serpin heparin cofactor II. J Biol Chem 1991; 266:704–709.
50. Itagaki S, McGeer PL, Akiyama H, Zhu S, Selkoe D. Relationship of microglia and astrocytes to the amyloid deposits of Alzheimer's disease. J Neuroimmunol 1989; 27:173–182.

# 12

# Transgenic Animals with the $\alpha$1AT Promoter

**WILFRIED DALEMANS, FRÉDÉRIC PERRAUD, DALILA ALI-HADJI, SOPHIE JALLAT, and ANDREA PAVIRANI**

Transgene
Strasbourg, France

## I. Introduction

Transcription control elements specific for hepatocytes are a prerequisite for targeting the expression of heterologous proteins to the liver of transgenic animals. Several promoters have been used to direct expression of transgenes to liver cells, e.g. those of the albumin, the alpha 1–antitrypsin ($\alpha$1AT), or the antithrombin III genes (1–11). Consistent with the fact that $\alpha$1AT (12,13) is one of the major secreted hepatic proteins, with plasma levels ranging from 1 to 3 mg/ml, the promoter of the $\alpha$1AT gene might be of choice for efficient, hepatospecific expression. The $\alpha$1AT promoter has been extensively studied, and liver-specific (14–23), macrophage-specific (24), and negative (25) *cis*-acting DNA sequence elements have been determined.

We have used a human $\alpha$1AT promoter fragment containing the hepatospecific elements to express heterologous proteins (26–28), including *onc* genes—*c-myc* and the SV40 T antigen (SV40TAg)—and hepatic proteins of therapeutic interest—human $\alpha$1AT or coagulation factor IX (FIX). The different transgenes were expressed either alone or in combination. Transgenic mice expressing *onc* genes developed hepatomas and tumor cells could subsequently be established as permanent cell lines. Moreover, the presence of a second transgene, coding for a human hepatic protein, led to efficient in vitro secretion of fully active proteins into the cell-culture supernatant.

## II. Transgenic Mice

### A. *Onc* Gene Expression

Different transgenic expression cassettes were generated using a human α1AT promoter fragment, contained in a *Kpn*I restriction fragment of 1.8 kilobases (kb). In the most successful experiments, the complete fragment which carried 1.5 kb of promoter sequences, the α1AT first noncoding exon, and 0.2 kb of the first intron was used (26,29). In other constructs, a polylinker was introduced into the first noncoding exon of the α1AT gene wherein heterologous genes could be inserted. This obviated the need of an intron acceptor splice site in the 5′ end of the transgene to be expressed. Both types of promoter constructs carried the necessary *cis*-acting sequence elements for hepatospecific expression (14–23), while being void of the macrophage-specific sequence element (24). Three *onc* gene sequences were linked to the α1AT promoter: the murine *c-myc* proto-oncogene (30,31), the SV40T antigen (Ag) (32), and the human *c-Ha-ras onc* gene (33) (see Table 1). In the case of the *c-myc* construct (pTG2984), the fusion between promoter and coding regions was done by joining the two fragments within their respective first noncoding introns, thereby generating a hybrid intron (Fig. 1a) (26). The SV40TAg construct (pTG4912; Fig. 1b) (28) was based on the above construct and thus contains the same hybrid intron. The *c-Ha-ras* transgene was cloned both in the intron-less promoter fragment (pTG2979) and in the hybrid intron-containing promoter (pTG3965).

**Table 1** Transgenic Mice with the α1AT Promoter

| Transgene | Denomination | No. of transgenic lines | Phenotype |
|---|---|---|---|
| Murine *c-myc* | TMTG2984 | 5 | Hepatoma |
| SV40TAg | TMTG4912 | 4 | Hepatoma |
| Human *c-Ha-ras* | TMTG2979 | 6 | No detectable mRNA transcripts |
| | (TG3965) | 0 | Lethality ? |
| Human α1AT | TMTG2984 | 5 | Secretion in the circulation (up to 2.5 mg/ml) |
| Human FIX | TMTG3962 | 1 | Secretion in the circulation (2–4 μg/ml) |
| Human FVIII | TMTG2998 | 6 | No secretion detectable in the circulation |

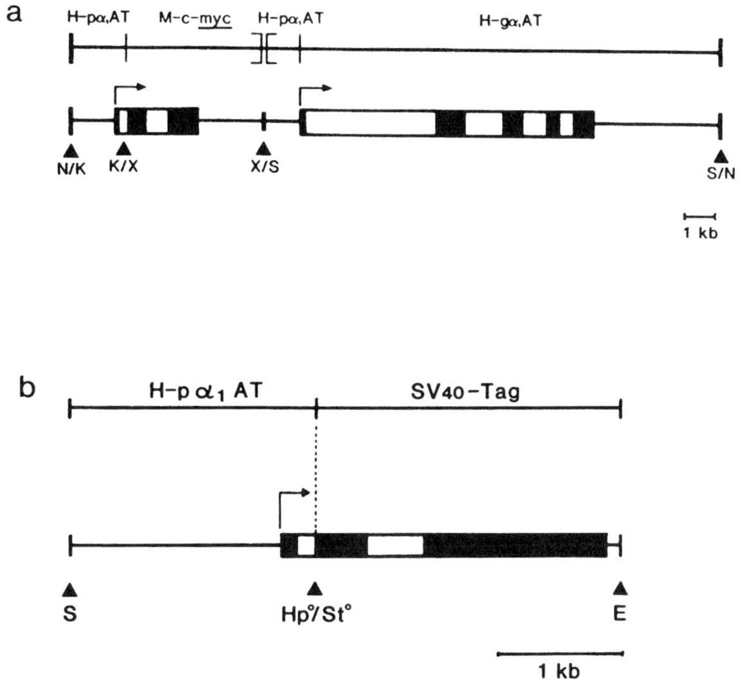


**Figure 1** Structure of (a) pTG2984- and (b) pTG4912-derived transgenes (H-pα1AT: human α1AT promoter; M-*c-myc*: murine *c-myc* coding exons 2 and 3; H-gα1AT: genomic copy of the human α1AT gene; SV40TAg: SV40 T antigen; N, K, X, S, $Hp^0$, $St^0$, E: restriction sites *Not*I, *Kpn*I, *Xho*I, *Sal*I, truncated *Hpa*I, truncated *Stu*I, *Eco*RI, respectively; black boxes: exons; white boxes: introns). (Adapted from Ref. 26.)

The expression of the respective transgenes led to tumorigenesis of the liver in the case of the construct containing *c-myc* and SV40TAg (1,8–10,26–38,34–36). Transgenic mice developed liver tumors (hepatomas) at the average age of 12 months in the case of both selected mouse lines expressing *c-myc* (TMTG2984; Ref. 26). The four mouse lines established with the SV40 transgene (TMTG4912) showed tumorigenesis in a broader time range, i.e., after 2.5–8 months. This was directly linked to the copy number of the transgenes, line 34 with the highest copy number having a tumor onset between 10 and 16 weeks of age. Both kinds of *onc* mice developed hepatomas in a reproducible way, displaying the phenotype for five (*c-myc*-derived) and 10 (SV40TAg-derived) generations, respectively. In the SV40TAg transgenic mice, fluctuations in the copy number of the transgene sequences were observed; since the SV40TAg sequence is known to be involved in the replication of the SV40 viral genome (32), a role of this protein might be accounted for. Histological analysis showed that the tumors were of epithelial origin (hepatocellular carcinomas) (26,28). However, the tumors in both types of mice presented morphological differences. SV40TAg-derived tumors consisted of multiple small foci covering the whole liver (Fig. 2B), whereas *c-myc*-derived tumors presented one or few large tumor nodules (Fig. 2A). Morphological examination of tumor development was performed on one of the SV40TAg mouse lines. Tumor formation was not preceded by visual hyperplasia of the liver, but tumor onset could be detected by the presence of a few small foci of tumor nodules. These results show that targeting of oncogene expression to hepatocytes can be efficiently done under control of the human α1AT promoter.

Expression of transgene transcripts under control of the α1AT promoter was examined by S1 nuclease mapping and shown to be specific to the liver of the transgenic mice (26). This was in contrast to data from other groups showing additional transgene transcription by the α1AT promoter in other tissues, such as the kidneys (2–8). The observed difference can possibly be explained by the length of the particular promoter fragment used (2–8), the site of integration (2), or the mouse strain employed (7,23,37–39). The expression level of endogenous murine *c-myc* seemed not to be influenced by the high expression level of transgenic *c-myc* (26). The SV40TAg transgene transcripts were also confined to the liver, but the expression level was low in all cases studied, although sufficient to elicit hepatoma development.

In contrast to the expression of the two *onc* genes described above, no tumors were observed in transgenic mice carrying either of the human *c-Ha-ras* transgene constructs. In the case of the first construct, Southern blot analysis

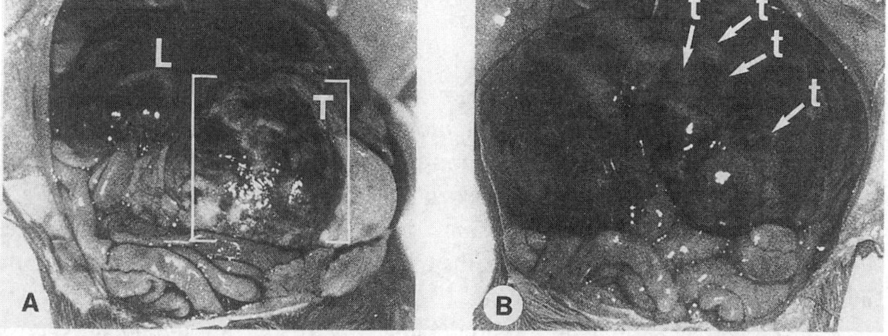


**Figure 2** Hepatomas in transgenic mice expressing *onc* genes under control of the human α1AT promoter. (A) Expression of murine *c-myc* (TMTG2984). L: liver; T: large tumor nodule. (B) Expression of SV40TAg (TMTG4912). t: small tumor nodules.

showed that the transgene sequences were not rearranged. Northern blot analysis of several transgenic lines demonstrated the absence of specific *c-Ha-ras* mRNAs, thus excluding a possible position effect. However, transient in vitro expression in human hepatoma-derived HepG2 cells showed transcription of *c-Ha-ras* mRNA from this construct. These results suggest that this particular combination of the α1AT promoter with the *c-Ha-ras* sequence is incapable of generating transgenic mRNA in vivo (see also Ref. 40). In the case of the DNA construct carrying the hybrid intron promoter fragment (pTG3965), no transgenic mice could be obtained. Since this construct was also shown to produce correctly processed *c-Ha-ras* mRNA transcripts, as shown in transient HepG2 transfection experiments, a lethality due to *c-Ha-ras* expression was suspected.

### B. Human Liver Protein Expression

Human liver proteins were expressed under control of the same α1AT promoter elements described above (see Table 1). As a first example, we used the homologous gene, i.e., human α1AT, under control of its own promoter. This construct, pTG2984 (see Fig. 1a), carried a double expression cassette containing the murine *c-myc* transgene (see above) and the human α1AT gene, both under control of the human α1AT promoter. Five transgenic mouse lines (TMTG2984) were generated; three of them expressed levels of human α1AT in the circulation (between 0.5 and 2.5 mg/ml), similar to the human physiological concentration. The transgenic line most studied, TMTG2984/7, contained approximately 20 copies of the transgene and expressed on average 1 mg/ml of human α1AT. During hepatoma development, a hypertrophy of the liver was manifest, and levels of circulating α1AT increased to 8 mg/ml. This suggests that the α1AT promoter is still active in the tumor cells, which is indirect evidence of their differentiated status. Interestingly, when the steady-state levels of mouse α1AT mRNA were compared to those of nontransgenic littermates a decrease was observed. This observation complements another report, in which lower levels of murine α1AT in transgenic mice expressing human α1AT were observed (41). This suggests the possible existence of a mechanism that controls and regulates the absolute amount of α1AT present in the circulation. Another possible explanation is titration of transcription factors in favor of the copy of the human gene; however, this is less likely, since total amounts (mouse plus human) of α1AT mRNA were higher in transgenic animals.

The second protein expressed under control of the α1AT promoter was human FIX (pTG3962). The expression cassette contained the same α1AT promoter that was described before and a genomic copy of the human FIX gene (27). When compared to human α1AT gene expression with serum levels up to 1 mg/ml (TMTG2984), FIX expression was significantly lower, with levels of 2–4 μg/ml in the circulation. In contrast, levels of secreted human FIX in transgenic mice containing the gene under control of its own FIX promoter were consistently higher, 25–40 μg/ml (27). Since in both cases a genomic copy of the FIX gene was used, intronic sequences were present and correct mRNA processing was thus expected. The specific interaction between both sequences—the α1AT promoter and the FIX gene—seems to be of importance, as was also observed in other heterologous expression constructs (27,40). A similar effect, i.e., inefficient in vivo interaction between two heterologous DNA sequences, *in casu* the α1AT promoter and a reporter gene, was already observed in the case of the human *c-Ha-ras* construct (pTG2979; see above).

A third hepatic protein of therapeutic interest that we attempted to express was human factor VIII (FVIII) (pTG2998). In this particular case, the promoter element lacking the intronic sequences coupled to the cDNA of the FVIII protein was used. Although the transgenic DNA was integrated without rearrangement, no FVIII could be detected in the circulation of transgenic mice. Northern blot analysis illustrated the absence of transgenic mRNA. Two possible explanations were offered for this absence of expression: 1) the specific combination between both sequences is unfavorable for correct RNA expression, as also indicated for the earlier described *c-Ha-ras* or 2) there is a need for, or at least a positive effect of, the presence of intronic sequences to permit efficient or correct processing of the transcripts (27,40,42). A similar observation was made when expression of the FIX cDNA under control of the same intron-less promoter segment was attempted.

Efficient expression from the human α1AT promoter (construct TG2984) was also obtained in transgenic rabbits (43).

## III. Transimmortalization

Continuous cell cultures could be established from tumor cells generated in *onc* gene–derived transgenic mice; we have previously termed this approach *transimmortalization* (26–28,44).

In early attempts to derive novel hepatic cell lines based on α1AT promoter-driven transgenic *c-myc* expression (TG2984 construct; see Fig. 1a), we were confronted with the phenomenon of cellular dedifferentiation (45–49). Whereas the establishment of immortalized cell cultures was easily achieved, cells rapidly lost their hepatocyte characteristics, as exemplified by the rapid shutoff of adult hepatic protein expression. The use of an adapted cell-culture protocol, in particular with respect to the composition of the culture medium proved to be essential in maintaining a differentiated cellular phenotype (26–28). Tumors elicited by α1AT promoter-driven *c-myc* or SV40TAg expression could be established as continuous, hepatocyte-derived cell cultures. *c-myc* tumor-derived cells grew slowly in the beginning of culture establishment, and cell viability in this stage of the culture could be maintained only by plating the cells as clusters. However, once adapted to in vitro culturing, they could further be plated as conventional cell lines. Cells had an epithelial cell appearance (Fig. 3A), and hepatic structures as tight junctions or bile canaliculi could be observed (28). SV40TAg tumor-derived cells (Fig. 3B) grew more rapidly in the initial stages of culture establishment, and could immediately be propagated as individual cells (28). Once cultures were established, both types of cell cultures grew in a comparable way. Electron microscopic analysis illustrated their adult hepatocyte character (28).

Long-term maintenance of the adult hepatocyte differentiation status was further confirmed by the analysis of hepatic marker protein expression (Table 2; 26–28). The predominant secreted protein characteristic for adult hepatocytes, albumin (35,45,48,49), was secreted from cell cultures of *onc* gene origin (Table 2), at levels comparable to those from, for example, the highly differentiated murine hepatoma cell line Hepa (50). The active expression of other murine marker proteins characteristic of differentiation—e.g., transferrin, gluthatione S transferase, and α1AT—was evidenced by RNA analysis (26–28). The activity of the α1AT promoter could be monitored through transgene expression. For TG2984-derived cell lines, both α1AT promoter-controlled expression cassettes were shown to be efficiently expressed (26). This was the case for the two homologous genes—human and murine α1AT (Table 2), each transcribed from its own promoter—as well as for the heterologous gene, *c-myc* transcribed from the human α1AT promoter. The secreted human α1AT was shown to be glycosylated (26), and preliminary results indicated that the secreted protein was active, as determined by inhibition of human elastase activity. The presence of mouse α1AT in the supernatant of these cell cultures complicated correct determination of the

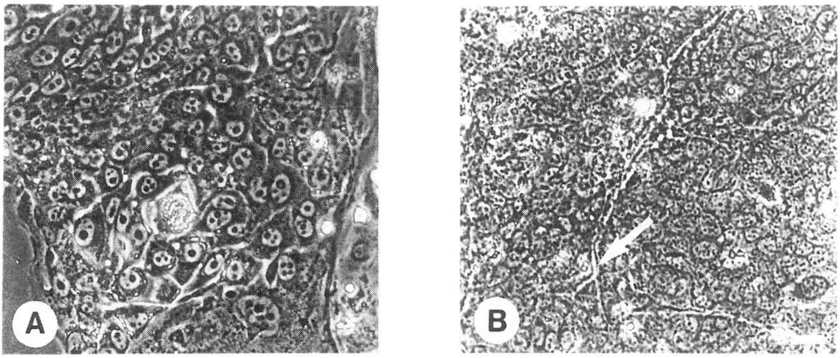


**Figure 3** Transimmortalized hepatic cell lines derived from (A) TMTG2984 or (B) TMTG4912 transgenic mice. The arrow (B) points toward tight junctions clearly visible when cells reached high density. Bar: 50 μm.

**Table 2** Example of Transimmortalized Cell Lines Derived from α1AT Promoter-Controlled *onc* Gene Expression

| Name | *onc* Gene | Derived from transgenic mouse | Secretion of hepatic proteins (μg/ml/24 hr) | | | Generation time (hr) |
|---|---|---|---|---|---|---|
| | | | Mouse albumin | Human α1AT | Human FIX | |
| TMhepTG2 | *c-myc* | TMTG2984/7 | 5 | 5 | — | 35 |
| TMhepTG10 | SV40TAg | TMTG4912/34 | 7 | — | — | 40 |
| TMhepTG39 | *c-myc* + SV40TAg | TMTG2984 × 4912 × 3960[a] | 15 | 4 | 0.35[b] | 60 |
| TMhepTG48 | *c-myc* + SV40TAg | TMTG2984 × 4912 × 3960[a] | 10 | 8 | 0.80[b] | 40 |

[a]TG3960 contains a human FIX genomic expression cassette under the control of the same α1AT promoter (27).
[b]Production was measured at high cell density.

specific activity of the human α1AT protein. In the TG4912 (SV40TAg-derived) cell lines, both α1AT promoters were also active. In general, α1AT promoter-driven transcripts were present in larger amounts in the transimmortalized cells than in the transgenic hepatocytes, in particular with respect to both *onc* genes. Active expression from the α1AT promoter was still present after long-term culturing, for up to 40 culture passages in the case of the TG2984-derived cell line TMhepTG2 (26,28). The most convincing proof for the differentiated hepatic phenotype was derived from data on transimmortalized cultures secreting human FIX (27). Human FIX was shown to have specific activity similar to that of plasma-derived FIX, illustrating the maintenance of the complex posttranslational processing activities characteristic of differentiated hepatocytes.

## IV. Conclusions and Prospects

The tissue-specific function of the human α1AT promoter was explored in transgenic mice. Targeted expression of *onc* genes to the liver of transgenic mice led to subsequent hepatoma development. Tumor cells could be established as differentiated hepatic cell lines. When genes coding for proteins of therapeutic interest, such as human α1AT or FIX, were included in the transgenic constructs, secretion of active human proteins could be detected in the circulation of transgenic mice as well as in the supernatants of the respective transimmortalized cell lines. These results illustrate the efficient and specific in vivo expression of genes under control of the human α1AT promoter. The presence of different α1AT promoters (murine and/or human), each driving specific genes in the same cell, provides an interesting model system for studying (cross-)regulation of α1AT promoters. The effect of intra- and extracellular effectors or agonists, as well as potential interactions between both α1AT promoters themselves or the respective genes they transcribe, can easily be monitored by means of the respective gene expression. Moreover, these studies can be conducted in vivo (with transgenic animals) as well as in vitro (with transimmortalized cell lines). In addition, such transgenic mice can also be model systems for hepatocellular carcinogenesis using different *onc* genes.

## Acknowledgments

We thank the late J. P. Lecocq for continuous interest and encouragement; M. Courtney for critical reading of the manuscript; R. G. Crystal for the generous gift of the human α1AT gene; all our collaborators and technicians, whose skillful work has been greatly appreciated; N. Monfrini for editorial help; and B. Heller for artwork. Work on FIX was supported by Institut Merieux, France.

## References

1. Sandgren EP, Quaife CJ, Pinkert CA, Palmiter RD, Brinster RL. Oncogene-induced liver neoplasia in transgenic mice. Oncogene 1989; 4:715–724.
2. Sifers RN, Carlson JA, Clift SM, DeMayo, FJ, Bullock DW, Woo SLC. Tissue specific expression of the human alpha-1-antitrypsin gene in transgenic mice. Nucleic Acids Res 1987; 15:1459–1475.
3. Kelsey GD, Povey S, Bygrave AE, Lovell-Badge RH. Species- and tissue-specific expression of human $\alpha_1$-antitrypsin in transgenic mice. Genes Dev 1987; 1:161–171.
4. Rüther U, Tripodi M, Cortese R, Wagner EF. The human alpha-1-antitrypsin gene is efficiently expressed from two tissue-specific promoters in transgenic mice. Nucleic Acids Res 1987; 15:7519–7529.
5. Carlson JA, Rogers BB, Sifers RN, Hawkins HK, Finegold MJ, Woo SLC. Multiple tissues express $\text{alpha}_1$-antitrypsin in transgenic mice and man. J Clin Invest 1988; 82:26–36.
6. Dycaico MJ, Grant SGN, Felts K, Nichols WS, Geller SA, Hager JH, Pollard AJ, Kohler SW, Short HP, Jirik FR, Hanahan D, Sorge JA. Neonatal hepatitis induced by $\alpha_1$-antitrypsin: a transgenic mouse model. Science 1988; 242:1409–1412.
7. Koopman P, Povey S, Lovell-Badge RH. Widespread expression of human $\alpha_1$-antitrypsin in transgenic mice revealed by in situ hybridization. Genes Dev 1989; 3: 16–25.
8. Shen R-F, Clift SM, DeMayo JL, Sifers RN, Finegold MJ, Woo SLC. Tissue-specific regulation of human α1-antitrypsin gene expression in transgenic mice. DNA 1989; 8:101–108.
9. Sepulveda AR, Finegold MJ, Smith B, Slagle BL, DeMayo JL, Shen R-F, Woo SLC,

Butel JS. Development of a transgenic mouse system for the analysis of stages in liver carcinogenesis using tissue-specific expression of SV40 large T-antigen controlled by regulatory elements of the human $\alpha$-1-antitrypsin gene. Cancer Res 1989; 49:6108–6117.

10. Butel JS, Sepulveda AR, Finegold MJ, Woo SLC. SV40 large T antigen directed by regulatory elements of the human alpha-1-antitrypsin gene. Intervirology 1990; 31: 85–100.
11. Dubois N, Bennoun M, Grimber G, Allemand I, Cavard C, Hasse J-F, Kamoun P, Briand P. Hepatocarcinogenesis in transgenic mice carrying the antithrombin III-SV40 T antigen. In: Mouse Molecular Genetics. Cold Spring Harbor, NY: Cold Spring Harbor Laboratory Press, 1988:46.
12. Carrell RW, Jeppsson J-O, Laurell CB, Brennan SO, Owen MC, Vaughan L, Boswell DR. Structure and variation of human $\alpha_1$-antitrypsin. Nature 1982; 298:329–334.
13. Crystal RG. The $\alpha_1$-antitrypsin gene and its deficiency states. Trends Genet 1989; 5:411–417.
14. Ciliberto G, Dente L, Cortese R. Cell-specific expression of a transfected human $\alpha_1$-antitrypsin gene. Cell 1985; 41:531–540.
15. De Simone V, Ciliberto G, Hardon E, Paonessa G, Palla F, Lundberg L, Cortese R. *cis*- and *trans*-acting elements responsible for the cell-specific expression of the human $\alpha$1-antitrypsin gene. EMBO J 1987; 6:2759–2766.
16. Courtois G, Morgan JG, Campbell LA, Fourel G, Crabtree GR. Interaction of a liver-specific nuclear factor with the fibrinogen and $\alpha_1$-antitrypsin promoters. Science 1987; 238:688–692.
17. Shen RF, Li Y, Sifers RN, Wang H, Hardick C, Tsai SY, Woo SLC. Tissue-specific expression of the human $\alpha_1$-antitrypsin gene is controlled by multiple cis-regulatory elements. Nucleic Acids Res 1987; 15:8399–8415.
18. Grayson DR, Costa RH, Xanthopoulos KG, Darnell JE Jr. A cell-specific enhancer of the mouse $\alpha$1-antitrypsin gene has multiple functional regions and corresponding protein-binding sites. Mol Cell Biol 1988; 8:1055–1066.
19. Monaci P, Nicosia A, Cortese R. Two different liver-specific factors stimulate *in vitro* transcription from the human $\alpha$1-antitrypsin promoter. EMBO J 1988; 7:2075–2087.
20. Li Y, Shen R-F, Tsai SY, Woo SLC. Multiple hepatic *trans*-acting factors are required for in vitro transcription of the human alpha-1-antitrypsin gene. Mol Cell Biol 1988; 8:4362–4369.
21. Ochoa A, Brunel F, Mendelzon D, Cohen GN, Zakin MM. Different liver nuclear proteins bind to similar DNA sequences in the 5′ flanking regions of three hepatic genes. Nucleic Acids Res 1989; 17:119–133.
22. Ryffel GU, Kugler W, Wagner U, Kaling M. Liver cell specific gene transcription *in vitro*: the promoter elements HP1 and TATA box are necessary and sufficient to generate a liver-specific promoter. Nucleic Acids Res 1989; 17:939–953.
23. Latimer JJ, Berger FG, Baumann H. Highly conserved upstream regions of the $\alpha_1$-antitrypsin gene in two mouse species govern liver-specific expression by different mechanisms. Mol Cell Biol 1990; 10:760–769.
24. Perlino E, Cortese R, Ciliberto G. The human $\alpha_1$-antitrypsin gene is transcribed from two different promoters in macrophages and hepatocytes. EMBO J 1987; 6:2767–2771.

25. De Simone V, Cortese R. A negative regulatory element in the promoter of the human α1-antitrypsin gene. Nucleic Acids Res 1989; 17:9407–9415.
26. Dalemans, W Perraud F, Le Meur M, Gerlinger P, Courtney M, Pavirani A. Heterologous protein expression by transimmortalized differentiated liver cell lines derived from transgenic mice. Biologicals 1990; 18:191–198.
27. Jallat S, Perraud F, Dalemans W, Balland A, Dieterle A, Faure T, Meulien P, Pavirani A. Characterization of recombinant human factor IX expressed in transgenic mice and in derived trans-immortalized hepatic cell lines. EMBO J 1990; 9:3295–3301.
28. Perraud F, Dalemans W, Gendrault J-L, Dreyer D, Ali-Hadji D, Faure T, Pavirani A. Characterization of trans-immortalized hepatic cell lines established from transgenic mice. Exp Cell Res 1991; 195:59–65.
29. Long GL, Chandra T, Woo SLC, Davie EW, Kurachi K. Complete sequence of the cDNA for human $\alpha_1$-antitrypsin and the gene for the S variant. Biochemistry 1984; 23:4828–4837.
30. Bernard O, Cory S, Gerondakis S, Webb E, Adams JM. Sequence of the murine and human cellular *myc* oncogenes and two modes of *myc* transcription resulting from chromosome translocation in B lymphoid tumours. EMBO J 1983; 2:2375–2383.
31. Alexander WS, Schrader JW, Adams JM. Expression of the *c-myc* oncogene under control of an immunoglobulin enhancer in Eμ-*myc* transgenic mice. Mol Cell Biol 1987; 7:1436–1444.
32. Stahl H, Knippers R. The simian virus 40 large tumor antigen. Biochim Biophys Acta 1987; 910:1–10.
33. Capon DJ, Chen EY, Levinson AD, Seeburg PH, Goeddel DV. Complete nucleotide sequences of the T24 human bladder carcinoma oncogene and its normal homologue. Nature 1983; 302:33–37.
34. Messing A, Chen HY, Palmiter RD, Brinster RL. Peripheral neuropathies, hepatocellular carcinomas and islet cell adenomas in transgenic mice. Nature 1985; 316: 461–463.
35. Paul D, Höhne M, Pinkert C, Piasecki A, Ummelmann E, Brinster RL. Immortalized differentiated hepatocyte lines derived from transgenic mice harboring SV40 T-antigen genes. Exp Cell Res 1988; 175:354–362.
36. Araki K, Hino O, Miyazaki J-I, Yamamura K-I. Development of two types of hepatocellular carcinoma in transgenic mice carrying the SV40 large T-antigen gene. Carcinogenesis 1991; 12:2059–2062.
37. Berger FG, Bauman H. An evolutionary switch in tissue-specific gene expression. J Biol Chem 1985; 260:1160–1165.
38. Latimer JJ, Berger FG, Baumann H. Developmental expression, cellular localization, and testosterone regulation of $\alpha_1$-antitrypsin in *Mus caroli* kidney. J Biol Chem 1987; 262:12641–12646.
39. Rheaume C, Latimer JJ, Baumann H, Berger FG. Tissue- and species-specific regulation of murine $\alpha_1$-antitrypsin gene transcription. J Biol Chem 1988; 263:15118–15121.
40. Koltunow AM, Gregg K, Rogers GE. Promoter efficiency depends upon intragenic sequences. Nucleic Acids Res 1987; 15:7795–7807.
41. Sifers RN, Rogers BB, Hawkins HK, Finegold MJ, Woo SLC. Elevated synthesis of

human $\alpha_1$-antitrypsin hinders the secretion of murinc $\alpha_1$-antitrypsin from hepatocytes of transgenic mice. J Biol Chem 1989; 264:15696–15700.
42. Brinster RL, Allen JM, Behringer RR, Gelinas RE, Palmiter RD. Introns increase transcription efficiency in transgenic mice. Proc Natl Acad Sci USA 1988; 85: 836–840.
43. Massoud M, Bischoff R, Dalemans W, Pointu H, Attal J, Schultz H, Clesse D, Stinnakre M-G, Pavirani A, Houdebine LM. Expression of active recombinant human $\alpha_1$-antitrypsin in transgenic rabbits. J Biotech 1991; 18:193–204.
44. Pavirani A, Skern T, Le Meur M, Lutz Y, Lathe R, Crystal RG, Fuchs J-P, Gerlinger P, Courtney M. Recombinant proteins of therapeutic interest expressed by lymphoid cell lines derived from transgenic mice. Bio/Technology 1989; 7:1049–1054.
45. Cassio D, Weiss MC, Ott M-O, Sala-Trepat JM, Friès J, Erdos T. Expression of the albumin gene in rat hepatoma cells and their dedifferentiated variants. Cell 1981; 27:351–358.
46. Clayton DF, Weiss M, Darnell JE Jr. Liver-specific RNA metabolism in hepatoma cells: variations in transcription rates and mRNA levels. Mol Cell Biol 1985; 5:2633–2641.
47. Clayton DF, Harrelson AL, Darnell JE Jr. Dependence of liver-specific transcription on tissue organization. Mol Cell Biol 1985; 5:2623–2632.
48. Isom H, Georgoff I, Salditt-Georgieff M, Darnell JE Jr. Persistence of liver-specific messenger RNA in cultured hepatocytes: different regulatory events for different genes. J Cell Biol 1987; 105:2877–2885.
49. Cereghini S, Blumenfeld M, Yaniv M. A liver-specific factor essential for albumin transcription differs between differentiated rat hepatoma cells. Genes Dev 1988; 2:957–974.
50. Ledford BE, Davis DF. Kinetics of serum protein secretion by cultured hepatoma cells. J Biol Chem 1983; 258:3304–3308.

# 13

# Chemistry and Biology of Secretory Leukoprotease Inhibitor

**DAVID F. CARMICHAEL**

Aerie Consulting Group
Boulder, Colorado

**KJELL OHLSSON**

University of Lund
Lund, Sweden
and Malmö General Hospital
Malmö, Sweden

## I. Introduction

The acid-stable, antiprotease activity of human secretory leukocyte protease inhibitor (SLPI) was first identified in seminal fluid (1) and later in the secretions of the nasal, bronchial, and cervical mucosa as well as those of the parotid gland (2). SLPI's physiological role appears to be that of antiprotease defense for these tissues against the enzymes of extravascular neutrophils (3). The involvement of activated oxygen species and nonspecific proteolysis in the pathogenic destruction of tissues within the respiratory tract and elsewhere is widely accepted. The presence of large amounts of proteolytic enzymes in purulent bronchial secretions is an old observation, as is the presence of plasma proteins, including alpha 1–antitrypsin (4,5). Leukocyte proteinases, like elastase, were identified as the major enzymes responsible for the proteolytic activity (5,6). In such respiratory pathologies, increased proteolytic activity and/or decreased protease inhibitory capacity result in a characteristic protease–inhibitor imbalance. In many chronic respiratory diseases, this imbalance is largely attributable to increased number and activation of neutrophils.

The etiology of the imbalance between proteases and their inhibitors is often complex and varies with the disease. Nonetheless, the presence of a protease–

inhibitor imbalance presents a common component in these pathologies. The use of natural protease inhibitors as therapeutics may have application in the treatment of many of these disease states. Clinical use of protease inhibitors are discussed elsewhere in this volume. The purpose of this chapter is to describe the chemistry and biology of SLPI.

Human secretory leukocyte protease inhibitor is a 107 amino acid, nonglycosylated, single-chain protein. The molecule is stabilized by extensive intrachain disulfide bonds. SLPI forms inhibitory complexes with a variety of serine proteases, including the pancreatic proteases trypsin and chymotrypsin; this inhibition was the basis for SLPI's discovery and subsequent purification. More noteworthy, from the perspective of SLPI's physiological role, is its ability to complex and inhibit the prominent proteolytic enzymes of the polymorphonuclear leukocyte, elastase, and cathepsin G.

## II. Purification and Characterization

### A. Purification

The description of serine protease inhibitory activity in mucosal secretions was made as early as 1965 by Haendle et al. (1). Subsequently, similar activities were partially purified and characterized from cervical mucosa, seminal plasma, nasal secretions, and bronchial mucosal secretions (2,3,7). The inhibitors isolated from each of these sources were acid-stable inhibitors of several serine proteases, but most notably of the major neutrophil proteases, elastase and cathepsin G (8). Olsson et al. (3) noted in 1977 that bronchial secretions contained a distinct acid-stable serine protease inhibitor not derived from inter-alpha-trypsin inhibitor. The similarities in physicochemical characteristics of a basic serine proteinase inhibitor from other mucosal sources were formally noted in 1978 by Schiessler et al. (8).

The concept of using naturally occurring inhibitors of leukocyte proteases in a therapeutic capacity kindled new interest in the proteins in the early 1980s. Thompson and Ohlsson (9) identified this same acid-stable inhibitor of leukocyte proteases from parotid secretions that later served as the source for the purification and complete amino acid sequence of SLPI. The following year, a revised sequence was published for the inhibitor from seminal plasma, confirming the identity of the proteins from these two sources (10).

The purification of SLPI from human parotid secretions was based on the observation that this fluid appeared to contain approximately 1 μg/ml of the inhibitor. The inhibitory activity was acid-stable and immunologically cross-reactive with that of the bronchial mucosa (9). The protein was immunologically distinct from the acid-stable inter-alpha-trypsin inhibitor described by Hochstrasser et al. (3,11–13). The purification and characterization, including the complete primary structure of SLPI, served as a point of comparison for protease inhibitors from other sources. The procedure depicted in Table 1 made use of the relatively basic isoelectric point of the protein (pI > 9.5) and low molecular weight (calculated 11,726) to yield material suitable for protein sequence determination. The observed primary structure of the protein is shown in Fig. 1 (9).

### B. Characterization

The sequence is composed of two roughly equal domains bearing a modest resemblance to the "Kazal"-type sequences defined for other protease inhibitors (Fig. 2). Each domain contains eight half-cystine residues that are completely disulfide-bonded. The protein is not glycosylated despite an N-linked consensus glycosylation sequence at residues asparagine-55 through threonine-57. As discussed below, the lack of glycosylation has allowed the use of prokaryotic expression systems for the large-scale production of the recombinant human SLPI molecule (rhSLPI), which is identical to the inhibitor originally isolated from parotid secretions.

## III. Complementary DNA and Genomic Structure

Based on the protein sequence information, complementary DNA clones were isolated from libraries of mRNA generated from human cervix and, later, parotid gland. The cDNA structure and corresponding protein sequence for SLPI are shown in Fig. 3. In addition to prescribing the protein structure observed in the isolated protein, the cDNA depicts a 25 amino acid prepeptide typical of secreted proteins (14).

The genomic clone containing the SLPI gene was found in a 3.8 kb Eco R1 fragment isolated from a lambda Charon 30 human genomic library. To obtain the complete sequence of the SLPI gene, fragments of the genomic clone were subcloned and sequenced according to the method of Sanger (15). Organization of

**Table 1** Purification of SLPI

| Step | Total vol. (ml) | Total protein (mg) | Total SLPI (mg) | Recovery (%) |
|---|---|---|---|---|
| Parotid secretion | 6000 | 5280 | 5.7 | 100 |
| SP-Sephadex C-50 | 75 | 736 | 4.6 | 81 |
| Sephadex G-50 | 18 | 4.9 | 4.0 | 70 |

Amount of SLPI determined by radioimmunoassay. Titration of granulocyte elastase with the isolated SLPI gave a final amount of purified inhibitor of 4.2 mg.
*Source*: Ref. 9.

**Figure 1** The complete amino acid sequence of SLPI presented in the standard one-letter code, in a manner that emphasizes the homologies between the first and second halves of the protein. The key peptides used to determine the sequence are adjacent to the sequence. N: Edman degradation of the undigested reduced carboxymethylated protein; S: submaxillary protease; LC: endoproteinase LysC; C: chymotrypsin; V: V8 protease. A dash indicates a positively identified residue; a dot indicates a residue presumed to be present in the peptide on the basis of amino acid composition but not positively identified. (From Ref. 9.)

the SLPI gene is depicted in Fig. 4 (16). The gene is composed of four exons with three intervening sequences. Each of the first three exons correspond roughly to a functional domain of a translated protein; exon 1 corresponding to the signal sequence for peptide secretion and exons 2 and 3 corresponding to the first and second structural domains. The fourth exon is composed primarily of three prime untranslated regions of the mature mRNA. Based on the organization of the SLPI gene, and the observed repeat domains in the translated protein, it was hypothesized that the trypsin and chymotrypsin inhibitory activities of SLPI resided in the N- and C-terminal domains, respectively (16).

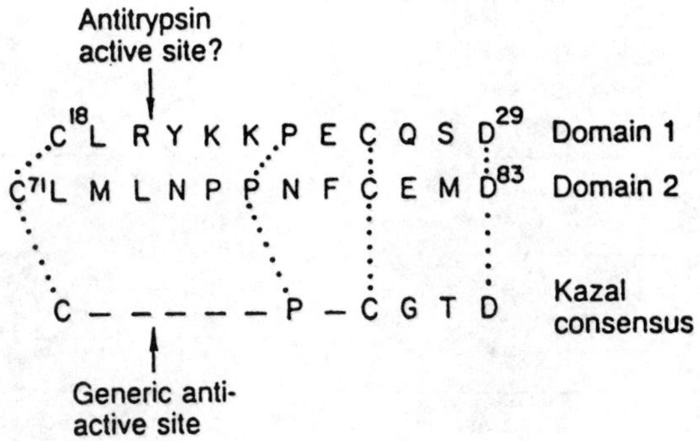


**Figure 2** Homology between residues 18–19 and 71–83 of SLPI and the consensus active-site region of Kazal protease inhibitors. (From Ref. 9.)

```
            1                                                    30
ATG   AAG   TCC   AGC   GGC   CTC   TTC   CCC   TTC   CTG   GTG   CTG   CTT   GCC   CTG
M     K     S     S     G     L     F     P     F     L     V     L     L     A     L
                                                                                  90
GGA   ACT   CTG   GCA   CCT   TGG   GCT   GTG   GAA   GGC   TCT   GGA   AAG   TCC   TTC
G     T     L     A     P     W     A     V     E     G     S     G     K     S     F
                                                        ^Signal Peptidase
                                                      120        cleavage site
AAA   GCT   GGA   GTC   TGT   CCT   CCT   AAG   AAA   TCT   GCC   CAG   TGC   CTT   AGA
K     A     G     V     C     P     P     K     K     S     A     Q     C     L     R
                        150                                                      180
TAC   AAG   AAA   CCT   GAG   TGC   CAG   AGT   GAC   TGG   CAG   TGT   CCA   GGG   AAG
Y     K     K     P     E     C     Q     S     D     W     Q     C     P     G     K
                                                      210
AAG   AGA   TGT   TGT   CCT   GAC   ACT   TGT   GGC   ATC   AAA   TGC   CTG   GAT   CCT
K     R     C     C     P     D     T     C     G     I     K     C     L     D     P
                        240                                                      270
GTT   GAC   ACC   CCA   AAC   CCA   ACA   AGG   AGG   AAG   CCT   GGG   AAG   TGC   CCA
V     D     T     P     N     P     T     R     R     K     P     G     K     C     P
                                                      300
GTG   ACT   TAT   GGC   CAA   TGT   TTG   ATG   CTT   AAC   CCC   CCC   AAT   TTC   TGT
V     T     Y     G     Q     C     L     M     L     N     P     P     N     F     C
                        330                                                      360
GAG   ATG   GAT   GGC   CAG   TGC   AAG   CGT   GAC   TTG   AAG   TGT   TGC   ATG   GGC
E     M     D     G     Q     C     K     R     D     L     K     C     C     M     G
                                                      390
ATG   TGT   GGG   AAA   TCC   TGC   GTT   TCC   CCT   GTG   AAA   GCT   TGA   ttc   ctg
M     C     G     K     S     C     V     S     P     V     K     A     END
                        420                                                      450
cca   tat   gga   gga   ggc   tct   gga   gtc   ctg   ctc   tgt   gtg   gtc   cag   gtc
                                                      480
ctt   tcc   acc   ctg   aga   ctt   ggc   tcc   acc   act   gat   atc   ctc   ctt   tgg
                        510                                                      540
gga   aag   gca   agc   aca   cag   cag   gtc   ttc   aag   aag   tgc   cag   ttg   atc
                                                      570
gaa   tgT   AAT   AAA   taa   acg   agc   cta   ttt   ctc   ttt   AAA   AAA   A
         polyadenylation signal
```

**Figure 3** Sequence of a parotid cDNA clone. Messenger RNA was purified from human parotid glands. Eight nanograms of cDNA ligated to *Eco*RI-digested and alkaline phosphatase–treated lambda gt10 was packaged in vitro (Vector Cloning Systems) and gave $7.7 \times 10^5$ recombinant phage when titered on *E. coli* C600 hflA. A clone was selected that hybridized to a 3.8 kb genomic fragment known to contain the coding region of SLPI.

Using constructed cDNA expression vectors, SLPI and SLPI variants have been produced in both prokaryotic and yeast expression systems. Expression in *E. coli* results in the production of a polypeptide chain identical in its sequence to the natural human inhibitor. The protein is accumulated intracellularly in an inactive form and can be partially recovered upon disruption of the cells. To establish the full specific activity and stability of the rhSLPI, the protein must be refolded. Production in *E. coli* and refolding provides virtually all of the rhSLPI available today (17,18).

Expression of active full- and half-length versions of SLPI in yeast has also been accomplished. Full-length SLPI expressed in *Saccharomyces cerevisiae*, using a common expression system and employing the invertase signal sequence,

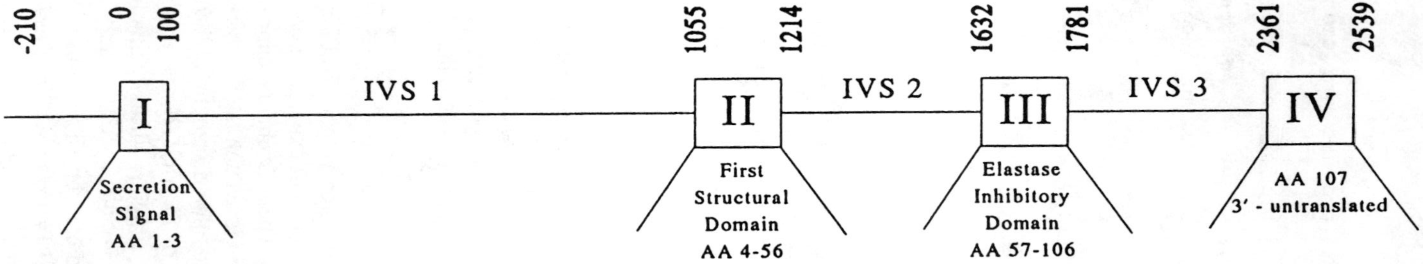


**Figure 4** Correlation of the functional domains of the SLPI protein with the organization of the SLPI gene. The top line shows the distance in base pairs from the proposed transcriptional initiation site. Each of the exons is contained within the boxed regions. IVS: intervening sequence; AA: amino acid positions in the mature protein. The precise length of the gene 5′ to the start of the protein-coding region is, as yet, undetermined. (From Ref. 14.)

resulted in both processed and unprocessed forms of SLPI, both of which remained associated with the cells. Complementary DNA expression of the second domain of SLPI in yeast produced a truncated version with elastase inhibitory activity. The lack of trypsin inhibitory activity in the 60 amino acid one-domain variant initially supported the hypothesis that the trypsin inhibitory function of SLPI was located in the N-terminal domain. Mutation analysis of rhSLPI produced in *E. coli*, however, later disproved this concept. Both trypsin and chymotrypsin inhibitory activities have been shown to reside in the C-terminal domain of rhSLPI.

## IV. Molecular Structure

The primary structure of SLPI is depicted in Fig. 1, which shows the twofold repeat homology indicative of separate domains. Based on similarities with other Kazal-type inhibitors, it was hypothesized that protease-interacting segments of the respective domains would be located between amino acids 18–29 in the N-terminal domain and 71–83 in the C-terminal domain. Using rhSLPI produced in *E. coli*, Grutter et al. (19) produced diffraction-quality crystals and obtained a three-dimensional structure for the molecule in complex with chymotrypsin. Based on the crystal structure of the SLPI chymotrypsin complex, Grutter assigned the P1 residue of the inhibitor enzyme complex to leucine 72 of the C-terminal domain.

The crystal structure of the SLPI chymotrypsin complex also served to unambiguously assign the disulfide-bonding pattern in rhSLPI. The secondary structure as assigned by this study is depicted in Fig. 5. In keeping with the intradomain disulfide bonding typical of Kazal inhibitors, the eight disulfide bonds with the SLPI molecule are constrained to four disulfides in each of the two separate domains.

Based on the analogies between Kazal inhibitors, the typical substrate specificity for interaction with the S1 site in trypsin, and the crystallographic studies of Grutter et al. (19), it was hypothesized that the trypsin inhibitory domain of SLPI would be located in the amino-terminal domain of SLPI. The most likely candidate for the P1 site in the substrate loop of this domain was arginine 20. Surprisingly, a series of mutational changes to the SLPI molecule reflected a dramatic insensitivity of this region to the inhibitory capacity of SLPI for trypsin. On the contrary, mutation of the C-terminal inhibitory loop dramatically affected the interaction of the SLPI with trypsin (20,21). A series of mutations of the putative enzyme interaction sites is depicted in Table 2. As can be seen, mutations of the P1 site, Leu-72, identified in the SLPI chymotrypsin complex to residues typifying P1 residues preferred in trypsin substrates, lower the inhibitory constant of SLPI for trypsin by several orders of magnitude. Mutation of the hypothesized enzyme inhibitory loop of the first domain was relatively without effect on the

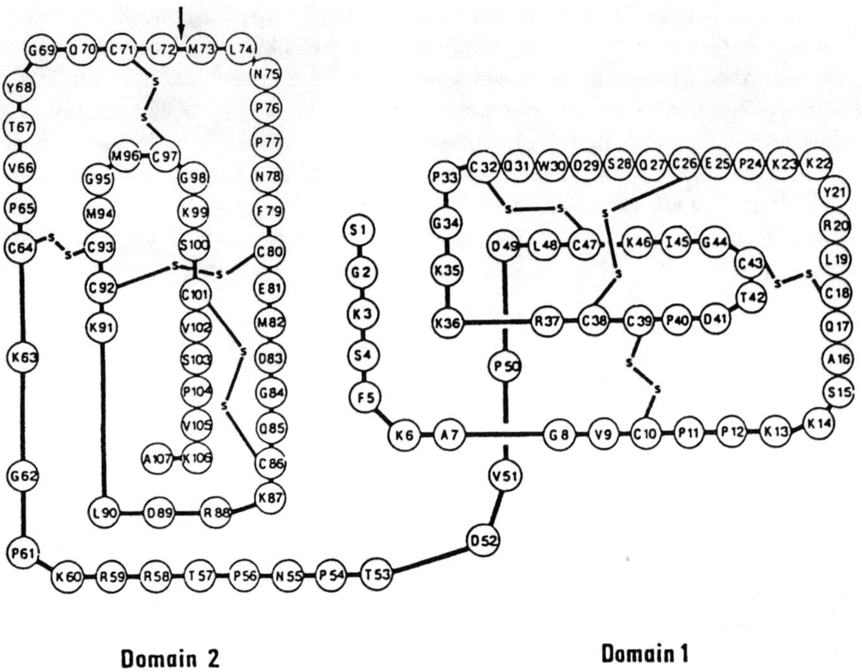


**Figure 5** Schematic representation of the secondary structure of SLPI as determined from x-ray diffraction studies.

**Table 2** Kinetic Dissociation Constants of SLPI Mutants

| Mutant | Chymotrypsin (nM) | Elastase (nM) | Trypsin (nM) |
|---|---|---|---|
| $Leu^{72}$ (wild-type) | 0.4 | 0.15 | 3.0 |
| $Gly^{72}$ | 700.0 | 6.5 | 1000.0 |
| $Phe^{72}$ | 0.01 | 70.0 | 0.3 |
| $Val^{72}$ | 27.0 | 0.4 | 110.0 |
| $Arg^{72}$ | 37.0 | >2500.0 | <0.001 |
| $Lys^{72}$ | 45.0 | 300.0 | <0.003 |
| $Gly^{73}$ | 65.0 | 0.4 | 950.0 |
| $Gly^{74}$ | 3.2 | 0.5 | 6.9 |
| $Gly^{20}$ | 0.5 | 0.5 | 4.5 |
| $Met^{20}$ | 0.1 | 0.1 | 2.0 |
| $Val^{20}$ | 0.1 | 0.1 | 3.8 |

*Source*: Adapted from ref. 20.

trypsin interaction. Chemical separation of the domains by acid hydrolysis of $Asp_{49}$–$Pro_{50}$ subsequently corroborated this result (22).

SLPI is sensitive to oxidative inactivation. Some site-directed mutagenesis has been used to study the effect of methionine oxidation on the inactivation of SLPI's inhibitory capacity. Rudolphus et al. (23) replaced methionine 73 within the enzyme-interaction loop with leucine, and found that the resultant protein was less susceptible to oxidative inactivation by a variety of chemical or cellular oxidative conditions. As in the above studies, the results of the oxidation-resistant variants of rhSLPI suggest that the inhibitory portion of the molecule is confined to the C-terminal domain.

## V. The Inhibitory Properties, Functional Role, and Turnover of SLPI

Ohlsson et al. (24) identified SLPI in parotid secretions and could show that it was present as a basic single-chain protein. We found the term secretory leukocyte proteinase inhibitor appropriate because it is secreted and inhibits leukocyte elastase and cathepsin G. SLPI was isolated from parotid secretions and used for peptide and amino acid sequencing (9) and cDNA sequencing (14). Native SLPI showed a $K_d$ of $2 \times 10^{-10}$ M for the elastase–SLPI complex and a $K_d$ of $5 \times 10^{-10}$ M for the cathepsin G–SLPI complex. The corresponding value for the SLPI complex with anionic human trypsin was determined to $4 \times 10^{-10}$ M (10). Despite the low $K_d$ value for the elastase–SLPI complex, both alpha 1-PI and alpha 2-M are able to rapidly dissociate and take over the elastase from this complex in vitro (25,26). The transfer of elastase from SLPI may also occur in vivo, at least at the alveolar level, where the molar level of alpha 1-PI is relatively high. This explains why SLPI is present only in its free form in human serum (27,28). When elastase–SLPI complexes reach the interstitial fluid and the blood circulation, the protease may exchange with the high amount of alpha 1-PI present. Elastase–alpha 1-PI complexes are regularly present in human blood (28). On the other hand, SLPI can effectively block the plasma protein digestion obtained when leukocyte elastase is added, or released from phagocytosing leukocytes, in excess of the available plasma proteinase inhibitors (29,30). Furthermore, SLPI, but not alpha 1-PI, has been shown to inhibit elastin-bound elastase (31). This capacity may be of biological importance for the preservation of the elastic lung tissues. SLPI has also recently been shown to inhibit mast-cell chymase and may thus also contribute to regulating the proteolytic enzymes of these cells, which are abundant in mucosal tissues (32). The data obtained for SLPI may be compared with those for another low-molecular-weight and acid-stable inhibitor, the pancreatic secretory trypsin inhibitor (PSTI), which is a potent trypsin inhibitor. The complexes between trypsin and PSTI are also rapidly dissociated on addition of human serum, the trypsin being taken over mainly by alpha 2-M (33).

SLPI is found in a number of secretions other than the bronchial mucus and parotid juice, including cervical mucus from the uterus and seminal plasma (34), nasal (35,36), and middle-ear secretions (37,38). Low concentrations (125 μg/L) of free SLPI are found in normal plasma (27), and these levels are increased 10-fold in patients suffering from pneumonia (39). The plasma level of SLPI does not increase after surgery or other trauma (26), indicating that SLPI is not an acute-phase reactant.

Following an intravenous injection of $^{125}$I-labeled native SLPI in human volunteers, a rapid initial clearance of both protein-bound and total plasma radioactivity (half-life 10 minutes) was seen (40). Later, the protein-bound radioactivity cleared more slowly (half-life 120 minutes) than the total radioactivity, indicating a progressive degradation of SLPI with release of radioactive fragments to plasma. After 54 hours, 80–96% of the radioactivity had been excreted in the urine, mainly as free $^{125}$I. No intact SLPI was found in the urine. Similar results were obtained after intravenous injection of $^{35}$S-labeled rSLPI in dogs. After killing at 3 hours, the kidneys contained more radioactivity per gram of tissue than any other parenchymal organ. A renal metabolism of SLPI is assumed, which is also supported by the finding of elevated serum levels of SLPI in uremic patients (40).

SLPI accounts for about 90% of the proteinase inhibitory capacity of normal bronchial secretions. In these, SLPI is found mainly in a free and active leukocyte elastase–binding form (41). Oxidized SLPI does not form stable complexes with leukocyte elastase (42). Complexes of SLPI with elastase are found in purulent bronchial secretions (39), which is consistent with the inhibitor exerting its protective effects locally rather than systematically. The total level of SLPI, free and complexed, is about 50 mg/L in the secretions. The ratio between free and complexed inhibitor varies with the purulency of the secretion. In the different secretions studied from respiratory (36,37,39) and genital tracts (34,43), the free inhibitor has also shown retained elastase-binding capacity. In patients with severe, acute bronchitis, however, free elastase activity is frequently seen in the purulent secretions of the respiratory tract (4–6,39).

## VI. Tissue Localizations of SLPI

The SLPI in bronchial mucus appears to be produced in the submucosal glands of the upper airways. Immunoreactive SLPI was originally localized to these structures using an indirect immunoperoxidase method (Fig. 6) (44). More recently, improved techniques have allowed increased resolution of morphological detail. SLPI production was localized to the serous cells of the submucosal glands of tracheal and bronchial mucosa (45–47). SLPI-producing cells have also been identified in the epithelium of the bronchioli in the so-called Clara cells (Fig. 7)

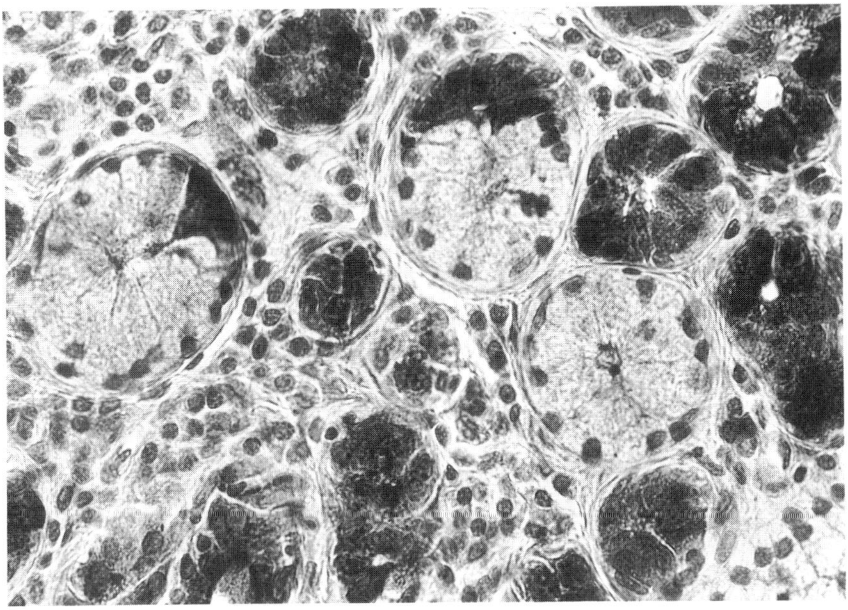

**Figure 6** Histological picture of a submucosal gland of human tracheal mucosa immunostained for SLPI. Note that only the serous portion of the gland, semilunar surrounding the negative mucus portions, reacts with the antibody and appears dark.

(48,49), suggesting that SLPI may have a role in protecting the distal respiratory tract from proteases. In vitro studies have shown that SLPI protects the ciliated epithelium from destruction by granulocyte proteases (50). Cigarette smoke inactivates SLPI in vitro (51), probably mainly via oxidation (42).

SLPI is present in effusions from acute and chronically infected middle ears at about 50 mg/L, as judged from a Mancini immunoassay (37). The inhibitor is largely free in chronic effusion with retained leukocyte elastase–binding capacity, but in acute otitis media it is present mainly in the form of a complex with proteinases (37). As indicated by the results of immunohistology of the tissues, SLPI is judged to be produced in the PAS-positive goblet-like cells of the surface epithelium and the submucosal glands and crypts (38). There are more of these cells and of cells containing SLPI in inflamed mucosa than in normal mucosa. Ciliated mucosal cells and stratified squamous epithelial cells are devoid of SLPI.

Undiluted nasal secretions contain levels of SLPI that range from 1 to 16 μmol/L; more than 90% was in a free and active form, while the rest was mainly in complex with leucocyte elastase (36). The highest concentration of alpha 1-PI noted in the same secretions was 0.6 μmol/L. Immunohistological examination of

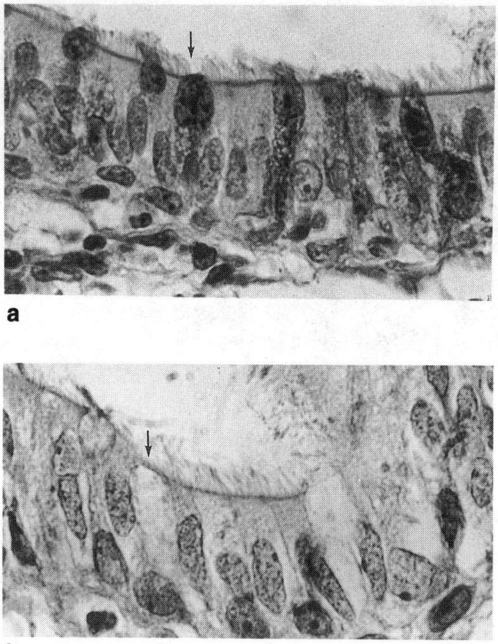

a

b

**Figure 7** (a) Human bronchiolar epithelium. Positive immunostaining for SLPI of the nonciliated secretory cells (arrow). (b) Control. Secretory cells (arrow).

the maxillary sinus mucosa indicates the presence of SLPI in the serous parts of the submucosal glands (44,46) and the PAS-positive goblet-like cells of the sinus mucosa.

SLPI is the only detectable leukocyte proteinase inhibitor in parotid secretions, and accounts for about 70% of the leukocyte proteinase–inhibiting capacity in mixed saliva. In the parotid secretions, all of the SLPI is free and active, but in mixed saliva about 15% is present in the form of a complex with leukocyte elastase (24). The proportion of the complexed form increases in periodontitis. SLPI is produced by the serous cells of the parotid (52) and submandibular glands (47,52), as judged from the results of immunohistological studies.

The location, structure, and pharmacology of SLPI argue that the physiological role of this protein is to buffer the extracellular protease–mediated effects of inflammatory leukocytes, especially neutrophils. In pathologies typified by large increases in the number of activated neutrophils in the affected organ, it may be therapeutically beneficial to supplement the endogenous protease inhibitory capacity with additional SLPI. The ability, through genetic engineering, to mass-produce rhSLPI has recently brought us to the point of testing this hypothesis in the clinic.

## References

1. Haendle H, Fritz H, Trautschold I, Werle E, Uber einen hormonabhangigen inhibitor fur proteolytische enzyme in mannlichen accessorischen geschlechtsdrusen und im sperma. Hoppe Seylers Z Physiol Chem 1965; 343:185–188.
2. Vogel R, Trautschold I, Werle E, eds. Natural Proteinase Inhibitors. New York: Academic Press, 1968.
3. Ohlsson K, Tegner H, Akesson U. Isolation and partial characterization of a low molecular weight acid stable protease inhibitor from human bronchial secretion. Hoppe Seylers Z Physiol Chem 1977; 358:583–589.
4. Opie EL. J Exp Med 1905; 7:316–334.
5. Lieberman J, Trimmer BM, Kurnic NB. Substrate specificity of protease activities in purulent sputum. Lab Invest 1965; 14:249–257.
6. Ohlsson K, Tegner H. Granulocyte collagenase elastase and plasma protease inhibitors. Eur J Clin Invest 1975; 5:221–227.
7. Wallner O, Fritz H. Characterization of an acid-stable proteinase in human cervical mucus. Hoppe Seylers Z Physiol Chem 1974; 355:709–715.
8. Schiessler H, Hochstrasser K, Ohlsson K. In: Havemmann K, Janoff A, eds. Neutral Proteases of Human Polymorphonuclearleucocytes. Baltimore: Urban and Schwarzenberg, 1978:197–207.
9. Thompson RC, Ohlsson K. Isolation, properties and complete amino acid sequence of human secretory leukocyte elastase. Proc Natl Acad Sci USA 1986; 83:6692–6696.
10. Heinzel R, Appelhans H, Gassen HG, Seemueller U, Arnhold M, Fritz H, Lottspeich F, Wiedenmann K, Machleidt W. In: Taylor JC, Mietmann CH, eds. Pulmonary Emphysema in Proteolysis. Orlando, FL: Academic Press, 1987:297–306.
11. Hochstrasser K, Reichert R, Schwarz R, et al. Isolierung und charakterisierung eines proteaseninhibitors aus menschluchen bronchialsekret. Hoppe Seylers Z Physiol Chem, 1972; 353:221–226.
12. Hochstrasser K, Reichert R, Heimburger N. Antigenic relationship between the human bronchial mucus inhibitor and plasma inter-alpha-trypsin inhibitor. Hoppe Seylers Z Physiol Chem 1973; 354:587–588.
13. Hochstrasser K, Relchert R, Werle E, Haenie H. In: Peters H, ed. Proteids of the Biological Fluids—20th Colloquium, 1973:417–424.
14. Ohlsson K, Rosengren M, Stetler G, Brewer M, Hale KK, Thompson RC. In: Taylor JC, Mittman C, eds. Pulmonary Emphysema and Proteolysis. New York: Academic Press, 1986:307–322.
15. Sanger F, Coulson AR. A rapid method for determining sequences in DNA by primed synthesis with DNA polymerase. J Mol Biol 1985; 94:441–448.
16. Stetler F, Brewer MT, Thompson RC. Isolation and sequence of a human gene encoding a potent inhibitor of leukocyte proteases. Nucleic Acids Res 1986; 14:7883–7896.

17. Seely RJ, Young MD. In: Georgiou G, De Bernandez-Clark E, eds. Protein Refolding. ACS Symposium Series. Vol 470. American Chemical Society, 1991:206–216.
18. Kohno T, Carmichael DF, Sommer A, Thompson RC. Refolding of recombinant proteins. Methods Enzymol 1990; 185:187–195.
19. Grutter M, Fendrich F, Huber R, Bode W. The 2.5 Å x-ray crystal structure of the acid stable proteinase inhibitor from human mucus secretions analyzed in its complex with bovine alpha-chymotrypsin. EMBO J 1988; 7:345–351.
20. Eisenberg SP, Hale KK, Heimdal P, Thompson RC. Location of the protease-inhibitory region of secretory leukocyte protease inhibitor. J Biol Chem 1990; 265: 7976–7981.
21. Meckelein B, Nikiforov T, Clemen A, Appelhans H. The location of inhibitory specificities in human mucus proteinase inhibitor (MPI): Separate expression of the COOH-terminal domain yields an active inhibitor of three different proteinases. Protein Eng 1990; 3:215–220.
22. Van-Seuningen I, Davril M. Separation of the two domains of human mucus proteinase inhibitor: inhibitory activity is only located in the carboxy-terminal domain. Biochem Biophys Res Commun 1991; 179:1587–1592.
23. Rudolphus A, Heinzel-Wieland R, Vincent VAMM, Saunders D, Steffens GJ, Dijkman JH, Kramps JD. Oxidation resistant variants of recombinant antileucoprotease are better inhibitors of human-neutrophil-elastase-induced emphysema in hamsters than natural recombinant antileucoprotease. Clin Sci 1991; 81:777–784.
24. Olsson M, Rosengren M, Tegner H, Ohlsson K. Quantitation of granulocyte elastase inhibitors in human mixed saliva and in pure parotid secretion. Hoppe Seylers Z Physiol Chem 1983; 364:1323–1328.
25. Gauthier F, Fryksmark U, Ohlsson K, Bleth JG. Kinetics of the inhibition of leukocyte elastase by the bronchial inhibitor. Biochim Biophys Acta 1982; 700:178–183.
26. Fryksmark U, Ohlsson K, Rosengren M, Tegner H. The studies on the interaction between leukocyte elastase, antileukoproteinase and the plasma proteinase inhibitors alpha 1-proteinase inhibitor and alpha 2-macroglobulin. Hoppe Seylers Z Physiol Chem 1983; 364:793–800.
27. Fryksmark U, Ohlsson K, Rosengren M, Tegner H. A radioimmunoassay for measurement and characterization of human antileukoprotease in serum. Hoppe Seylers Z Physiol Chem 1981; 362:1273–1277.
28. Ohlsson K, Olsson AS. Immunoreactive granulocyte elastase in human serum. Hoppe Seylers Z Physiol Chem 1978; 359:1531–1539.
29. Bjork P, Axelsson L. Bergenfeldt M, Ohlsson K. Influence of plasma protease inhibitors and the secretory leucocyte protease inhibitor on leucocyte elastase-induced consumption of selected plasma proteins in vitro in man. Scand J Clin Lab Invest 1988; 48:205–211.
30. Axelsson L, Linder C, Ohlsson K, Rosengren M. The effect of the secretory leukocyte protease inhibitor on leukocyte proteases released during phagocytosis. Biol Chem Hoppe Seyler 1988; 369:89–93.
31. Bruch M, Bieth JG. Influence of elastin on the inhibition of leucocyte elastase by alpha 1-proteinase inhibitor and bronchial inhibitor: Potent inhibition of elastin-bound elastase by bronchial inhibitor. Biochem J 1986; 238:269–273.

32. Fritz H. Human mucus proteinase inhibitor (human MPI), human seminal inhibitor-I (HUSI-I) antileukoprotease (ALP), secretory leukocyte protease inhibitor (SLPI). Biol Chem Hoppe Seyler, 1988; 369:79–82.
33. Eddeland A, Ohlsson K. Purification and immunochemical quantification of human pancreatic secretory trypsin inhibitor. Scand J Clin Lab Invest 1978; 38:261–267.
34. Schliessler H, Arnhold M, Ohlsson K, Fritz H. Inhibitors of acrosin and granulocyte proteinases from human genital tract secretions. Hoppe Seylers Z Physiol Chem 1976; 357:1251–1260.
35. Hochstrasser K, Haendle H, Reichert R, Werle E. Uber vorkommen und eigenschaften eines proteaseininhibitors in menschlichem nasensekret. Hoppe Seylers Z Physiol Chem 1971; 352:954–958.
36. Fryksmark U, Jannert M, Ohlsson K, Tegner H, Wihl JA. Secretory leukocyte protease inhibitor in normal, allergic and virus induced nasal secretions. Rhinology 1989; 27:97–103.
37. Carlsson B, Lundberg C, Ohlsson K. Protease inhibitors in middle ear effusions. Ann Otol Rhinol Laryngol (St Louis) 1981; 90:38–41.
38. Carlsson B, Ohlsson K. Localization of antileukoprotease in middle ear mucosa. Acta Otolaryngol (Stockholm) 1983; 95:111–116.
39. Fryksmark U, Prellner T, Tegner H, Ohlsson K. Eur J Respir Dis (Copenhagen) 1984; 65:201–209.
40. Bergenfeldt M, Bjork P, Ohlsson K. The elimination of secretory leukocyte protease inhibitor (SLPI) after intravenous injection in dog and man. Scand J Clin Lab Invest 1980; 50:729–737.
41. Tegner H. Quantitation of human granulocyte protease inhibitors in non-purulent bronchial lavage fluids. Acta Otolaryngol (Stockholm) 1978; 85:282–289.
42. Kramps JA, Willems LNA, Franken C, Dijkman JH. Antileukoprotease: its role in the human lung. Biol Chem Hoppe Seyler 1988; 369:83–87.
43. Casslen B, Rosengren M, Ohlsson K. Localization and quantitation of a low molecular weight proteinase inhibitor, antileukoprotease, in the human uterus. Hoppe Seylers Z Physiol Chem 1981; 362:953–961.
44. Tegner H, Ohlsson K. Localization of a low molecular weight protease inhibitor to tracheal and maxillary sinus mucosa. Hoppe Seylers Z Physiol Chem 1977; 358:425–429.
45. Ohlsson K. Interactions between granulocyte proteases and protease inhibitors in the lung. Bull Eur Physiopathol Respir 1980; 16:209–222.
46. Fryksmark U, Ohlsson K, Polling A, Tegner H. Distribution of antileukoprotease in upper respiratory mucosa. Ann Otol Rhinol Laryngol (St Louis) 1982; 91:268–271.
47. Kramps JA, Franken C, Meijer CJLM, Dijkman JD. Localization of low molecular weight protease inhibitor in serous secretory cells of the respiratory tract. J Histochem Cytochem (Baltimore) 1981; 29:712–719.
48. Ohlsson K, Fryksmark U, Ohlsson M, Tegner H. Interaction of granulocyte proteases with inhibitors in pulmonary disease. Adv Exp Med Biol 1984; 167:299–312.
49. de Water R, Willems LNBA, van Muljen GNP, Franken C, Fransen JAM, Dijkman JH, Kramps JA. Ultrastructural localization of bronchial antileukoprotease in central and peripheral human airways by a gold-labeling technique using monoclonal antibodies. Am Rev Respir Dis 1986; 133:882–890.

50. Ohlsson K, Bergenfeldt M, Bjork P. Functional studies of human secretory leukocyte protease inhibitor. Adv Exp Med Biol 1988; 240:123–131.
51. Ohlsson K, Fryksmark U, Tegner H. The effect of cigarette smoke condensate on alpha 1-antitrypsin, antileukoprotease and granulocyte elastase. Eur J Clin Invest 1980; 10:373–379.
52. Ohlsson M, Fryksmark U, Polling A, Tegner H, Ohlsson K. Localization of antileukoprotease in the parotid and the submandibular salivary glands. Acto Otolaryngol (Stockholm) 1984; 98:147–151.

# Part Three

## CLINICAL MANIFESTATIONS

# 14

# Laboratory Diagnosis of α1AT Deficiency

**MARK BRANTLY**

Pulmonary–Critical Care Medicine Branch
National Heart, Lung, and Blood Institute
National Institutes of Health
Bethesda, Maryland

## I. Introduction

The laboratory diagnosis of alpha 1–antitrypsin (α1AT) deficiency began in 1963 when C. B. Laurell and S. Eriksson, using a combination of paper electrophoresis, agar-gel electrophoresis, and immunoelectrophoresis, determined the association of familial emphysema with the absence of the alpha 1–globulin band (1). The use of starch-gel electrophoresis to evaluate the electrophoretic polymorphism in the prealbumin region led to the identification of the multiallelic Pi (protease inhibitor) system. Subsequently, these techniques were replaced by isoelectric focusing (IEF) of serum in polyacrylamide gels, which provides better α1AT band resolution (2). The development of immobilized pH gradients (IPG) in the early 1980s further increased the resolution between minor pH differences to 1/100 of a pH unit, making it possible to separate variants that have only minor pH differences (3). The cloning and DNA sequencing of the α1AT cDNA, and later the genomic segment, provided the DNA-sequence information necessary to identify practically the genotypes of individuals (4,5).

## II. Current Approach to the Laboratory Diagnosis of α1AT Deficiency

The current approach to the laboratory diagnosis of α1AT deficiency includes using a combination of the serum α1AT level and the α1AT IEF pattern at pH 4–5. Careful storage and transport of serum or plasma are critical to the accurate identification of α1AT phenotypes, particularly rare alleles with questionable stability at room temperature. In this context, our laboratory routinely encourages transport of samples on wet ice for clot tubes or whole blood, or on dry ice for serum or plasma. To prevent degradation of samples in the laboratory, samples should be divided into small working volumes and stored at temperatures at or below −70°C (6).

## III. Determination of Serum α1AT Antigenic Concentration

The α1AT concentration is typically determined by radial immunodiffusion, nephelometry, or rocket immunoelectrophoresis. Since all are immunologically based indirect methods of determining the α1AT concentration within a pool of proteins, accuracy of all these assays is based on the reference serum used to compare with unknown samples (6). Until very recently, clinical standards used to evaluate serum α1AT concentrations tended to overestimate the actual concentration of α1AT by as much as 35% (7). Additionally, standards among laboratories tended to vary substantially (7). To increase the reproducibility and accuracy of α1AT serum concentration determination, our laboratory, in conjunction with the USA α1AT Deficiency Registry, developed a serum standard based on purified α1AT (7). Utilizing this standard and isoelectric focusing, ranges and mean α1AT serum concentrations were established for the common phenotypes (see Fig. 4 in Chapter 4) (7).

Screening of large populations of individuals for α1AT deficiency has become practical with the development of automated fluorescent-based assays based on either function or actual level. However, caution must be exercised when interpreting the α1AT concentration in neonates because their mean α1AT levels at the time of birth are substantially below those of adults. In 200 neonates studied utilizing cord blood, 175 (87.5%) were PI*M, 6 (3%) PI*MZ, 16 (8%) PI*MS, and 3 (1.5%) were rare PI types. The average α1AT level of all neonates, regardless of PI type, was 23.8 ± 5.5 μM, normal PI*M 23.8 ± 5.2 μM, PI*MZ 14.3 ± 1.7 μM, and PI*MS 19.2 ± 4.8 μM. Comparison of normal adult α1AT serum levels (normal 32.7 ± 8.7 μM) to those of neonates reveals significant differences by two tailed *t*-test ($p < 0.0001$). Thus, in the context that α1AT serum levels are significantly lower in neonates than in adults, population screening for α1AT deficiency utilizing neonatal screening should be based on norms established specifically for neonates (8).

Finally, nephelometric assays commonly used by most clinical laboratories on occasion significantly overestimate serum α1AT concentration because of interference of lipids or hemoglobin. In this context, when samples appear turbid or hemolyzed, radial immunodiffusion or rocket immunoelectrophoresis may provide the most accurate result (6).

## IV. Quantification of α1AT Concentration by Neutrophil Elastase Inhibitory Capacity

As the major protease inhibitor in the serum, α1AT is responsible for the majority of the trypsin and elastase inhibitory capacity. Several studies have demonstrated an excellent correlation between the antigenically determined amount of α1AT and the "functional" amount of α1AT present in sera. Studies using trypsin or porcine elastase inhibitory capacity have largely been abandoned by most investigators and replaced by the more specific substrate, neutrophil elastase. Because alpha 2–macroglobulin also contributes to serum inhibition of neutrophil elastase, most assays now include methylamine to inactivate alpha 2–macroglobulin prior to assaying for neutrophil elastase inhibitory capacity. The antineutrophil elastase capacity is quantified by titrating increasing amounts of serum against a fixed amount of titrated standard of purified human neutrophil elastase (Athens Research and Technology). After incubation at 24°C for 30 minutes, the residual elastase activity is measured as absorbance at 410 nm, using the neutrophil elastase substrate methoxy-succinyl-ala-ala-pro-val-nitroanilide (Sigma Chemical) (6,9).

## V. Determination of α1AT Phenotypes by Isoelectric Focusing

Currently, the most practical method for identification of α1AT phenotypes utilizes separation of α1AT variants according to their differences in isoelectric point using thin-layer IEF gels over the pH range of 4–5 with or without immunoblot (Fig. 1). Routine IEF is performed on thin-layer polyacrylamide gels prepared on 0.5 mm U-frame 125 × 260 mm glass plates from 4.70% acrylamide, 0.15% bis, 9.85% glycerol, 3.6% of ampholytes pH 4.2–4.9, 1.2% of ampholytes pH 4–5, and 0.58 mM N-(2-acetamido)-2-aminoethanesulfonic acid (ACES). Polymerization is obtained by adding 6.55 μl/ml of a 10% ammonium persulfate solution and 1 μl/ml of N,N,N′, tetramethylethylenediamine (TEMED) (Bio-Rad). Anolyte is prepared from 25 mM L-aspartic acid and L-glutamic acid, and catholyte is prepared from 0.25 M glycine. Electrophoresis strips are soaked with their respec-

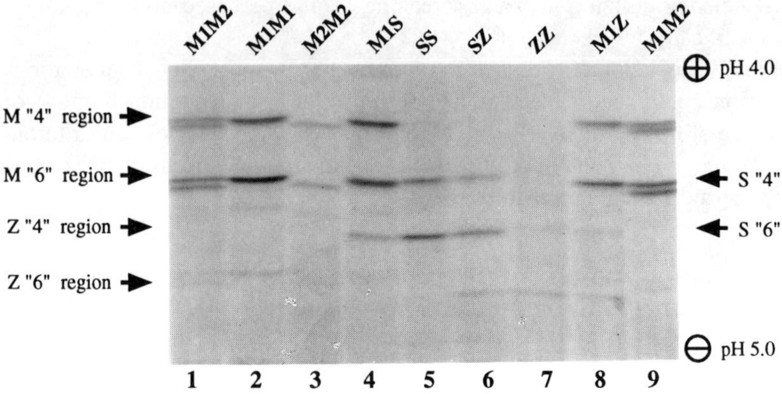


**Figure 1** Thin-layer polyacrylamide gel electrophoresis of α1AT variants. (Top) α1AT phenotypes. (Left) M″4″, M″6″, Z″4″, and Z″6″ major band migration areas. (Right) S″4″ and S″6″ major band migration areas. (See Fig. 1 in Chapter 4 for details on band identification.) Anode (+), pH 4.0. Cathode (−), pH 5.0. Lanes 1–3 and 9 are normal phenotypes. Lane 7 (ZZ) is the most common deficient variant. Lane 5 (SS) is a common deficiency phenotype associated with slightly reduced α1AT levels. Lanes 8 (M1Z) and 4 (M1S) are heterozygous for deficient variants. Lane 6 (SZ) is heterozygous for two common deficiency alleles. Migration-pattern differences are due largely to amino acid substitutions in the mature α1AT protein that alter the net charge of α1AT, hence changing the isoelectric point (pI) (the point at which net charge on the protein is zero and the protein cannot migrate farther in an electric field).

tive solutions. Prior to running the samples, the gel is prefocused for 1 hour at 2000 volts, 75 milliamps, and 5 watts. Serum proteins are reduced with 0.05 M dithiothreitol (DTT) and 8 μl of serum is applied to sample application pads. Samples are electrophoresed for 3 hours at 2000 volts, 75 milliamps, and 10 watts on a Multiphor II (Pharmacia-LKB) system horizontal water bed at 10.5°C. The gels are fixed for 30 minutes at room temperature in an 11.5% trichloroacetic acid (TCA), 0.16 M 5-sulfosalicylic acid solution and stained with a 0.25% w/v Coomassie blue G250 (Bio-Rad) solution dissolved in 37.9% ethanol, 12.1% glacial acetic acid destaining solution at 65°C for approximately 3 minutes (6, 10–12).

Immunoblot may be necessary when there are reduced amounts of stainable α1AT or if there is concern as to whether Coomassie-stained bands on the gel are indeed α1AT. Immunoprint fixation can be accomplished using standard IEF or IPG by making a "print" or "blot" of the gel prior to fixation by overlaying a 0.45 μ nitrocellulose membrane for 15 minutes. The membrane is then "blocked" with 3% gelatin (Bio-Rad) in Tris-buffered saline (20 mM Tris, 500 mM NaCl, pH 7.5) and incubated in the presence of 1/100 dilution of rabbit antihuman α1AT for 30 minutes (Accurate Chemical & Scientific Corp.). The gel is washed for 30 minutes in Tris-buffered saline, and incubated with gold conjugate (Bio-Rad); the membrane can then be fixed or silver lactate (Bio-Rad) can be added for further enhancement of faint bands (6,10–14).

To further accentuate the separation among α1AT variants, immobilized pH gradient (IPG) IEF gel can be utilized (Fig. 2). To accomplish this, gels are prepared on 0.5 mm U-frame 200 × 258 mm glass plates with 3.74% acrylamide, 0.16% bis, 12.5% glycerol w/v, 20.1 mM buffering immobiline pK 4.6, and 10.5 mM nonbuffering immobiline pK 9.3. The gels are polymerized with 1 μl/ml of a 40% ammonium persulfate solution and 0.6 μl/ml of TEMED (Bio-Rad). The polymerized gel is treated sequentially with 25% glycerol and 20% glycerol solutions for 30 minutes. Prior to electrophoresis, the gel is immersed in a 25% glycerol, 0.25% ampholytes pH 4–5 solution for 90 minutes. Electrophoresis strips are soaked with their respective solutions. Anolyte solution is composed of 10 mM glutamic acid and the catholyte solution is composed of 10 mM NaOH. Serum proteins are reduced with 0.05 M DTT and 20 μl of reduced serum sample is applied directly onto gel. The gel is prerun at 300 volts, 15 milliamps, and 5 watts for 1 hour, after which the conditions are changed to 5000 volts, 15 milliamps, and 5 watts and the run is continued for 18 hours. The IPG gel is fixed for 1 hour at room temperature in 11.5% TCA, 0.16 M 5-sulfosalicylic acid

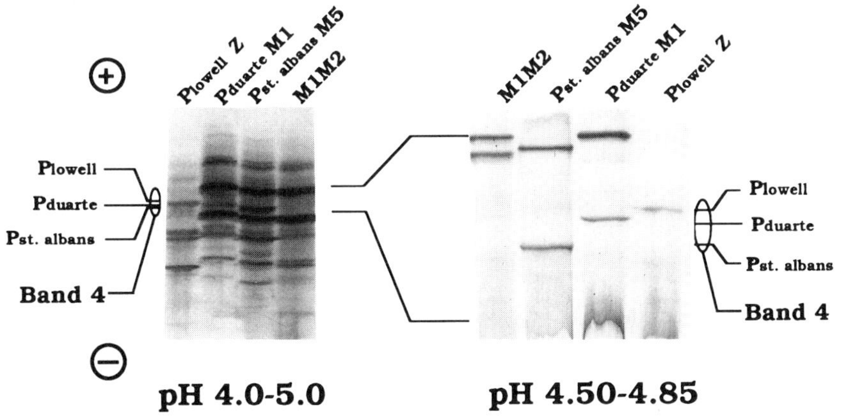


**Figure 2** Comparison of α1AT resolution on ampholyte and immobilized pH gradients. (Left) ampholyte isoelectric gel of P variants, pH range 4.0–5.0. (Right) immobilized pH gradient of P variants, pH range 4.50–4.85. Top, anode (+); bottom, cathode (−). Right and left, circled: the major 4 bands of $P_{lowell}$, $P_{duarte}$, and $P_{st.\ albans}$.

solution and stained with 0.5% w/v Coomassie blue dissolved in 37.9% ethanol and 12.1% glacial acetic acid at 65°C for approximately 5 minutes (3,11).

High-quality standards are essential to accurate identification of phenotypes. Our laboratory standards include PI*M1M2, PI*SZ, and PI*Z samples on each of our gels and we routinely repeat unknown samples twice on the same gel to assure a reproducibility of the migration pattern. Standard IEF under the conditions described above are able to differentiate the normal variants PI*M1, M2, and M3. Separation of the PI*M4 and M5 most often require IPG gel electrophoresis, which distinguishes subtle differences in migration (Fig. 2).

## VI. Pedigree Analysis to Determine α1AT Variants

Analysis of very low-level or nonexpressing α1AT variants can be substantially enhanced by using family studies to determine the presence and transmission of an allele that is not identified by standard protein-detection methods. Furthermore, confirmation of the presence of an abnormal allele in a kindred adds power to the accuracy of the diagnosis of any one individual since the same parental alleles can be examined in several different combinations.

## VII. Molecular Approaches to the Identification of α1AT Alleles

### A. DNA Sequence Analysis of α1AT Variants

By 1988, 14 α1AT variants had been determined by gene or protein sequencing; as of 1995 there are at least 51 characterized variants (Tables 1–3 in Chapter 4). This growth in the number of genotypically defined variants is due largely to the use of DNA sequencing and the application of the polymerase chain reaction to unknown variants. One successful approach has been to utilize genomic DNA as a template for generation of double-strand DNA utilizing PCR amplification. Using this approach, leukocytes obtained from the proband's whole blood is used for the preparation of high-molecular-weight genomic DNA using Plasmagel (Cellular Products) leukocyte separation reagent followed by serial treatment with proteinase K and then by extraction with phenol, chloroform, precipitation in ethanol, and resuspension in 10 mM Tris, 1 mM ethylenediaminetetraacetic acid (EDTA). Amplification of exons Ic–V and intron flanking regions, including regulatory, splice-junction, and polyadenylation regions, is accomplished using genomic DNA as a template, with oligonucleotides flanking key elements of the α1AT gene (Fig. 3 and Table 1). The PCR reaction is accomplished using Thermus Aquaticus (Taq) DNA polymerase (Perkin-Elmer) in a DNA thermal cycler (Perkin-Elmer) for 30 cycles at 94°C for 1 minute, 54°C for 2 minutes, and 72°C for 3 minutes. Double-strand PCR products are separated by agarose-gel electrophoresis, ex-

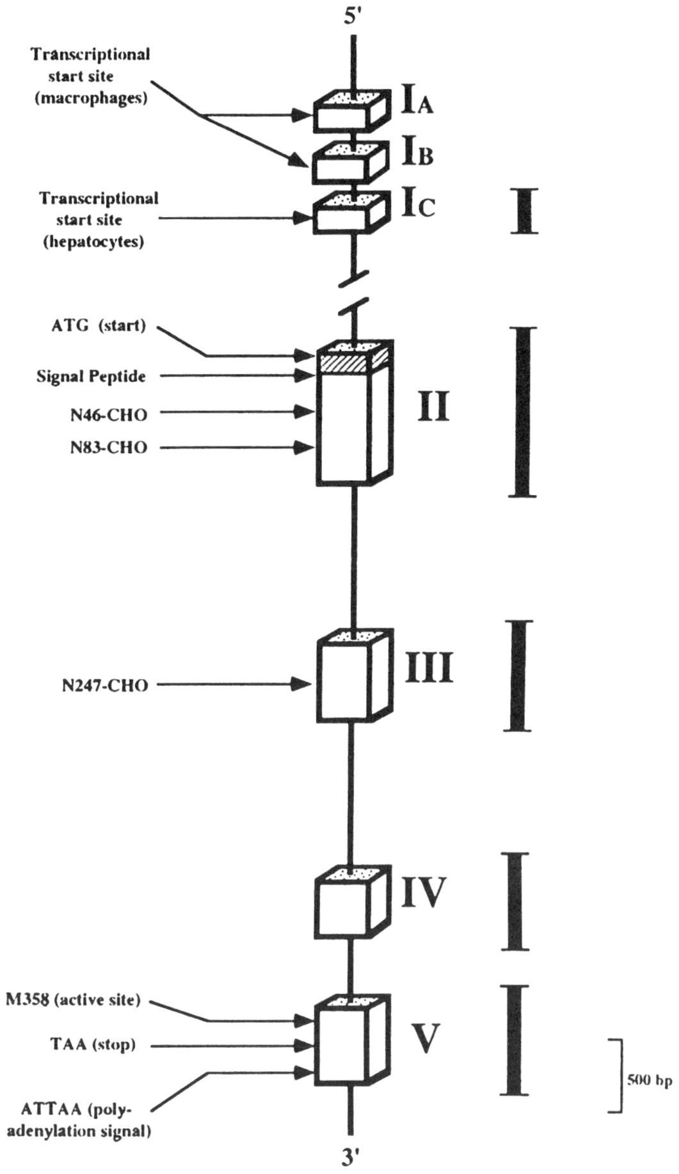


**Figure 3** DNA-sequencing strategy for novel α1AT variants. Boxes represent exons (IA–V), and vertical lines between boxes represent introns. (Left) regions of importance in gene and protein expression. (Right) dark vertical bars denote regions of the α1AT gene that are amplified and sequenced. Reference distance (500 bp) at lower right.

**Table 1** α1AT Exon PCR Primers

| Primer[a] | Sequence[b] | Exon[c] | Direction[d] |
|---|---|---|---|
| PC1M | CTACCAGTGGAACAGCCACTAAGGAT | I | 5′ |
| PC1P | CCCTGCACCTCAGCAGGCGGATAC | I | 3′ |
| NSP1M | TCTGCAGTGAGAGCAGAGGGCCAG | I | 5′ |
| NSP1P | CTCCAGAACCCCTCGCAGTGAAAG | I | 3′ |
| 2M3 | ACGTGGTGTCAATCCCTGATCACTG | II | 5′ |
| PC2P | GAGTTCAAGAACTGATGGTTTGAG | II | 3′ |
| NSP2M | GTCATCATGTGCCTTGACTCGGGCCT | II | 5′ |
| NSP2P | CTATGGGAAACAGCTCAGGCTGGTTG | II | 3′ |
| PC3M | CATGGTTTCTTATTCTGCTACACT | III | 5′ |
| 3PE1 | GAGACCTTTACCTCCTCACCCTGGGA | III | 3′ |
| NSP3M | CTTCCAAACCTTCACTCACCCCTGGT | III | 5′ |
| NSP3P | GTCCTCATGGAGCATGGACGGCG | III | 3′ |
| PC4M | CACTTGCACTGTGGTGGGTCCCAG | IV | 5′ |
| PC4P | TTCTTCCCTACAGATACCATGG | IV | 3′ |
| NSP4M | GCTGTGCCATGCCTTGAATTTC | IV | 5′ |
| NSP4P | CAAGGTCGTCAGGGTGATCTC | IV | 3′ |
| PC5M | GAGCCTTGCTCGAGGCCTGGGATC | V | 5′ |
| 5P3 | CAGAGAAAACATGGGAGGGATTTACA | V | 3′ |
| NSP5M | CTTACAACGTCTCTCTGCTTC | V | 5′ |
| NSP5P | CAGATCACATGCAGGCAGGGAC | V | 3′ |

[a]NSP indicates a nested primer.
[b]Sequence is written 5′ → 3′.
[c]Indicates which exon is amplified.
[d]5′ = 5′ upstream primer; 3′ = 3′ downstream primer.

tracted, and then used as a template for the generation of single-stranded DNA by means of the asymmetric primer extension method (Table 2) (11,17). PCR-generated single-stranded DNA is then purified using Centricon 30 (Amicon) and used as a template for either sense or antisense DNA sequencing by dideoxy-chain termination using Sequenase (United States Biochemical). [$^{35}$S]-labeled DNA is separated on a standard 6% polyacrylamide, 8 M urea gel, dried, and autoradiographed (11,15–18).

Using this general approach allows for direct sequencing of both α1AT alleles simultaneously and makes it particularly easy to identify heterozygotes since there are two bands at the level of the gene mutation, as is illustrated by sequencing the PI*M1P$_{duarte}$ individual (Fig. 4).

### B. Rapid Genotypical Identification of α1AT Genes

Once the sequence is known for a specific mutation, it is possible to identify most of these mutations rapidly using either allele-specific amplification (ASA) or

**Table 2** α1AT Sequencing Primers

| Primer | Sequence[a] | Exon[b] | Direction[c] |
|---|---|---|---|
| E1M1 | CTGCAGTGAGAGCAGAGG | I | 5′ |
| E1MO | TCGGTAAGTGCAGTGGAA | I | 5′ |
| E1p1 | AACCCCTCGCAGTGA | I | 3′ |
| E1P2 | TTAAGCAGTGGATCCAGA | I | 3′ |
| E2M1 | CCTTGACTCGGGCCT | II | 5′ |
| E2M2 | CAGAAGACAGATACATCC | II | 5′ |
| 2M9 | CTACAGCCTTTGCAATGC | II | 5′ |
| E2M4 | TCCAGCTGACCACCG | II | 5′ |
| E2M5 | CAGATCAACGATTACGTG | II | 5′ |
| E2p1 | TGGGAAACAGCTCAG | II | 3′ |
| E2P2 | TCCCTTGAGTACCCT | II | 3′ |
| E2P3 | AACTTATCCACTAGC | II | 3′ |
| E2P4 | GCATTGCAAAGGCTGTAG | II | 3′ |
| E2P5 | TATAGGCTGAAGGCGA | II | 3′ |
| E3M1 | TCACTCACCCCTGG | III | 5′ |
| E3M2 | GGCATGTTTAACATCC | III | 5′ |
| E3P1 | ATGGCTAAGAGGTGT | III | 3′ |
| E3P2 | CCTTCACGGTGGTCA | III | 3′ |
| E4M1 | AACAAGAAGACCTG | IV | 5′ |
| E4M2 | AGCAATGGGGCTGAC | IV | 5′ |
| E4P1 | CTACAGATACCATGG | IV | 3′ |
| E4P2 | AGTTGACCCAGGACGC | IV | 3′ |
| E5M1 | GCCTTACAACGTGTCT | V | 5′ |
| E5M2 | AATGATTGAACAAAAT | V | 5′ |
| E5P1 | AGAAAACATGGGAGGG | V | 3′ |
| E5P2 | TTCACCACTTTTCCC | V | 3′ |

[a]Sequence is written 5′ → 3′.
[b]Indicates in which exon the primer is located.
[c]5′ = 5′ upstream primer; 3′ = 3′ downstream primer.

PCR-based restriction-fragment-length polymorphism analysis. Limitations of these methods are based on the generation or loss of a restriction site in the case of restriction-fragment-length polymorphism (RFLP) analysis or the absence of extensive reiteration of sequence at the mutation site in the case of allele-specific amplification. Additionally, the products of digestion or amplification need to be easily identified by gel electrophoresis.

One of the most useful techniques for quickly identifying genotypical differences is ASA. To use ASA in the identification of a genotype, two primers are designed that differ only at their 3′ end and reflect the base difference between the two alleles. To begin efficient amplification, DNA Taq polymerase requires

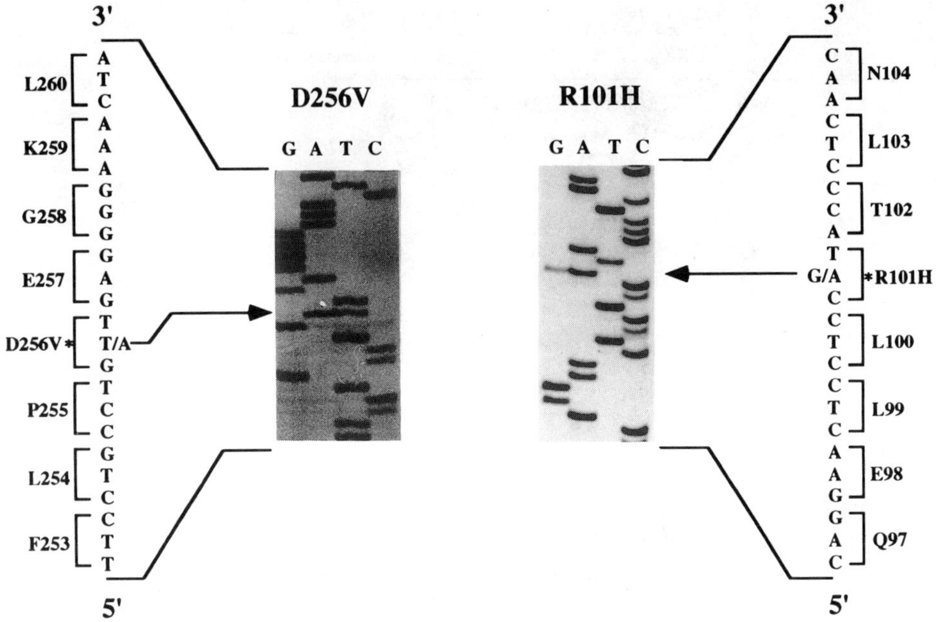


**Figure 4** DNA sequencing gel of the novel variant $p_{duarte}$. Autoradiograms of α1AT $P_{duarte}$ DNA sequence. Above each autoradiogram is the amino acid substitution and above each lane are the bases represented (G, A, T, and C). On the outside of each autoradiogram is the DNA sequence with the predicted one-letter-code amino acid sequence. The bold arrow denotes the base substitution and the asterisk (*) represents the amino acid substitution. The $P_{duarte}$ allele differs from the common normal M1(V213) allele by two point mutations, which in turn result in two amino acid substitutions. They include a mutation in exon III in codon D256(GAT)→V256(GTT) and a mutation in exon II in codon R101(CGT)→H101(CAT).

complete complementarity between the 3′ end of the primer and its complement. In addition, a common primer is designed to be 3′ to the primers located at the mutation site and should be far enough from the mutation site to be identified by gel electrophoresis following amplification. Using this general approach, it is possible to identify several α1AT alleles, including the most common deficiency allele, PI*Z (Fig. 5 and Table 3) (18).

Identification of RFLPs involves the amplification of all or a portion of the exon containing the mutation, digesting the amplified DNA fragment with the appropriate restriction endonuclease and separating the digested fragments according to their molecular mass in agarose. One example of this approach is the

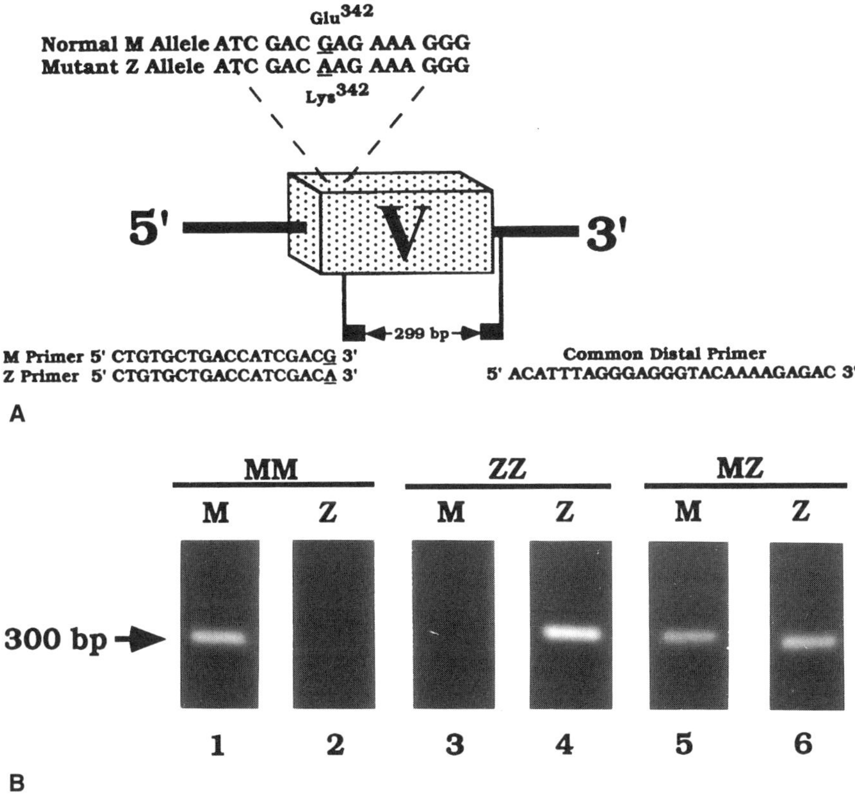


**Figure 5** Detection of the α1AT Z genotype by allele-specific amplification. (A) Schematic of Z α1AT gene allele-specific amplification. The box depicts exon V of the α1AT gene. Above exon V, the DNA sequence surrounding the Z mutation compared with the sequence of the normal M allele. By using the polymerase chain reaction and proximal primers that differ at the 3′ end terminating with the site of the mutation, in combination with a common distal primer, amplification of the specific allele (M or Z) occurs only when there is an identical match in an individual's gene sequence surrounding the mutation site. When there is an exact match at the 3′ end, a DNA fragment of 299 bp is amplified that can be identified by gel electrophoresis. (B) Agarose gel of allele-specific amplified DNA fragments separated by electrophoresis from individuals with the MM (lanes 1 and 2), ZZ (lanes 3 and 4), and MZ (lanes 5 and 6) genotypes. The specific primers used are shown above the lanes (M or Z), right, approximate molecular weight in base pair (bp). The normal MM individual has a 300 bp fragment only with the M primer (lane 1). The deficient ZZ individual shows a 300 bp fragment only with the Z primer (lane 4). The heterozygous individual has 300 bp fragments with both the M and Z primers (lanes 5 and 6).

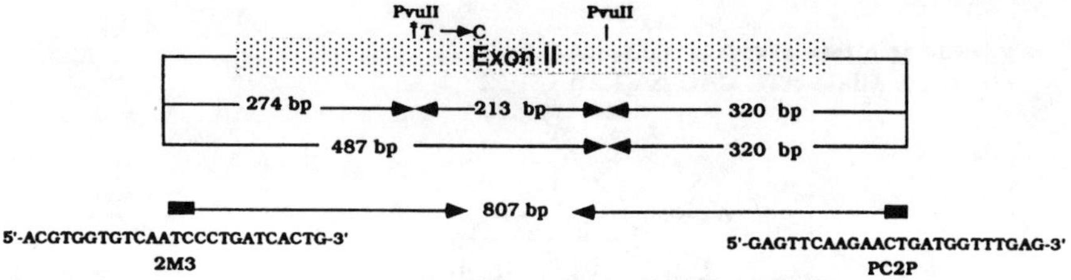
PvuII
T → C
PvuII
Exon II
274 bp
213 bp
320 bp
487 bp
320 bp
807 bp
5'-ACGTGGTGTCAATCCCTGATCACTG-3'
2M3
5'-GAGTTCAAGAACTGATGGTTTGAG-3'
PC2P

A

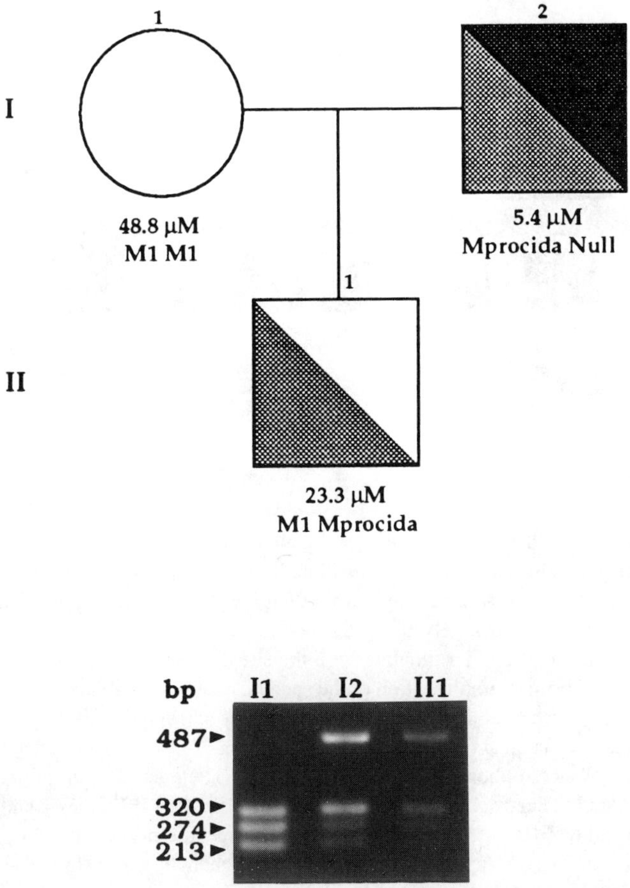
1
2
I
48.8 μM
M1 M1
5.4 μM
Mprocida Null
1
II
23.3 μM
M1 Mprocida
bp
I1
I2
II1
487
320
274
213

B

identification of the $M_{procida}$ allele using the loss of the restriction endonuclease site PvuII (Fig. 6). Alleles that can be identified by RFLP include $M_{procida}$, M1(V213), M1(A213), M3, and $QO_{new\ hope}$ (19).

## VIII. Strategies for Identifying Novel α1AT Variants

The easiest way to identify novel α1AT alleles is by first defining the variant at the protein level. Any changes in the pI of the protein are likely due to changes in the amino acid sequence and hence localize the mutation to the exons. Carbohydrate abnormalities often observed in carbohydrate-deficiency disorders, hepatic disorders, and cystic fibrosis may significantly alter the migration pattern of α1AT by virtue of their effect on the attachment and/synthesis of charged carbohydrate side chains.

In individuals suspected of being carriers for a null allele, our laboratory first screens for known null mutations using ASA and then directly sequences exon V, the location of the mutational hotspot for PI*clayton, bolton, and saarbruecken. If this screening approach does not identify known null mutations or very-low-α1AT-level variants, we proceed to sequence all exons and exon–intron junctions (Fig. 3). Other approaches include the use of single-strand conformational polymorphism and denaturing gradient-gel electrophoresis (20,21). Both these techniques have the advantage of quickly screening all critical gene segments, but in general they are best suited for screening larger numbers of individuals for potential mutations.

---

**Figure 6** Detection of the α1AT $M_{procida}$ genotype using a restriction-fragment-length polymorphism. (A) Schematic map of exon II cut with the restriction endonuclease PvuII. Shaded region represents exon II; above it are the 2 PvuII restriction endonuclease sites of the normal α1AT gene sequence. Inheritance of the $M_{procida}$ allele is associated with the loss of a PvuII site (*) because of the substitution of a thymidine for a cytosine (T→C) (Table 2 in Chapter 4). Below exon II are the predicted sizes of DNA fragments with (closest to Exon II) PvuII cut site and without the PvuII cut site. At the bottom are the primers and overall size of the fragment amplified by polymerase chain reaction prior to digestion with PvuII. (B) Identification of the $M_{procida}$ allele in a pedigree using agarose-gel electrophoresis of exon II digested with PvuII. (Top) two-generation pedigree (I, II). Below each individual is the α1AT level in μM and the α1AT genotype. Lightly shaded region is $M_{procida}$ allele; white are normal alleles; and darkly shaded area represents a null allele. (Bottom) Agarose gel with DNA fragments separated by molecular weight. Top of gel, individuals by pedigree number; left, molecular weight (bp) of digested PvuII-digested DNA. Individual I1 is homozygous for Leu41; family members I2 and II1 have one Leu41 and one Pro41 allele (see Table 2 and Fig. 3 in Chapter 4 for details about the $M_{procida}$ variant).

**Table 3** α1AT Allele-Specific Amplification Primers

| ASA primer | ASA primer sequence[a] | Distal primer sequence[b] | PCR product size (bp) | α1AT allele[b] |
|---|---|---|---|---|
| NHK-N | CCTCTGTGACCCCGGAGA | ACTTGCACTGTGGTGGGTCCCAG | 210 | hong kong |
| NHK-M | CCTCTGTGACCCCGGAGG | | | |
| Bel-W | TGGACCAGGTGACCACCGTGA | GACCTTTACCTCCTCACCCTGGGA | 290 | bellingham |
| Bel-M | TGGACCAGGTGACCACCGTGT | | | |
| Mat-N | AGCTGCTGGGGCCATGTTTTTA | AGAAAACATGGGAGGGATTTACA | 515 | mattawa |
| Mat-M | AGCTGCTGGGGCCATGTTTTTT | | | |
| Z-N | CTGTGCTGAACCATCGACG | ACATTTAGGGAGGGTACAAAAGGC | 299 | Z |
| Z-M | CTGTGCTGAACCATCGACA | | | |
| Trast-N | TTCCCCTCTCTCCAGGCAAATG | GAGACCTTTACCTCCTCACCCTGA | 515 | trastevere |
| Trast-M | TTCCCCTCTCTCCAGGCAAATA | | | |
| GF-W | CAAGAAACAGATCAACGATTC | GAGTTCAAGAACTGATGGTTTGAG | 200 | granite falls |
| GF-M | CAAGAAACAGATCAACGATTG | | | |

[a]Sequence is written 5′ to 3′, the "wild-type" allele specific amplification (ASA) primer is listed first for each pair, underlined bases correspond to the single-base mutational differences of the α1AT wild-type and mutant alleles.
[b]Indicates the name of the α1AT allele identified by the corresponding ASA primers.

## IX. Conclusion

Identification of the α1AT-deficient individual begins most often with a high index of suspicion in the office or at bedside and is confirmed in the laboratory. Advances in the identification of α1AT variants, both phenotypically and genotypically, provide the clinician and the basic researcher with powerful tools to identify and better understand this inherited disease.

## References

1. Laurell C, Eriksson S. The electrophoretic α1-globulin pattern of serum in α1-antitrypsin deficiency. Scand J Clin Laboratory Invest 1963; 15:132–140.
2. Fagerhol MK. The Pi-system: Genetic variants of serum alpha-1-antitrypsin. Series Haematologica 1968; 1(1):153–161.
3. Gorg A, Postel W, Weser J, Patutschnick W, Cleve H. Improved resolution of PI (alpha 1-antitrypsin) phenotypes by a large-scale immobilized pH gradient. Am J Hum Genet 1985; 37(5):922–930.
4. Kurachi K, Chandra T, Degen SJ, et al. Cloning and sequence of cDNA coding for alpha 1-antitrypsin. Proc Natl Acad Sci USA 1981; 78(11):6826–6830.
5. Long GL, Chandra T, Woo SL, Davie EW, Kurachi K. Complete sequence of the cDNA for human alpha 1-antitrypsin and the gene for the S variant. Biochemistry 1984; 23(21):4828–4837.
6. Talamo R, Bruce R, Langley C, et al. Alpha-1-antitrypsin Laboratory Manual. Department of Health Education and Welfare pub. no. NIH 78-1420. Bethesda, MD: National Institutes of Health, 1978:1–129.
7. Brantly ML, Wittes JT, Vogelmeier CF, Hubbard RC, Fells GA, Crystal RG. Use of a highly purified alpha 1-antitrypsin standard to establish ranges for the common normal and deficient alpha 1-antitrypsin phenotypes. Chest 1991; 100(3):703–708.
8. Birrer P, Rundquist B, Wirtz-Sommer C, Brantly M. Establishment of an accurate normal range of serum alpha-1-antitrypsin concentration in cord blood of healthy newborns. Am Rev Resp Dis 1992; 145:A342.
9. Wewers M, Casolaro M, Sellers S, et al. Replacement therapy for alpha-1-antitrypsin deficiency associated with emphysema. N Engl J Med 1987; 316:1055–1062.
10. Constans J, Viau M, Gouaillard C. PiM4: an additional PiM subtype. Hum Genet 1980; 55:119–121.
11. Hildesheim J, Kinsley G, Bissell M, Pierce J, Brantly M. Genetic diversity from a limited repertoire of mutations on different common allelic backgrounds: α1-antitrypsin deficiency variant $P_{duarte}$. Hum Mutation 1993; 2:221–228.
12. Kueppers F. Determination of alpha 1-antitrypsin phenotypes by isoelectric focusing in polyacrylamide gels. J Lab Clin Med 1976; 88(1):151–155.
13. Arnaud P, Wilson GB, Koistinen J, Fudenberg HH. Immunofixation after electrofocusing: improved method for specific detection of serum proteins with determination of isoelectric points. I. Immunofixation print technique for detection of alpha-1-protease inhibitor. J Immunol Methods 1977; 16(3):221–231.

14. Boutin B, Ferg S, Arnaud P. The genetic polymorphism of alpha 2-HS glycoprotein: Study by ultrathin-layer isoelectric focusing and immunoblot. Am J Hum Genet 1985; 37:1098–1105.
15. Holmes MD, Brantly ML, Fells GA, Crystal RG. Alpha 1-antitrypsin $W_{bethesda}$: molecular basis of an unusual alpha 1-antitrypsin deficiency variant. Biochem Biophys Res Commun 1990; 170(3):1013–1020.
16. Holmes MD, Brantly ML, Curiel DT, Weidinger S, Crystal RG. Characterization of the normal alpha 1-antitrypsin allele $V_{munich}$: a variant associated with a unique protein isoelectric focusing pattern. Am J Hum Genet 1990; 46(4):810–816.
17. Holmes MD, Brantly ML, Crystal RG. Molecular analysis of the heterogeneity among the P-family of alpha-1-antitrypsin alleles. Am Rev Respir Dis 1990; 142(5):1185–1192.
18. Okayama H, Holmes MD, Brantly ML, Crystal RG. Characterization of the coding region of the normal M4 alpha-1-antitrypsin gene. Biochem Biophys Res Comm 1989; 162(3):1560–1570.
19. Takahashi H, Nukiwa T, Satoh K, et al. Characterization of the gene and protein of the alpha-1-antitrypsin "deficiency" allele $M_{procida}$. J Biol Chem 1988; 263(30):15528–15534.
20. Billingsley G, Cox D. Rare deficiency alpha-1-antitrypsin variants: current status and SSCP analysis. Am J Hum Gen 1994; 55(3):A212.
21. Dubel JR, Finwick R, Hejtmancik JF. Denaturing gradient gel electrophoresis of the alpha 1-antitrypsin gene: application to prenatal diagnosis. Am J Med Genet 1991; 41(1):39–43.

# 15

# Clinical Manifestations of α1AT Deficiency

**NOEL G. McELVANEY**

Pulmonary and Critical Care Medicine Branch
National Heart, Lung, and Blood Institute
National Institutes of Health
Bethesda, Maryland

**RONALD G. CRYSTAL**

The New York Hospital–Cornell Medical Center
New York, New York

## I. Introduction

Alpha 1–antitrypsin (α1AT) deficiency, one of the most common lethal hereditary disorders affecting Caucasians of European descent, is characterized by a marked reduction in serum levels of α1AT and a high risk for the development of emphysema by ages 30–40 years (1–5). There is also a lesser risk for the development of liver disease (3,5,6) and, very rarely, individuals with α1AT deficiency develop panniculitis (1,3,7). α1AT deficiency was first noted in Sweden in 1963, when Laurell and Eriksson described five individuals lacking an alpha 1–globulin band in electrophoretic analysis of serum, three of whom had significant pulmonary disease. Although the allelic frequency of the Z mutation, the most common mutation associated with the deficiency state, is between 0.01 and 0.02 in North American Caucasians (3,8–12) and 0.02 and 0.03 in northern Europeans (3,13,14), the number of individuals definitively diagnosed with α1AT deficiency in these regions is far short of expected, suggesting that many individuals with the condition are either undiagnosed or misdiagnosed.

Much still needs to be learned about the natural history and clinical course of this disease, but there is no doubt that α1AT deficiency is associated with decreased survival (15,16). This decreased survival is particularly apparent in individuals with α1AT deficiency who have symptoms and/or a history of cigarette smoking and is mainly due to impaired lung function. The destructive lung disease associated with α1AT deficiency results in a greater than normal annual decline of lung function, including the forced expiratory volume in 1 second ($FEV_1$) and diffusing capacity, resulting eventually in death from either respiratory failure or its cardiovascular completions (13,15).

## II. Lung Disease Associated with α1AT Deficiency

### A. Epidemiology of Emphysema in α1AT Deficiency

The emphysema associated with α1AT deficiency is mainly a disease of Caucasians in their third to fourth decade, the majority of whom have a history of cigarette smoking (2,16,17–19). Most studies show a preponderance of males (2,16,17–19), but this probably reflects the fact that more males than females smoke cigarettes, and the disparity is changing as smoking increases among females. α1AT deficiency is rare among southern Europeans (Z allelic frequency 0.009) and among African Americans (Z allelic frequency 0.004), and is almost unknown among Asian populations (20–23). It is estimated that α1AT deficiency accounts for approximately 2% of the cases of emphysema seen by clinicians in the United States (24).

### B. Phenotypes Associated with α1AT Deficiency

While the normal serum α1AT levels range from 20 to 53 μM [in individuals homozygous for the M allele (25)], an α1AT level <11 μM is associated with a high risk for the development of emphysema. Over 20 α1AT alleles associated with this severity of α1AT deficiency have been described (4,5), but the most common, accounting for over 95% of the total, is the Z allele. Individuals homozygous for the Z allele usually have an α1AT level in the region of 5 μM (25) and are at risk for the development of emphysema, liver disease, and panniculitis (3–7).

The next most common allele associated with deficiency is the S allele, which, although more common than the Z allele (allelic frequency 0.02–0.04), is not as often associated with α1AT deficiency. This is because S homozygotes have serum levels of α1AT sufficient to protect the lung. However, if the S allele is inherited in combination with the Z allele, serum levels may range from 10 to 23 μM (25), and approximately 10% of these individuals develop emphysema, particularly if they have a history of smoking (2,5). The remainder of the deficiency alleles (see Refs. 3–5) are extremely rare.

There is still some dispute as to whether individuals heterozygote with the MZ or MS phenotypes are prone to develop emphysema. Studies into this question have usually been of two types. First, several studies have asked what the α1AT phenotype is of individuals with emphysema. These studies generally show no difference in the incidence of the MS phenotype in individuals with emphysema compared to the normal population, but have occasionally shown an increased incidence of the MZ phenotype in the emphysema population (26–28). Second, there are studies directed at the evaluation of pulmonary function tests in individuals with MS or MZ phenotype. These studies generally show little difference between these two groups and the normal control populations (29–31). While the disparity between these two different types of study are confusing, the general consensus is that MS and MZ individuals carry little increased risk for the development of emphysema, particularly if they do not smoke.

### C. Clinical Features of α1AT Deficiency in the Lung

Symptoms suggestive of emphysema in α1AT deficiency usually become apparent between the third and fourth decade (2,3,5,19). Occasionally symptoms can begin in the early teens or as late as 50–60 years of age, but this is uncommon (2,3,19). Usually, individuals with a history of cigarette smoking develop symptoms at an earlier age than nonsmokers, with a mean age of diagnosis approximately one decade earlier than in nonsmokers (16). The usual presenting symptoms are shortness of breath; wheezing, with or without upper-respiratory-tract infection; cough; sputum production; and frequent chest infections (2,3,19). There is often a history of "allergies" or "asthma," and as many as 25% of adults with α1AT deficiency have reactive airway disease (19,32–34), which seems to be more common in those with severe disease. The reasons for this reactive-airways component are unclear but may be related to the lack of protease protection in the lungs of these individuals. In this regard, both human polymorphonuclear neutrophils and rat peritoneal macrophages have been shown to synthesize and release platelet-activating factor, a potent mediator of inflammation and bronchoconstriction following stimulation by proteases such as neutrophil elastase, an effect that is inhibited by addition of α1AT (35). Furthermore, compared to normal macrophages, macrophages from α1AT-deficient individuals release more leukotriene B4, a potent mediator of inflammation and a product of arachidonic-acid metabolism (36).

On examination, the physical signs in clinically apparent α1AT-deficiency emphysema are similar to those in non-α1AT-deficiency emphysema. Occasionally, the decreased breath sounds may be most marked in the lower-lung regions in α1AT deficiency, but, in general, lung auscultation does not help in identifying α1AT-deficiency-associated emphysema. The chest is large, with an increased anterior–posterior diameter, poorly moving diaphragm on inspiration, and distant heart sounds (2,3,19). Expiratory wheeze is heard in about 15–20% of individuals (32–34).

### D. Morphology of the Lungs in α1AT Deficiency

The morphological changes in the lungs of individuals with α1AT deficiency are not pathognomonic. Classically, there is diffuse panacinar emphysema with enlargement of the airspaces distal to the terminal bronchioles. There may be lower-lobe predominance of these changes, but often the whole lung is involved (13,37).

### E. Chest Roentgenogram

Chest roentgenography classically shows hyperinflation with an anterior diaphragmatic angle greater than 90 degrees on lateral view and an increased retrosternal airspace (>3.5 cm; see Fig. 1). Decreased lung markings are present, mainly in the lower zones, consistent with loss of vascularity, and lung destruction (2,13,19,38–40), in contrast to the preponderance of upper-zone disease in non-α1AT-deficiency emphysema. A decreased cardiothoracic ratio (<0.5) is also common, along with convexity of the main pulmonary artery (19,40). Bullae may be present in as many as 50% of symptomatic adults with α1AT deficiency (2,3,19).

### F. Lung Function

Lung function tests at time of presentation are typical of emphysema (2,13,19, 34,41). Both $FEV_1$ and forced vital capacity (FVC) are decreased, typically with a markedly decreased $FEV_1$-to-FVC ratio. The flow–volume curves are usually abnormal, with marked decrease in flow with decreasing lung volumes, typically evidenced by coving of the expiratory portion of the curve. Slow vital capacity is usually mildly reduced and usually greater than FVC (2,19). Lung-volume measurements typically show increased total lung capacity (TLC) and residual volume. TLC as measured by body plethysmography is usually greater than that measured by helium dilution (19), which is consistent with the concept that these individuals have areas of lung that are poorly ventilated. Diffusing capacity is moderately reduced. Arterial blood gases show mild hypoxemia, and mild hypocarbia with a normal pH (1,2–5,19,34). As the disorder progresses, and $FEV_1$ becomes severely reduced, $CO_2$ retention occurs.

### G. Ventilation–Perfusion Scanning

Ventilation-perfusion (V/Q) scanning dramatically illustrates the basilar predilection of α1AT deficiency, particularly in its early to middle manifestations (Fig. 2).

---

**Figure 1** Chest roentgenograms of an individual with α1AT deficiency. (A) posteroanterior view showing hyperinflation, increased lucency in both bases and decreased cardiothoracic ratio. (B) lateral view showing flattened diaphragms, increased retrosternal airspace, and increased anterior diaphragmatic angle.

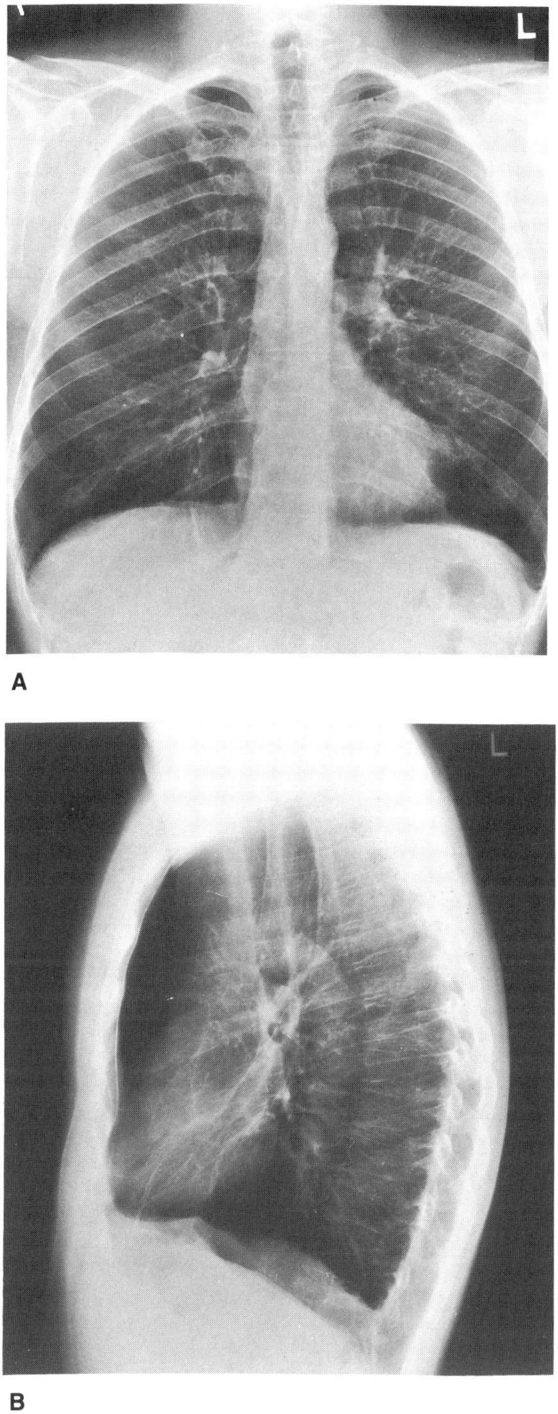


A

B

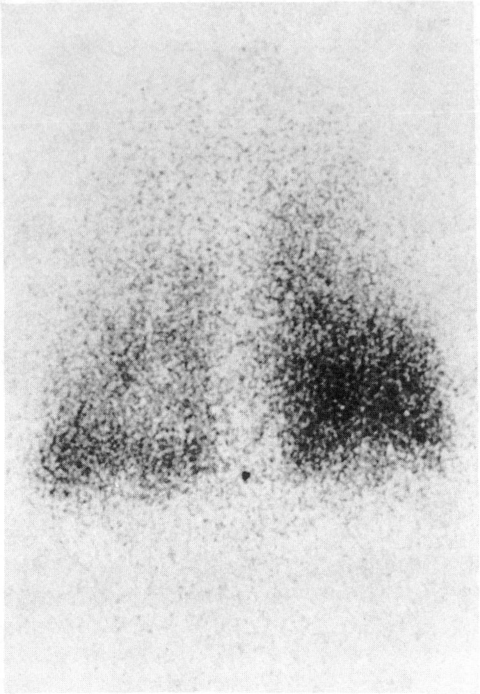

A

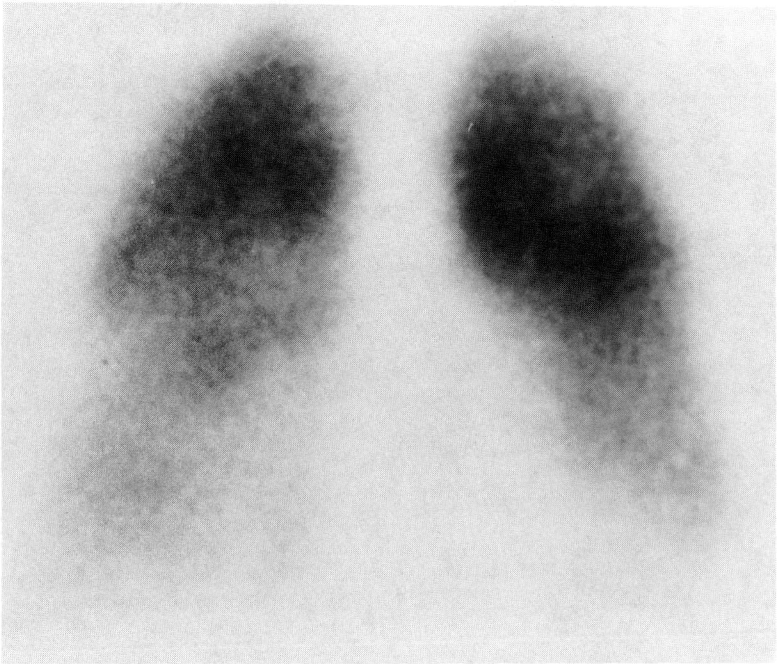

B

Typically, the V/Q scan shows symmetrical distribution of $^{133}$xenon throughout all zones of the lung during the equilibrium phase followed by a symmetrical delay in washout, most prominent in the lung bases and midzones (19,42). A symmetrical loss of pulmonary arterial perfusion is also found, most marked in the bases (19,42–44). V/Q scanning may be a useful tool in detection of early changes associated with α1AT deficiency, as even individuals with relatively normal lung function may have abnormal V/Q scans (43,44). One drawback with this method, however, is the difficulty in differentiating between holdup of radioactive tracer in the washout phase due to lung destruction and that due to bronchoconstriction.

### H. Chest Computed Tomography

Chest computed tomography (CT) scanning is rapidly gaining favor as a useful modality in the diagnosis of emphysema and may be useful for detecting the early pulmonary manifestations of α1AT deficiency (44,45). The classic findings in individuals with α1AT deficiency are loss of parenchymal markings, large airspaces, and bullae (Fig. 3). CT scans have some advantages over V/Q scans in detecting early changes in α1AT deficiency in that the parenchymal abnormalities on CT scan can be more readily specified as lung destruction than in V/Q scanning. The emphysematous changes seen on CT scan can also be quantified, and the rest of the lung parenchyma can be evaluated for evidence of non-α1AT-related lung problems. A number of studies have shown the utility of CT scanning in detecting lung parenchymal abnormalities in individuals with α1AT deficiency prior to pulmonary-function abnormalities or symptomatic deterioration (44,45). Furthermore, in individuals with pulmonary-function abnormalities, there are close correlations between $FEV_1$ (% predicted) or DLCO (% predicted) and emphysema "scores" generated from CT scans (44,45).

### I. Pulmonary Circulation

The pulmonary circulation is also adversely affected by α1AT deficiency. Pulmonary hypertension occurs due to loss of alveolar capillary bed, particularly in those with advanced pulmonary disease. This is corroborated by the high number of abnormal perfusion scans in this population (19,42–44) and the increased incidence of right-heart strain and right-axis deviation on electrocardiography (19,46). Pulmonary angiography shows a paucity of arborization and decreased

---

**Figure 2** Ventilation and perfusion scintigraphic scans of the chest of an individual with α1AT deficiency. The patient is viewed from the back in both scans. (A) $^{133}$Xe scan 3 minutes after washout. Whereas in normal individuals the radioactive tracer would be gone, in α1AT deficiency there is retention of gas in areas of lung destruction, mainly in the lower lung zones. (B) $^{99m}$Tc-macroaggregated albumin scan in the same individual. There is decreased perfusion of the lung bases secondary to lung destruction, with diversion of blood flow to the upper zones.

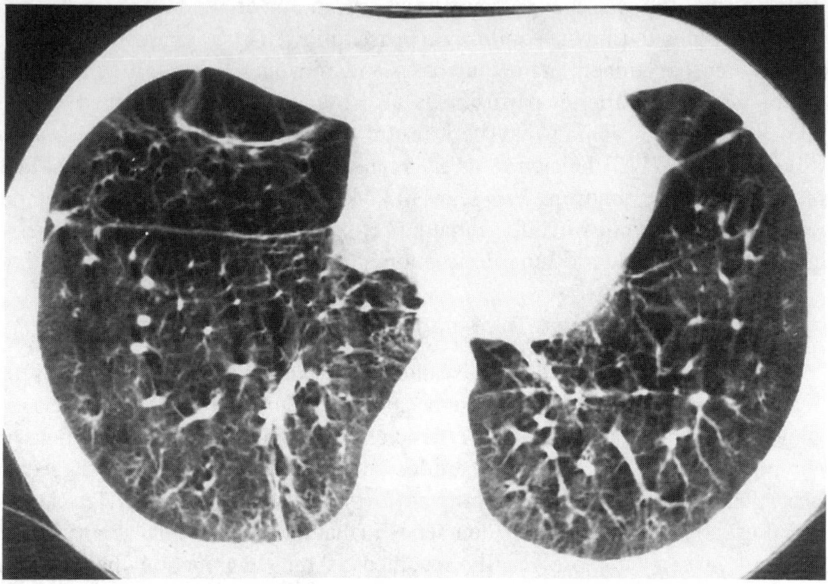

**Figure 3** Thin-section computed axial tomography scan of the chest of an individual with α1AT deficiency. There is widespread destruction, evidenced by large areas of hypolucency and bulla formation bilaterally.

pulmonary capillary blood flow, consistent with the observation of increased pulmonary-artery pressure and right-ventricular work (47).

### J. Exercise

Individuals with α1AT deficiency and evidence of lung impairment usually complain of difficulty with even mild to moderate amounts of exercise. The most striking exercise abnormality in these individuals is that of gas exchange. While in normal individuals the $Pao_2$ may not change, or slightly increase, on exercise, individuals with α1AT deficiency show markedly decreased $Pao_2$ and increased alveolar–arterial oxygen difference even with mild exercise. In one study, the estimated $Pao_2$ at 1 L/min $O_2$ consumption (mild work) was 41 torr (48). These changes occurred at such low levels of $O_2$ demand that none of the individuals became acidotic at the maximal work achieved, presumably because the patients were able to meet the exercise-imposed increase in $O_2$ demand by extracting more $O_2$ from blood (cardiac output is not limiting at these exercise levels). However, with higher levels of exercise, the low $Pao_2$ in these patients will cause $O_2$ delivery to be insufficient to meet demand, resulting in acidosis.

Individuals with α1AT deficiency have increased respiratory rates at rest, and on mild exercise rapidly reach >80% of their predicted maximal voluntary ventilation, suggesting that problems with ventilation could become a limiting factor at higher work levels. As might be expected with a condition associated with airflow problems, the ratio of dead space to tidal volume ($V_D/V_T$) is increased at rest in individuals with α1AT deficiency (48). While this ratio decreases with exercise in normal individuals (49,50), in individuals with α1AT deficiency it may occasionally increase or, more commonly, remain abnormally high, even at maximal exercise levels (48). Because individuals with α1AT deficiency usually have mild hypocarbia at rest and continue to have hypocarbia on moderate exercise, given their likely ventilatory limitation at higher work levels, due to a reduced tidal volume and an inability to improve the $V_D/V_T$ ratio, it is likely that they might not be able to remove $CO_2$ if greater demands are placed on the system. However, such ventilatory limitations are usually theoretical, as the exercise capacity in these individuals is so markedly reduced even at mild exercise levels.

### K. Lung Disease and Cigarette Smoking

Cigarette smoking has an important adverse effect on the lung disease associated with α1AT deficiency (2,13,15,18,51). In a Swedish study of α1AT-deficient individuals with a history of smoking, it was found that only 30% and 18% of females and males, respectively, were alive at age 55 (15), compared to 98% of nonsmoking females and 65% of nonsmoking males. Consistent with these observations, in a study in the United States in which almost all the subjects had a history of smoking, α1AT-deficient adults with pulmonary symptomatology had a 52% probability of survival to 50 years and only a 16% probability of survival to 60 years, compared to a cumulative probability of survival for adults in the total population (age >20 years, combined male and female data for 1980) of 92% survival to 50 years and 85% survival to 60 years (19). The reduced life expectancy for individuals with this condition who smoke is further emphasized by a study in Britain (2) showing, with multiple regression analysis, that smoking was the only factor of importance in the progress of this condition; other factors—such as age, sex, and occupational exposure to dust and fumes—were not.

## III. Liver Disease Associated with α1AT Deficiency

The association between α1AT deficiency and liver disease was first reported by Sharp and colleagues in 1969 (52). Although all the initial cases were in children, it soon became apparent that the liver disease could also affect adults (3,6). α1AT deficiency, which is now recognized as the most common hereditary liver disease, occurs in some form in approximately 10% of all neonates with the Z homozygous form of α1AT deficiency (53,54). The incidence of clinically relevant liver disease in adults with α1AT deficiency is not clear. In adults cirrhosis associated with α1AT deficiency may occur without any preceding history of childhood liver disease (3,6,55). In one study of autopsy records from over 35,000 recorded autopsies, 17 patients with α1AT deficiency were found (6); of these, eight had cirrhosis and five had hepatocellular carcinoma. As might be expected, the clinical syndromes associated with the liver disease in α1AT deficiency in children differ from the manifestations in adults.

### A. Clinical Manifestations of α1AT Deficiency in Children

In children, α1AT deficiency usually presents as a neonatal hepatitis syndrome with cholestasis, although hepatomegaly without jaundice has been reported. About 45% of affected neonates are small for gestational age, suggesting some intrauterine effects of the α1AT deficiency state (3,54,55). Physical signs of cholestasis appear between 4 days and 2 months after birth and can last for up to 8 months. The cholestasis can be severe enough to cause acholic stools, and the disease is easily confused with biliary atresia (3,55). Spontaneous clinical regression is common and usually occurs before 6 months of age, although mild biochemical abnormalities can persist (3,54,55). In a minority of the neonates who develop liver disease in association with α1AT deficiency, the disease does not subside but goes on to cirrhosis and liver failure (53,54,56). Overall, cirrhosis occurs in approximately 3% of individuals with α1AT deficiency, representing about 20–30% of the neonates who develop cholestasis (53–56). In the majority of these children, there is progressive liver failure, resulting in death unless corrected by liver transplantation.

### B. Clinical Manifestations of α1AT Deficiency in Adults

In adults, the spectrum of disease associated with α1AT deficiency varies from mild to severe (6). The early liver disease manifests with liver function test abnormalities and histological evidence of hepatitis and fibrosis. This can progress to cirrhosis and hepatic failure with portal hypertension. Often the diagnosis of α1AT deficiency is unsuspected at the time of histological and immunochemical evaluation of liver disease. In adults, once cirrhosis develops there is frequently rapid progression to death within 2 years of diagnosis (6). Adults with α1AT deficiency are also at increased risk for development of hepatocellular carcinoma, which may occur with or without concomitant cirrhosis (57–59); this predisposition is greater in men (60).

### C. Morphology of Liver Disease in α1AT Deficiency

The constant finding in the liver disease associated with α1AT deficiency is the accumulation of α1AT within hepatocytes, regardless of whether the condition is in children or adults. This manifests as intracytoplasmic inclusion bodies found mainly in periportal hepatocytes (61–65). These inclusion bodies appear as oval globules of different sizes and shapes with hematoxylin and eosin staining. These globules are periodic acid-Schiff-positive and diastase-resistant. The content of the globules is α1AT as shown by immunohistochemical evaluation, while electron microscopy shows that most of the accumulated α1AT lies within the cisterna of the rough endoplasmic reticulum.

### D. α1AT Phenotypes Associated with Liver Disease

As noted previously, there are more than 20 "at-risk" alleles associated with a deficiency state of α1AT. While the lung disease in α1AT deficiency is clearly related to decreased levels of α1AT and thus decreased antiprotease protection in the lung, the pathogenesis of the liver disease is less clear. If the liver disease in α1AT deficiency is the result of proteolytic attack in a fashion similar to that in the lung disease, one would expect that all the different α1AT alleles causing α1AT deficiency would be associated with an increased risk for liver disease. This is not the case. The only proven α1AT alleles associated with liver disease are the Z and $M_{malton}$ alleles (3,5,66–70), and, in fact, individuals with the null-null α1AT phenotype, despite having no α1AT in serum, have no liver disease. The fact that both the Z and $M_{malton}$ alleles are associated with intracellular accumulation of α1AT strongly suggests that the liver disease associated with α1AT deficiency is due to intracellular accumulation of α1AT rather than to extracellular attack.

The mechanisms for this intracellular accumulation remain unclear. Most of the work aimed at elucidating this question has been done on the Z allele, with which it has been suggested that there is a slowing of the rate of folding of α1AT polypeptide and/or a change in tertiary structure in the rough endoplasmic reticulum (71–73). While there are many theoretical ways in which abnormal folding of α1AT may affect secretion and lead to accumulation, they remain unproven as yet (74–78). Furthermore, while the mechanism of intracellular accumulation is not yet fully understood, neither is the process by which α1AT accumulation causes hepatocyte damage, although it is assumed that "mass effect" produced by engorgement of the RER may produce the damage.

### E. Correlation Between Liver Disease and Lung Disease

The liver disease in α1AT deficiency differs markedly from the lung disease in its pathogenesis and also in the spectrum of alleles responsible. Despite this, however, the majority of liver disease and lung disease associated with α1AT deficiency occurs in Z homozygote individuals (2–5). Interestingly, significant lung and liver disease rarely coexist in the same individual (4,5). Furthermore, while the factors that modulate the lung disease in these individuals is reasonably well understood, especially with regard to the effects of cigarette smoking, much remains to be learned about the factors that modulate α1AT-related liver disease. The fact that all Z homozygous individuals develop liver disease suggests a complex pathogenesis, as do the facts that males with α1AT deficiency develop liver disease more often than females (6) and that breastfeeding in the neonatal period may offer some protection against liver disease in children (79). In this regard, the major histocompatibility locus antigen B5 seems to confer protection against liver disease, while DR3 increases susceptibility (80). Furthermore, if liver disease occurs in association with α1AT deficiency, there seems to be an increased risk for the second child to develop liver disease (81).

## IV. Skin Disease with α1AT Deficiency

A distinct form of ulcerative panniculitis develops in a subgroup of individuals with α1AT deficiency. This was first described in 1972, and to date most of the individuals described have been Z homozygotes although a number have been MZ or of unknown phenotype (3,7). Biopsy of the affected areas show neutrophilic panniculitis, adjacent lymphohistiocytic panniculitis, and extensive necrosis (7,82). The condition seems to affect males and females equally, and at any age. The majority of the lesions occur on the trunk and proximal extremities and are characterized by ulceration and accompanying systemic symptoms including fever. Traumatic induction is noted in a large percentage of cases. The reason for this association between α1AT and panniculitis is unknown, but, interestingly, the skin lesions—even in their most severe form—may respond favorably to α1AT-replacement therapy (7), suggesting that a lack of antiprotease defenses is associated with the pathogenesis of the panniculitis. The other therapeutic agent used to good effect is dapsone, which can be used in conjunction with α1AT-replacement therapy (7).

## References

1. Gadek JE, Crystal RG. $\alpha_1$-antitrypsin deficiency. In: Stanbury JB, Wyngaarden JB, Frederickson DS, Goldstein JI, Brown MS, eds. The Metabolic Basis of Inherited Disease. 5th ed. New York: McGraw-Hill, 1982:1450–1467.
2. Tobin MJ, Cook PJL, Hutchison DCS. Alpha$_1$-antitrypsin deficiency: the clinical and physiological features of pulmonary emphysema in subjects homozygous for Pi type Z. Br J Dis Chest 1983; 77:14–27.
3. Cox DW. α1-antitrypsin deficiency. In: Scriver CR, Beaudet AL, Sly WS, Valle D, eds. The Metabolic Basis of Inherited Disease. New York: McGraw-Hill, 1989:2409–2437.
4. Crystal RG, Brantly ML, Hubbard RC, Curiel DT, States DJ, Holmes MD. The α1-antitrypsin gene and its mutations: clinical consequences and strategies for therapy. Chest 1989; 95:196–208.
5. Crystal RG. α1-antitrypsin deficiency, emphysema, and liver disease: Genetic basis and strategies for therapy. J Clin Invest 1990; 85:1343–1352.

6. Eriksson S, Carlson J, Velez R. Risk of cirrhosis and primary liver cancer in $\alpha_1$-antitrypsin deficiency. N Engl J Med 1986; 314:736–739.
7. Pittelkow MR, Sith KC, Daniel WP. Alpha-1-antitrypsin deficiency and panniculitis: perspectives on disease relationship and replacement therapy. Am J Med 1988; 84: 80–86.
8. Pierce JA, Eradio B, Dew TA. Antitrypsin phenotypes in St. Louis. JAMA 1975; 231: 1609–1612.
9. Kueppers F, Christopherson MJ. Alpha-1-antitrypsin: further genetic heterogeneity revealed by isoelectric focusing. J Hum Genet 1978; 30:359–365.
10. Dykes DD, Miller SA, Polesky HF. Distribution of $\alpha_1$-antitrypsin variants in a US white population. Hum Hered 1984; 34:308–310.
11. Silverman EK, Miletich JP, Pierce JA, Sherman LA, Endicott SK, Broze GJ, Campbell EJ. Alpha$_1$-antitrypsin deficiency: high prevalence in the St. Louis area determined by direct population screening. Am Rev Respir Dis 1989; 140:961–966.
12. Spence WC, Morris JE, Pass K, Murphy PD. Molecular confirmation of alpha$_1$-antitrypsin genotypes in newborn dried blood specimens. Biochem Med Met Biol 1993; 50:233–240.
13. Eriksson S. Studies in $\alpha_1$-antitrypsin deficiency. Acta Med Scant 1965; 177 (suppl): 1–85.
14. Laurell CB, Sveger T. Mass screening of newborn Swedish infants for $\alpha_1$ antitrypsin deficiency. Am J Hum Genet 1975; 27:213–217.
15. Larsson C. Natural history and life expectancy in severe $\alpha_1$-antitrypsin deficiency, Pi Z. Acta Med Scand 1978; 204:345–351.
16. Kueppers F, Black LF. $\alpha_1$-antitrypsin and its deficiency. Am Rev Respir Dis 1974; 110:176–194.
17. Black LF, Kueppers F. Alpha$_1$-antitrypsin and its deficiency in nonsmokers. Am Rev Respir Dis 1978; 117:421–428.
18. Buist AS, Burrows B, Eriksson S, Mittman C, Wu M. The natural history of air-flow obstruction in PiZ emphysema: Report of a NHLBI workshop. Am Rev Respir Dis 1983; 127 (suppl):43–45.
19. Brantly ML, Paul LD, Miller BH, Falk RT, Wu M, Crystal RG. Clinical features and history of the destructive lung disease associated with alpha-1-antitrypsin deficiency of adults with pulmonary symptoms. Am Rev Respir Dis 1988; 138:327–336.
20. Santos Rosa MA, Robalo Cordeiro AJA. Alpha-1-proteinase inhibitor phenotypes in Portuguese population. Eur J Respir Dis 1986; 69 (suppl 146):167–173.
21. Evans HE, Bognacki NS, Perrott LM, Glass L. Prevalence of alpha$_1$-antitrypsin Pi types among newborn infants of different ethnic backgrounds. J Pediatr 1977; 90: 621–624.
22. Ying Q-L, Zhang M-L, Liang C-C, Chen L-C, Chen L-F, Huang Y-W, Wang R-X, Zhang N-J, Li H-J, Liu S-S, Gao EX. Alpha-1-antitrypsin types in five Chinese national minorities. Hum Genet 1985; 71:225–226.
23. Ohtani H, Saito M. Alpha-1-antitrypsin: frequencies of PiM subtypes and serum concentration in the Japanese population. Hum Hered 1985; 35:62–64.
24. Morse JO. Alpha$_1$-antitrypsin deficiency. N Engl J Med 1978; 299:1045–1048, 1099–1105.
25. Brantly ML, Wittes JT, Vogelmeier CF, Hubbard RC, Fells GA, Crystal RG. Use of a

highly purified $\alpha_1$-antitrypsin standard to establish ranges for the common normal and deficient $\alpha_1$-antitrypsin phenotypes. Chest 1991; 100:703–708.
26. Cox DW, Hoeppner VH, Levison H. Protease inhibitors in patients with chronic obstructive lung disease: the alpha$_1$-antitrypsin heterozygote controversy. Am Rev Respir Dis 1976; 113:601–606.
27. Shigeoka JW, Hall WJ, Hyde RW, Schwartz RH, Mudholkar GS, Speers DM, Lin CC. The prevalence of alpha$_1$-antitrypsin heterozygotes (Pi MZ) in patients with obstructive pulmonary disease. Am Rev Respir Dis 1976; 114:1077–1084.
28. Leiberman J, Winter B, Sastre A. Alpha$_1$-antitrypsin P$_1$-types in 965 COPD patients. Chest 1986; 89:370–373.
29. Cole RB, Nevin NC, Blundell C, Merrett JD, McDonald JR, Johnston WP. Relation of alpha$_1$-antitrypsin phenotype to the performance of pulmonary function tests and to the prevalence of respiratory illness in a working population. Thorax 1976; 31: 149–157.
30. Morse JO, Lebowitz MD, Knudson RJ, Burroes B. Relation of protease inhibitor phenotypes to obstructive lung disease in a community. N Engl J Med 1977; 296: 1190–1194.
31. Buist AS, Sexton GJ, Azam A-MH, Adams BE. Pulmonary function in heterozygotes for alpha$_1$-antitrypsin deficiency: a case-control study. Am Rev Respir Dis 1979; 120:759–766.
32. Jones MC, Thomas GO. $\alpha$1-antitrypsin deficiency and pulmonary emphysema. Thorax 1971; 26:652–661.
33. Black LF, Hyatt RE, Stubbs SE. Mechanism of airflow limitation in chronic obstructive pulmonary disease associated with $\alpha$1-antitrypsin deficiency. Am Rev Respir Dis 1972; 105:891–899.
34. Rawlings W, Kreiss P, Levy D, Cohen B, Menkes H, Brashears S, Permutt S. Clinical, epidemiologic, and pulmonary function studies in $\alpha$1-antitrypsin-deficient subjects of PiZ type. Am Rev Respir Dis 1976; 114:945–953.
35. Camussi G, Tetta C, Bussolino F, Baglioni C. Synthesis and release of platelet activating factor is inhibited by plasma alpha 1-proteinase inhibitor or alpha 1-antichymotrypsin and is stimulated by proteinases. J Exp Med 1988; 168:1293–1306.
36. Hubbard RC, Fells G, Gadek J, Pacholok S, Humes J, Crystal RG. Neutrophil accumulation in the lung in alpha 1-antitrypsin deficiency: spontaneous release of leukotriene B4 by alveolar macrophages. J Clin Invest 1991; 88:891–897.
37. Thurlbeck WM, Henderson JA, Fraser RG, Bates DV. Chronic obstructive lung disease: a comparison between clinical roentgenologic, functional and morphologic criteria in chronic bronchitis, emphysema, asthma and bronchiectasis. Medicine (Baltimore) 1970; 49:81–145.
38. Varpela E, Salorinne Y. Respiratory disease profile in 22 patients with alpha$_1$-antitrypsin deficiencies. Scand J Respir Dis 1974; 89 (suppl):251–260.
39. Hepper NGG, Muhm JP, Sheehan WX, Kueppers F, Offord KP. Roentgenographic study of chronic obstructive pulmonary disease by alpha 1-antitrypsin phenotype. Mayo Clin Proc 1978; 53:166–172.
40. Gishen P, Saunders AJS, Tobin MJ, Hutchison DCS. Alpha$_1$-antitrypsin deficiency:

the radiological features of pulmonary emphysema in subjects of $P_i$ type Z and $P_i$ type SZ: a survey by the British Thoracic Association. Br J Dis Chest 1983; 77: 14–27.
41. Eriksson S, Berven H. Lung function in homozygous $alpha_1$-antitrypsin deficiency: studies in patients with severe disease. In: Mittman C, ed. Pulmonary Emphysema and Proteolysis. New York: Academic Press, 1972:7–24.
42. Fallat RJ, Powell MR, Kueppers F, Lilker E. $^{133}Xe$ ventilatory studies in $\alpha_1$-antitrypsin deficiency. J Nucl Med 1979; 20:917–922.
43. Simon TR, McElvaney NG, Feuerstein I, Hubbard RC, Crystal RG. Quantitative comparison of V-Q and CT for identifying emphysema in α1-antitrypsin deficiency. J Nucl Med 1989; 30:10.
44. McElvaney NG, Feuerstein I, Simon TR, Hubbard RC, Crystal RG. Comparison of the relative sensitivity of routine pulmonary function tests, scintigraphy, and computed axial tomography in detecting "early" lung disease associated with α-1-antitrypsin deficiency. Am Rev Respir Dis 1989; 139:A122.
45. Rienmuller RK, Behr J, Kalender WA, Schatzl M, Altmann I, Merin M, Beinert T. Standardized quantitative high resolution CT in lung diseases. J Comput Assist Tomogr 1991; 15:742–749.
46. Guenter CA, Welch MH, Russel TR, Hyde RM, Hammarsten JF. The pattern of lung disease associated with $alpha_1$-antitrypsin deficiency. Arch Intern Med 1968; 122: 254–257.
47. Stein PD, Leu JD, Welch MH, Guenter CA. Pathophysiology of the pulmonary circulation in emphysema associated with $alpha_1$-antitrypsin deficiency. Circulation 1971; 1053:227–239.
48. Keogh BA, Lakatos E, Price D, Crystal RG. Importance of the lower respiratory tract in oxygen transfer: Exercise testing in patients with interstitial and destructive lung disease. Am Rev Respir Dis 1984; 129 (suppl):S76–S80.
49. Wasserman K, Whipp BJ. Exercise physiology in health and disease. Am Rev Respir Dis 1975; 112:219–249.
50. Jones NL, Campbell EJ. Clinical Exercise Testing. Philadelphia: WB Saunders, 1982.
51. Janus ED, Phillips NT, Carrell RW. Smoking, lung function and $alpha_1$-antitrypsin deficiency. Lancet 1985; i:152–154.
52. Sharp HL, Bridges RA, Krivit W, Freier EF. Cirrhosis associated with alpha-1-antitrypsin deficiency: a previously unrecognized inherited disorder. J Lab Clin Med 1969; 72:934–939.
53. Sveger T. Liver disease in alpha-1-antitrypsin deficiency detected by screening of 200,000 infants. N Engl J Med 1976; 294:1316–1321.
54. Sveger T. The natural history of liver disease in α1-antitrypsin deficient children. Acta Pediatr Scand 1988; 77:847–851.
55. Birrer P, McElvaney NG, Chang-Stroman LM, Crystal RG. $\alpha_1$-antitrypsin deficiency and liver disease. J Inher Metab Dis 1991; 14:512–525.
56. Psacharopoulos HT, Mowat AP, Cook PJL, Carlile PA, Portmann B, Rodeck CH. Outcome of liver disease associated with α1-antitrypsin deficiency (PiZ). Arch Dis Child 1983; 58:882–887.

57. Eriksson S, Haegerstrand I. Cirrhosis and malignant hepatoma in α1-antitrypsin deficiency. Acta Med Scand 1974; 193:451–458.
58. Govindarajan S, Ashcavi M. Peters RL. α-1-antitrypsin phenotypes in hepatocellular carcinoma. Hepatology 1981; 1:628–631.
59. Sparos L, Tountas Y, Chapuis-Cellier C, Theodoropoulos G, Trichopoulos D. Alpha-1-antitrypsin levels and phenotypes and hepatitis B serology in liver cancer. Br J Cancer 1984; 49:567–570.
60. Cox DW, Smyth S. Risk for liver disease in adults with α1-antitrypsin deficiency. Am J Med 1983; 74:221–227.
61. DeLellis R, Balogh K, Merk F, Chirife A. Distinctive hepatic cell globules in adult α1-antitrypsin deficiency. Arch Pathol 1972; 94:308–316.
62. Feldmann G, Bignon J, Chahinian P, Degott C, Benhamou J. Hepatocyte ultrastructural changes in α1-antitrypsin deficiency. Gastroenterology 1974; 74:1214–1224.
63. Palmer PE, DeLellis RA, Wolfe HJ. Immunohistochemistry of liver in α1-antitrypsin deficiency. Am J Clin Pathol 1974; 64:350–354.
64. Talbot IC, Mowat AP. Liver disease in infancy: histological features and relationship to α1-antitrypsin phenotype. J Clin Pathol 1975; 28:559–563.
65. Roberts EA, Cox DW, Medline A, Wanless IR. Occurrence of alpha-1-antitrypsin deficiency in 155 patients with alcoholic liver disease. Am J Clin Pathol 1984; 82: 424–427.
66. Perlmuter DH. Liver disease associated with alpha 1-antitrypsin deficiency. Prog Liver Dis 1993; 11:139–165.
67. Perlmutter DH, Kay RM, Cole FS, Rossing TH, Van Thiel D, Colten HR. The cellular defect in α1-proteinase inhibitor (α-1-Pi) deficiency is expressed in human monocytes and in xenopus oocytes injected with human liver mRNA. Proc Natl Acad Sci USA 1985; 82:6918–6921.
68. Brantly M, Toshihiro N, Crystal RG. Molecular basis of alpha-1-antitrypsin deficiency. Am J Med 1988; 84:13–31.
69. Carlson JA, Rogers BB, Sifers RN, Finegold MJ, Clift SM, DeMayo FJ, Bullock DW, Woo SLC. Accumulation of PiZ α1-antitrypsin causes liver damage in transgenic mice. J Clin Invest 1989; 83:1183–1190.
70. Curiel DT, Holmes MD, Okayama H, Brantly ML, Vogelmeier C, Travis WD, Stier LE, Perks WH, Crystal RG. Molecular basis of the liver and lung disease associated with the α1-antitrypsin deficiency allele $M_{malton}$. J Biol Chem 1989; 264:13938–13945.
71. Brantly M, Courtney M, Crystal RG. Repair of the secretion defect in the Z form of α1-antitrypsin by addition of a second mutation. Science 1988; 242:1700–1702.
72. McCracken AA, Kruse KB, Brown JL. Molecular basis for defective secretion of the Z variant of human alpha-1-proteinase inhibitor: secretion of variants having altered potential for salt bridge formation between amino acids 290 and 342. Mol Cell Biol 1989; 9:1406–1414.
73. Sifers RN, Hardick CP, Woo SLC. Disruption of the 290–342 salt bridge is not responsible for the secretory defect of the PiZ α1-antitrypsin variant. J Biol Chem 1989; 264:2997–3001.

74. Ananthan J, Goldberg AL, Voellmy R. Abnormal proteins serve as eukaryotic stress signals and trigger the activation of heat shock genes. Science 1986; 232:522–524.
75. Kozutsumi Y, Segal M, Normington K, Gething M-J, Sambrook J. The presence of malfolded proteins in the endoplasmic reticulum signals the induction of glucose-related proteins. Nature 1988; 332:462–464.
76. Perlmutter DH, Schlesinger MJ, Pierce JA, Campbell EJ, Rothbaum RJ, Schwartz AL. Induction of the stress response in α1-antitrypsin deficiency. Trans Assoc Am Phys 1988; 101:33–41.
77. Perlmutter DH, Schlesinger MJ, Pierce JA, Punsal PI, Schwartz AL. Synthesis of stress proteins is increased in individuals with homozygous PiZZ α1-antitrypsin deficiency and liver disease. J Clin Invest 1989; 84:1555–1561.
78. Sifers RN, Finegold MJ, Woo SLC. Alpha-1-antitrypsin deficiency: accumulation or degradation of mutant variants within the hepatic endoplasmatic reticulum. Am J Respir Cell Moll Biol 1989; 1:341–345.
79. Udall JN, Dixon M, Newman AP, Wright JA, James B, Bloch KJ. Liver disease in α1-antitrypsin deficiency. J Am Med Assoc 1985; 253:2679–2682.
80. Doherty DG, Donaldson PT, Whitehouse DB, Mieli-Vergani G, Duthie A, Hopkinson DA, Mowat AP. HLA phenotypes and gene polymorphisms in juvenile liver disease associated with α1-antitrypsin deficiency. Hepatology 1990; 12:218–223.
81. Cox DW, Mansfield T. Prenatal diagnosis of alpha-1-antitrypsin deficiency and estimates of fetal risk for disease. J Med Genet 1987; 24:52–59.
82. Su WPD, Smith KC, Pittelkow MR, Winkelmann RK. Alpha-1-antitrypsin deficiency panniculitis: a histopathologic and immunopathologic study of four cases. Am J Dermatopathol 1987; 9:483–490.

# 16

# Lung Function and $\alpha$1AT Deficiency

**ALAN F. BARKER, RAY G. D'SILVA, and A. SONIA BUIST**

Oregon Health Sciences University
Portland, Oregon

## I. Introduction

This chapter reviews pulmonary function data supporting the development of premature emphysema in alpha 1-antitrypsin ($\alpha$1AT)-deficient individuals. Individuals with homozygous $\alpha$1AT deficiency develop pulmonary dysfunction similar to that seen with cigarette-smoking-induced chronic obstructive pulmonary disease (COPD). The studies that form this data base have mostly involved small numbers of patients, and few are population-based. They may not reflect accurately the range of physiological function associated with $\alpha$1AT deficiency. Central to the interpretation of these studies is the method of ascertainment of $\alpha$1AT individuals. $\alpha$1AT-deficient patients detected because of respiratory symptoms or from a pulmonary clinic typically have airflow obstruction. These patients are considered index cases. Individuals detected by screening of asymptomatic populations or relatives of $\alpha$1AT-deficient individuals have no or mild airflow obstruction; they are considered nonindex cases (1).

Spirometry in $\alpha$1AT-deficient individuals will be emphasized, as these tests are performed most often and are reproducible and frequently reported. The spirometric abnormalities include reductions in expiratory flow rates ($FEV_1$ and $FEF_{25-75}$) and a normal or slightly reduced forced vital capacity (FVC). The reduced $FEV_1/FVC$ is consistent with obstructive impairment. These physiological changes are primarily due to loss of elastic recoil from parenchymal disease (emphysema) and narrowed or tortuous airways (2). The reduced elastic recoil pressure and increased compliance allow for lung hyperinflation with increases in residual volume and total lung capacity (3). Gas exchange is impaired, with reductions in the diffusing capacity DLCO (4) and widening of the alveolar–arterial gradient for oxygen (4,5).

Important features of homozygous α1AT-deficient individuals to be stressed include: 1) relatively normal spirometry in children and young adults who have never smoked, 2) accelerated decline in lung function with age in never-smokers, 3) the powerful negative influence of cigarette smoking on pulmonary function, and 4) role of airway hyperresponsiveness as assessed by changes in pulmonary function after an aerosol bronchodilator.

## II. Pulmonary Function in $P_iZ$ Children

Existing data indicate that lung function is normal in most $P_iZ$ children up to age 18, suggesting that lung growth and development are not impaired. Studies are available on children without clinical liver disease. The best data come from a series of 25 $P_iZ$ children identified in the course of a statewide newborn-screening program in Oregon between 1971 and 1974 (6); repeat pulmonary function measurements are available to age 18. The first study included 19 $P_iZ$ and 3 $P_iSZ$ children 3–7 years of age compared to sex-, height-, age-, and weight-matched controls. Pulmonary function included maximal expiratory flow at FRC and FRC by rebreathing helium. No differences in any of the tests were noted between the α1AT-deficient individuals and controls (7). The same α1AT-deficient children were restudied at ages 12–18 with spirometry, lung volumes, and DLCO. All values were normal except in two individuals with a reduced $FEV_1$ that improved to normal after an aerosol bronchodilator (8). This study is important because it is truly population-based and not selective, and because longitudinal information is available.

The few case reports suggesting lung disease in children with α1AT deficiency are complicated by accompanying cirrhosis (9,10), other lung diseases (measles, pneumonia) (11), and lack of phenotyping for confirmation (12).

## III. Lung Function in Adult $P_iZ$ Never-Smokers

Studies have consistently shown that pulmonary function is well preserved in early adult life in nonsmoking $P_iZ$ homozygous individuals; however, pulmonary function from nonsmoking $P_iZ$ individuals aged 50–70 years will show airflow obstruction. Pulmonary function has been reported in fewer than 80 $P_1Z$ never-smokers over the age of 30. These reports have been from small cross-sectional studies of very different groups, for example, patients from a pulmonary clinic (13), participants identified by community screening for α1AT deficiency (1), surveys of α1AT patients (14,15), and an α1AT-deficiency registry (16).

One of the earliest of these studies, reported in 1978 by Black and Kueppers (13), included 22 $P_iZ$ individuals; four had confounding pulmonary diseases such as tuberculosis, and four were family members under age 30 with normal pulmonary function, leaving 14 (mean age was 62 years) for analysis. All 14 had some abnormality of lung function consistent with COPD, but the data are hard to compare with those from other studies because $FEV_1$ was not reported. Only the FVC, $FEF_{25-75}$, maximal breathing capacity (MBC), and DLCO are given, but these are consistent with airflow obstruction. Twelve of the 14 individuals had a $FEF_{25-27} < 1$ L/min; 9 of 13 had a reduced MBC; 10 of 11 had a reduced DLCO (13).

Other studies of α1AT-deficient never-smokers have provided data that are often conflicting. Silverman and colleagues (1) included 12 never-smokers (aged 11–64 years) in their report of 52 $P_iZ$ individuals identified by community screening of blood donors, as relatives of $P_iZ$ individuals, or from an α1AT typing laboratory. The mean $FEV_1$ of the 12 nonsmokers was 86.3%. Only three of those 12 had $FEV_1$s below 65% (1). The small number of subjects over the age of 40 years (seven subjects) and the variety of ascertainment methods limit the conclusions that can be drawn from this report. In contrast, a survey of British physicians who provided pulmonary function from their $P_iZ$ patients included 34 never-smokers (14). Airflow obstruction was observed but many individuals were symptomatic. The results from this survey are summarized in Table 1.

**Table 1** Pulmonary Function in $P_iZ$ Never-Smokers

| | No. | Mean $FEV_1$% predicted: Pre-BD[a] | Mean $FEV_1$% predicted: Post-BD[a] | Mean age (yr) |
|---|---|---|---|---|
| Index cases | | | | |
| Males | 7 | 42 | 52 | 53 |
| Females | 11 | 56 | 56 | 60 |
| Nonindex cases | | | | |
| Males | 6 | 63 | 74 | 51 |
| Females | 10 | 82 | 87 | 56 |

[a]Bronchodilator aerosol.
*Source*: Ref. 14.

Males had mean lower $FEV_1$% predicted than females. The effect of ascertainment is noted because index cases had reduced $FEV_1$s as compared to non-index cases (14).

Janus and colleagues from New Zealand (15) performed a chart review of individuals of European descent with α1AT deficiency, detected from their clinical pathology laboratory. There were 13 never-smokers with a mean age of 60 years and mean $FEV_1$ of 77% predicted. A Danish registry included eight never-smokers with a median age of 55 and median $FEV_1$ of 85% predicted (16).

In conclusion, these studies in nonsmokers give credence to the hypothesis that α1AT deficiency causes premature airflow obstruction, but it is not detectable by pulmonary function alone before the sixth or seventh decade.

## IV. Cigarette Smoking and Lung Function

Cigarette smoking is the most important risk factor for the development of COPD in individuals with normal $P_iM$ phenotype. Cigarette smoking is also the most important risk factor for the development and progression of COPD in individuals with severe hereditary α1AT deficiency and $P_iZ$ phenotype. Cross-sectional studies clearly demonstrate severe obstructive impairment in smokers. Table 2 summarizes the studies documenting this reduction in $FEV_1$ in current or former cigarette smokers. In each of these reports the individuals with the normal pulmonary function were also the youngest. These cross-sectional data are consistent with the notion that cigarette smoking is an additive or multiplicative risk factor with severe hereditary α1AT deficiency for the development of clinically significant COPD.

## V. Airway Hyperresponsiveness

Initially it was thought that α1AT deficiency affected only the lung parenchyma, causing a panlobular form of emphysema. The airways were thought to be

**Table 2** Spirometry in $P_iZ$ Individuals: Cross-Sectional Studies

| Ref. | No. of subjects | Mean age, yr (range) | Mean $FEV_1$% predicted (range) |
|---|---|---|---|
| Brantley et al. (4) | 112 | 45 (16–71) | 34 (10–100) |
| Silverman et al. (1) | 40 | 42 (19–58) | 47 (15–120) |
| Janus et al. (15) | 22 | 44 (20–68) | 37 (10–120) |
| Tobin et al. (14) | 75M/33F | 48 (21–78) | 33 (not available) |

uninvolved except insofar as they became narrowed and tortuous as a consequence of the loss of tethering of the alveoli. More recently, it has been recognized that symptoms of cough and wheezing suggesting airway hyperresponsiveness are present in an appreciable proportion of individuals with severe hereditary α1AT deficiency. The presumed mechanism is that elastases affect the airways as well as the interstitium, perhaps causing inflammation and narrowing in addition to the indirect effect resulting from loss of elastic recoil. Indeed, it is now recognized that some individuals with α1AT deficiency are initially diagnosed as having asthma. In various studies, the prevalence of a history or previous diagnosis of asthma ranges from 4 to 45% (1,4,14,17,18). A British Thoracic Association survey of physicians provided spirometry before and after a bronchodilator aerosol. In 164 individuals the mean $FEV_1$ was 42% predicted improving to 45% predicted after an aerosol bronchodilator. The mean FVC was 75% predicted, improving to 85% predicted after aerosol bronchodilator. No information about current medications was provided, so the small changes in $FEV_1$ and FVC are difficult to interpret (14).

## VI. Longitudinal Pulmonary Function in $P_iZ$ Individuals

Recognizing the intra- and interindividual variance in pulmonary function measurements, it is difficult to quantitate the decline in lung function with accuracy without relatively frequent measurements over several years. Nevertheless, there is some consistency in the estimates. In contrast to the age-related decline in lung function seen in nonsmokers without α1AT deficiency ($FEV_1$ decline of 15–20 ml/year) (19), nonsmoking $P_iZ$ individuals have a 60–105 ml annual decline in $FEV_1$. Smokers with the $P_iZ$ phenotype have a 80–150 ml annual decline in $FEV_1$.

Five reports provide at least two pulmonary function studies over time in $P_iZ$ individuals (4,15,20,21,22). One was a retrospective study from New Zealand that reported rates of decline by smoking habit in $P_iZ$ individuals tested at least twice between 1970 and 1983. There was an 80 ml ± 38 ml/year decline in $FEV_1$ in seven nonsmokers, 316 ml ± 80 ml/year decline in six smokers, and 61 ml ± 43 ml/year in eight ex-smokers (15). An American–Swedish survey included 30 subjects from the United States and 41 from Sweden with initial mean ages of 45 years (U.S.) and 47 years (Sweden). The average number of months of follow-up pulmonary function was 36 months for American subjects and 47 months for the Swedish subjects; smokers and ex-smokers were combined (20). The mean annual decline in $FEV_1$ was 102 ml/year in American subjects and 94 ml/year in Swedish subjects. These declines are remarkably similar, considering that these were clinical data contributed by investigators in both countries, not data collected for research purposes by one center.

Another retrospective analysis involved 80 $P_iZ$ individuals from Malmo,

Sweden, who had at least two measurements of $FEV_1$ between 1963 and 1982. Ex-smokers showed a 80 ml/year decline in $FEV_1$ compared to 60 ml/year in never- and current smokers. Current smokers were 9 years younger than never- and ex-smokers, emphasizing the importance of age in the decline of $FEV_1$ (21).

Of 101 subjects from Copenhagen who participated in a Danish registry, 80 individuals were followed annually for several years. The average annual decline in $FEV_1$ was 110 ml in 11 never-smokers (median age 51), 140 ml in 29 current smokers (median age 44), and 80 ml in 40 ex-smokers (median age 45) (22). The exact duration of follow-up and lack of annual $FEV_1$ data makes this report hard to interpret.

Prospective data are available from patients referred to the National Institutes of Health with COPD. These individuals were followed for a short period, but the data are prospective and came from the same laboratory and pulmonary-function-evaluation equipment. Twenty-four patients (smokers and nonsmokers combined) were studied at least three times at a minimum of 1-year intervals. The average decline in $FEV_1$ was 51 ml/year. This lower rate of decline in $FEV_1$, compared to the other studies, may reflect standardization of testing in a single laboratory, the fact that the patients with follow-up had lower initial $FEV_1$ (<30%), a learning effect, or a short time interval for follow-up (4).

In conclusion, all individuals with α1AT deficiency have an accelerated decline in pulmonary function as assessed by the longitudinal measurement of $FEV_1$. Cessation of cigarette smoking may slow this decline.

## VII. Summary of Pulmonary Function Impairment in $P_iZ$ Individuals

Although the pulmonary-function data on $P_iZ$ individuals are limited, several conclusions seem reasonable. Pulmonary-function impairment is usually not detectable before age 30–35 years. In never-smoking α1AT-deficient individuals, the $FEV_1$ declines faster than in nondeficient α1AT individuals, probably comparable to a smoker with a normal α1AT level. Impairment sufficient to cause symptoms will generally be delayed until approximately age 50 years. α1AT-deficient individuals who smoke cigarettes will have symptoms and impairment noted 10–20 years earlier (age 30–40 years). These observations are usually significant enough to warrant a diagnostic evaluation of α1AT deficiency in individuals aged 30–50 years with dyspnea and obstructive pulmonary-function impairment.

## VIII. Lung Function in Heterozygotes

The problem of ascertainment bias is illustrated in the debate about whether premature COPD or pulmonary dysfunction occurs in α1AT-deficient heterozygotes ($P_iMZ$, MS, SZ). Early studies reporting lung function suggested that the $P_iMZ$ phenotype was associated with airflow obstruction (23–29). Population-based studies did not confirm this observation (30,31). It seems very likely that the association reported in the earlier studies was a result of ascertainment bias because study participants were mainly cigarette smokers in hospitals or attending COPD clinics.

Pulmonary-function studies from community populations or asymptomatic family members ($P_iZ$ parents) have been compared to data from matched controls. Those cross-sectional studies, summarized in Table 3, suggest no difference between $P_iMZ$ or $P_iMS$ subjects and $P_iMM$ controls. A single study of nonsmoking heterozygotes reported abnormalities in maximal flow rates at several lung volumes. Comparing 15 nonsmoking $P_iMM$, MZ, and MS adults, the $FEV_1$ percentages were normal and identical in all groups; the mean $V_{75}$, $V_{50}$, and $V_{25}$ were significantly lower in the $P_iMZ$ group than in the $P_iMM$ and $P_iMS$ groups (40).

Two longitudinal studies add credence to the lack of obstructive impairment in $P_iMZ$ nonsmoking individuals. Eriksson et al. (41) studied 80% of a cohort of 53 men with the $P_iMZ$ phenotype on two occasions 6 years apart and found no significant difference in the mean annual decline in $FEV_1$ in $P_iMZ$ and $P_iMM$ nonsmokers (38 ml/year vs. 51 ml/year). In contrast, there was a significantly greater rate of $FEV_1$ decline in $P_iMZ$ smokers than in $P_iMM$ smokers (75 ml/year vs. 53 ml/year). This single observation suggests that smoking and intermediate α1AT deficiency may interact to prematurely reduce lung function. In another study, reported by Horton et al. (42), 28 MZ residents of rural Oklahoma identified from a random population survey had pulmonary function measured 7 years apart. Their spirometry was compared to that of $P_iMM$ controls matched for age, sex, race, and smoking background. There was no significant difference between $P_iMM$ and $P_iMZ$ individuals in FVC or $FEV_1$ in 1971 or at restudy in 1978.

In addition to cigarette smoking, particulate air pollution may adversely affect pulmonary function in individuals at risk for COPD. Two studies reported conflicting results of occupational dust exposure in $P_iMZ$ individuals. Horne et al. (43) reported pulmonary function in 28 $P_iMZ$ and 28 $P_iMM$ grain workers matched for smoking status, age, and length of employment in the grain elevators. The $FEV_1$% predicted and $FEV_1$/FVC% were significantly ($p < 0.05$) lower (but not in abnormal range) in the $P_iMZ$ grain workers ($FEV_1$, 94 ± 15% predicted; $FEV_1$/FVC, 76 ± 11%) as compared to $P_iMM$ grain workers ($FEV_1$, 104 ± 12% predicted; $FEV_1$/FVC, 80 ± 7%). Chan-Yeung et al. (44) reported studies from British Columbia of 1133 men employed in sawmills or grain elevators. There were 1011 with $P_i$ MM, 91 with MS, and 31 with MZ. There were no significant differences between mean $FEV_1$, FVC, or $FEV_1$/FVC in any of the groups, irrespective of smoking habits. The differing results in these studies may reflect different study designs, different exposures to dust (the mean duration of exposure was 15 years in the Horne study and 10 years in the Chan-Yeung study), or the absence of severely affected individuals from the workforce.

**Table 3** Pulmonary Function in $P_iMZ$ Heterozygotes

| Ref. | No. of heterozygotes | No. of controls | Age (yr) | $FEV_1/FVC$ | DLCO | Static recoil | Description of controls | Patient source |
|---|---|---|---|---|---|---|---|---|
| Gelb et al. (32) | 10 NS | 0 | 27–56 | N | N | N | — | $P_iZ$ parents |
| Larsson et al. (33) | 24 S<br>15 NS | 24; $P_iMM$<br>15 | 50<br>50 | N and[a]<br>N and[a] | —<br>— | N[a]<br>↓ | Matched for sex, weight, and smoking | Screen of men aged 50, Malmo |
| McDonagh et al. (34) | 8 NS<br>16 S | 38<br>38 | 25–66<br>25–66 | [a]<br>[a] | [a]<br>[a] | [a]<br>[a] | Matched for age, sex, smoking, and $P_iM$ | Random population, Tucson |
| Bruce et al. (35) | 143 | 143; $P_iMM$ | 25–64 | [a] | [a] | [a] | Matched for age, sex, and smoking | 6 centers, U.S. |
| Buist et al. (36) | 21 NS<br>13 S | 21 NS<br>13 S | 20–39 | [a] | | | Matched for age, sex, and smoking; no $P_i$ performed on controls | $P_iZ$ parents |
| Webb et al. (37) | 18 | 442 | >21 | [a] | | | $P_i$ match only | |
| Morse et al. (38,39) | 88 | 2637 | 6–96 | N and[a] | [a] | | $P_i$ match only | Tucson community |
| Morse et al. (39) | 208 | 2637 | 6–96 | N and[a] | | | $P_i$ match only | Tucson community |
| Webb et al. (37) | 30 | 442 | 7–21 | N and[a] | | | $P_i$ match only | multiphasic clinic, Monroe County, NY |

NS: nonsmoker; S: smoker; N: normal.
[a]No difference between controls and heterozygotes.

The only other heterozygote group studied is the $P_iSZ$. These individuals are of interest because their α1AT levels are 30–40% of normal and usually lower than those in MZ individuals (50–70% of normal). A British multicenter survey included 25 SZ heterozygotes. All 11 male index smokers, mean age 61 years, and one nonsmoker had obstructive impairment with a mean $FEV_1$ of 39% predicted. Of the four female index cases, two were aged 22 years, with normal pulmonary function; one was aged 50 years, with severe obstruction; and the single nonsmoker, aged 63 years, had a normal $FEV_1$. Of the nonindex SZ cases aged 25–67 (seven smokers, three nonsmokers), only one (a smoker) had a reduced $FEV_1$ (45). This single survey suggests that the SZ phenotype may well be associated with an accelerated decline in lung function, but that cigarette smoking is likely to be an additional risk factor.

Summarizing the heterozygote controversy, it seems likely that the risk in the heterozygotic individual is related to the actual serum level of α1AT, those with SZ phenotype being at greatest risk and those with MZ and MS phenotype at least risk. The $P_iMZ$ phenotype alone in the absence of other risk factors does not appear to predispose to early development of COPD. When it comes to the combined effects of cigarette smoking and partial α1AT deficiency, the evidence from population-based studies is that $P_iMZ$ individuals are at no greater risk for developing COPD than $P_iMM$ smokers.

## IX. Airway Hyperresponsiveness in Heterozygotes

Because of the possibility of asthma or airway hyperresponsiveness in $P_iZ$ homozygotes, the same concern has been raised in heterozygotes. Bronchoprovocation studies have been used as a means of detecting airway hyperresponsiveness. In an age-matched study of methacholine responsiveness in 34 $P_iMZ$ and 31 $P_iMM$ men, 35% of both groups showed airway hyperresponsiveness (≥15% fall in $FEV_1$). All but one of the positive tests in both groups were in smokers, suggesting that smoking, rather than the $P_iMZ$ phenotype, was associated with bronchial reactivity (46).

Individuals with the S allele have been examined in two different patient populations. Among Puerto Rican patients attending medical clinics in New York City, Colp and coworkers (47) reported an increased prevalence of symptoms of asthma and atopic manifestations (positive skin tests, high IgE levels) in heterozygotic MS and MV phenotypes as compared to MM. In spite of these histories and the presence of atopy, the $FEV_1$s were not different in the MM, MS, and MV groups. Townley et al. (48) compared bronchial reactivity to methacholine in individuals with MM, MS, and MZ phenotypes. The 36 individuals with the MS phenotype had a mean area under a methacholine dose-response curve that was smaller than seen in 419 MM and 34 MZ individuals. Smoking prevalence was the same in each phenotype group (48).

**Table 4** Spirometry in $P_i$ Null Individuals

| Author | Subject | Age (yr) | $FEV_1$ (% predicted) | FVC (% predicted) | DLCO (% predicted) |
|---|---|---|---|---|---|
| Cox | 1 (proband) | 31 | 1.14 (50) | 2.26 (66) | 13 (57) |
| | | 38 | 0.52 (19) | 1.17 (34) | |
| | 2 (sister) | 24 | 2.56 (71) | 3.59 (93) | 17 (75) |
| | | 31 | 1.97 (65) | 3.15 (89) | 21 (77) |
| | 3 (sister) | 17 | 2.55 (68) | 4.10 (100) | 18 (72) |
| | | 24 | 2.28 (62) | 3.75 (96) | 22 (76) |
| Muensch | 1 | 40 | 1.58 (69) | 3.8 (128) | 24 (70) |
| | 2 | 38 | 0.40 (18) | 1.24 (42) | 7.8 (41) |
| Garver | | 35 | (42) | (92) | (58) |

In summary, individuals with the MZ phenotype do not appear to have increased airway hyperresponsiveness compared to MM individuals. A single study suggests that airway hyperresponsiveness exists in $P_i$MS individuals. It is uncertain whether α1AT deficiency and the S allele contribute to the genesis of asthma.

## X. Null Homozygotes

Information about this very rare deficiency comes from case reports. Three members of one family with no α1AT detected (<1% detected by electroimmunoassay) and no bands on immunofixation isoelectric focusing have been reported with pulmonary function performed at two ages. All had reduced $FEV_1$% predicted and DLCO at an early age with substantial decrements in $FEV_1$% predicted in two of the three individuals after 7 years of follow-up (Table 4) (49).

Two other case reports also showed obstructive impairment, but the individuals were older and the impairment was similar to that seen in $P_i$Z phenotypes (50,51).

## References


1. Silverman EK, Pierce JA, Province MA, Rao DC, Campbell EJ. Variability of pulmonary function in alpha$_1$-antitrypsin deficiency: clinical correlates. Ann Intern Med 1989; 111:982–991.
2. Black LF, Hyatt RE, Stubbs SE. Mechanism of expiratory airflow limitation in chronic obstructive pulmonary disease associated with $\alpha_1$-antitrypsin deficiency. Am Rev Respir Dis 1972; 105:891–901.

3. Eidelman DH, Ghezzo H, Kim WD, Hyatt RE, Cosio MG. Pressure-volume curves in smokers: Comparison with alpha$_1$-antitrypsin deficiency. Am Rev Respir Dis 1989; 139:1452–1458.
4. Brantley ML, Paul LD, Miller BH, Falk RT, Wu M, Crystal RG. Clinical features and history of the destructive lung disease associated with alpha$_1$-antitrypsin deficiency of adults with pulmonary symptoms. Am Rev Respir Dis 1988; 138:327–336.
5. Levine BW, Talamo RC, Shannon DC, Kazemi H. Alteration in distribution of pulmonary blood flow—an early manifestation of alpha$_1$-antitrypsin deficiency. Ann Intern Med 1970; 73:397–401.
6. O'Brien ML, Buist NRM, Murphey WH. Neonatal screening for alpha$_1$-antitrypsin deficiency. J Pediatr 1978; 92:1006–1010.
7. Buist AS, Adams BE, Azzam AH, Sexton GJ. Pulmonary function in young children with alpha$_1$-antitrypsin deficiency. Am Rev Respir Dis 1980; 122:817–822.
8. Wall M, Moe E, Eisenberg J, Powers M, Buist N, Buist AS. Long-term follow-up of a cohort of children with alpha$_1$-antitrypsin deficiency. J Pediatrics 1990; 116:248–251.
9. Hird MF, Greenough A, Mieli-Vergani G, Mowat AP. Hyperinflation in children with liver disease due to alpha$_1$-antitrypsin deficiency. Pediatr Pulmonol 1991; 11: 212–216.
10. Glasgow JFT, Lynch MJ, Hercz A, Levison H, Sass-Kortsale A. Alpha$_1$-antitrypsin deficiency in association with both cirrhosis and chronic obstructive lung disease in two sibs. Am J Med 1973; 54:181–194.
11. Talamo RC, Levison H, Lynch MJ, et al. Symptomatic pulmonary emphysema in childhood associated with hereditary alpha$_1$-antitrypsin deficiency and elastase inhibitor deficiency. J Pediatr 1971; 79:20–26.
12. Houstek J, Copova M, Zapletal A, Tomasova H, Samanek M. Alpha$_1$-antitrypsin deficiency in a child with chronic lung disease. Chest 1973; 64:773–776.
13. Black LF, Kueppers F. Alpha$_1$-antitrypsin deficiency in non-smokers. Am Rev Respir Dis 1978; 117:421–428.
14. Tobin MJ, Cook PJL, Hutchison DCS. Alpha$_1$-antitrypsin deficiency: the clinical and physiological features of pulmonary emphysema in subjects homozygous for features $P_i$ type Z: A survey by the British Thoracic Association. Br J Dis Chest 1983; 77: 14–27.
15. Janus ED, Phillips NT, Carrell RW. Smoking, lung fung function and alpha$_1$-antitrypsin deficiency. Lancet 1985; i:152–154.
16. Evald T, Dirksen A, Keittelmann S, Viskum K, Kols-Jensen A. Decline in pulmonary function in patients with $\alpha_1$-antitrypsin deficiency. Lung 1990; suppl:579–585.
17. Makino S, Chosy L, Valdivia E, Reed CE. Emphysema with hereditary alpha$_1$-antitrypsin deficiency masquerading as asthma. J Allergy 1970; 46:40–48.
18. Larsson C. Natural history and life expectancy in severe alpha 1 antitrypsin deficiency, $P_iZ$. Acta Med Scand 1978; 204:345–351.
19. Knudson RJ, Lebowitz MD, Holberg CJ, Burrows B. Changes in the normal maximal expiratory flow-volume curve with growth and aging. Am Rev Respir Dis 1983; 127: 725–734.
20. Buist AS, Burrows B, Eriksson S, Mittman C, Wu M. The natural history of air-flow obstruction in PiZZ emphysema. Am Rev Respir Dis 1983; 127:S43–45.

21. Wu MC, Eriksson S. Lung function, smoking and survival in severe alpha$_1$-antitrypsin deficiency, PiZZ. J Clin Epidemiol 1988; 41:1157–1165.
22. Viskum K, Kok-Jensen A. Criteria for $\alpha_1$-antitrypsin substitution. Lung 1990; suppl:586–591.
23. Cox DW, Hoeppner VH, Levison H. Protease inhibitors in patients with chronic obstructive pulmonary disease: the alpha$_1$-antitrypsin heterozygote controversy. Am Rev Respir Dis 1976; 113:601–606.
24. Barnett TB, Gottovi D, Johnson AM. Protease inhibitors in chronic obstructive pulmonary disease. Am Rev Respir Dis 1975; 111:587–593.
25. Kueppers F, Donhardt A. Obstructive lung disease in heterozygotes for alpha$_1$ antitrypsin deficiency. Ann Intern Med 1974; 80:209–212.
26. Kozarevic D, Laban M, Buimir M, Vojvodic N, Roberts A, Gordon T, McGee DL. Intermediate alpha$_1$-antitrypsin deficiency and chronic obstructive pulmonary disease in Yugoslavia. Am Rev Respir Dis 1978; 117:1039–1043.
27. Cooper DM, Hoeppner V, Cox D, et al. Lung function in alpha$_1$-antitrypsin heterozygotes (Pi type MZ). Am Rev Respir Dis 1974; 110:708–766.
28. Bartmann K, Fooke-Achterrath M, Koch G, Nagy I, Schutz I, Weis E, Ziershi M. Heterozygosity in the P$_i$-system as a pathogenetic cofactor in chronic obstructive pulmonary disease (COPD). Eur J Respir Dis 1985; 66:284–296.
29. Lieberman J, Winter B, Sastre A. Alpha$_1$-antitrypsin P$_i$-types in 965 COPD patients. Chest 1986; 89:370–373.
30. Shigeoka JW, Hall WJ, Hyde RW, Schwartz RH, Mudholkar GS, Speers DM, Lin CC. The prevalence of alpha$_1$-antitrypsin heterozygotes (P$_i$ MZ) in patients with obstructive pulmonary disease. Am Rev Respir Dis 1976; 114:1077–1084.
31. Gulsvik AM, Fagerhol MK. Alpha$_1$-antitrypsin phenotypes and obstructive lung disease in the city of Oslo. Scand J Respir Dis 1979; 60:267–274.
32. Gelb AF, Klein E, Lieberman J. Pulmonary function in non-smoking subjects with alpha$_1$-antitrypsin deficiency (MZ phenotype). Am J Med 1977; 62:93–98.
33. Larsson C, Eriksson S, Dirksen H. Smoking and intermediate alpha$_1$-antitrypsin deficiency and lung function in middle-aged men. Br Med J 1977; 2:922–925.
34. McDonagh DJ, Nathan SP, Knudson RJ, Lebowitz MD. Assessment of alpha$_1$-antitrypsin deficiency heterozygosity as a risk factor in the etiology of emphysema. J Clin Invest 1979; 63:299–309.
35. Bruce RM, Cohen BH, Diamond EL, Fallat RJ, Knudson RJ, Lebowitz MD, Mittman C, Patterson CW, Tochman MS. Collaborative study to assess risk of lung disease in P$_i$MZ phenotype subjects. Am Rev Respir Dis 1984; 130:386–390.
36. Buist AS, Sexton GJ, Azzam AH, Adams BE. Pulmonary function in heterozygotes for alpha$_1$-antitrypsin deficiency: A case control study. Am Rev Respir Dis 1979; 120:759–766.
37. Webb DR, Hyde RW, Schwartz RH, Hall WJ, Condemi JJ, Townes PL. Serum alpha$_1$-antitrypsin variants: Prevalence and clinical spirometry. Am Rev Respir Dis 1973; 108:918–925.
38. Morse JO, Lebowitz MD, Knudson RJ, Burrows B. A community study of the relation of alpha$_1$-antitrypsin levels to obstructive lung disease. N Engl J Med 1975; 292: 278–281.

39. Morse JO, Lebowitz MD, Knudson RJ, Burrows B. Relation of protease inhibitor phenotypes to obstructive pulmonary diseases in a community. N Engl J Med 1977; 296:1190–1194.
40. Hall WJ, Hyde RW, Schwartz RH, Mudholkar GS, Webb DR, Chaubey VP, Townes PL. Pulmonary abnormalities in intermediate $alpha_1$-antitrypsin deficiency. J Clin Invest 1976; 58:1069–1077.
41. Eriksson S, Lindell SE, Wiberg R. Effects of smoking and intermediate $alpha_1$-antitrypsin deficiency ($P_i$ MZ) on lung function. Eur J Respir Dis 1985; 67:279–285.
42. Horton FO, Mackenthun AV, Anderson PS Jr, Patterson CW, Hammarsten JF. $Alpha_1$-antitrypsin heterozygotes (Pi type MZ): A longitudinal study of the risk of development of chronic air flow limitation. Chest 1980; 77:261–264.
43. Horne SL, Tennent RK, Cockcroft DW, Cotton DJ, Dosman JA. Pulmonary function in Pi M and MZ grainworkers. Chest 1986; 89:795–799.
44. Chan-Yeung M, Ashley MJ, Corey P, Maledy H. $P_i$ phenotypes and the prevalence of chest symptoms and lung function abnormalities in workers employed in dusty industries. Am Rev Respir Dis 1978; 117:239–245.
45. Hutchison DCS, Tobin MJ, Cook PJL. $Alpha_1$-antitrypsin deficiency: clinical and physiological features in heterozygotes of $P_i$ type SZ. Br J Dis Chest 1983; 77:28–34.
46. Kabiraj MU, Simonsson BG, Groth S, Bjorklung A, Bulow K, Lindell SE. Bronchial reactivity, smoking, and $alpha_1$-antitrypsin. Am Rev Respir Dis 1982; 126:864–869.
47. Colp C, Talavera W, Goldman D, Green J, Multz A, Lieberman J. Profile of bronchospastic disease in Puerto Rican patients in New York City: A possible relationship to $\alpha_1$-antitrypsin variants. Arch Intern Med 1990; 150:2349–2354.
48. Townley RG, Southard JG, Radford P, Hopp RJ, Bewtra AK, Ford L. Association of MS $P_i$ phenotype with airway responsiveness. Chest 1990; 98:594–599.
49. Cox DW, Levinson H. Emphysema of early onset associated with a complete deficiency of $alpha_1$-antitrypsin (null homozygotes). Am Rev Respir Dis 1988; 137: 371–375.
50. Muensch H, Gaidulis L, Kueppers F, So SY, Escano G, Kidd VJ, Woo SLC. Complete absence of serum $alpha_1$-antitrypsin in conjunction with an apparently normal gene structure. Am J Hum Genet 1986; 38:898–907.
51. Garver RI, Mornex JF, Nukiwa T, Brantly M, Courtney M, LeCoca JP, Crystal RG. $Alpha_1$-antitrypsin deficiency and emphysema caused by homozygous inheritance of non-expressing $alpha_1$ antitrypsin genes. N Engl J Med 1986; 314:762–766.

# 17

# Reactive Airways Disease and $\alpha$1AT Deficiency

**ROBERT J. FALLAT**

California Pacific Medical Center
San Francisco, California

## I. Introduction

Chronic obstructive pulmonary disease (COPD) is commonly recognized as a triad of chronic bronchitis, emphysema, and asthma. The majority of patients in more advanced forms of the disease have elements of all three, with the asthma component defined by the degree of response to bronchodilators. Patients with severe alpha 1–antitrypsin ($\alpha$1AT) deficiency have been generally categorized as the prime example of the "pink puffer," or pure emphysematous patient. This generalization is flawed, as discussed in this chapter when epidemiological and clinical reviews are discussed.

Reactive airways disease (RAWD) is generally defined on a functional basis as either a significant reversibility of airway obstruction in response to bronchodilators or, alternatively, as bronchial hyperresponsiveness (BHR) to nonspecific agents such as methacholine, histamine, cold air, or exercise. Both of these characteristics have been described with COPD, although it may simply be a reflection of reduced airway diameter (1–3). Asthma is characterized by reversibility and BHR even when airway mechanics are normal or nearly so. Clearly, the mechanisms for this responsive and acutely changing condition are quite distinct from the chronic changes associated with chronic bronchitis, and irreversible changes of emphysema. Asthma has been characterized as having a mild long-term course without development of chronic bronchitis or emphysema (4,5), but others have suggested that BHR may correlate with the development of COPD even in patients without α1AT deficiency (6,7).

Protein antiprotease imbalance has received wide attention and acceptance as a mechanism for alveolar injury and emphysema, as reviewed elsewhere in this and other texts (8). Many proteases are clearly present and active in the airways, but the association between α1AT deficiency and airways disease—in particular, RAWD or asthma—is not clear. In this chapter, I first review the broad range of proteases and antiproteases known to be present in the airways, and the theoretical and experimental basis for the role of proteases and antiproteases in RAWD. The epidemiological and clinical evidence for an association between asthma or RAWD and the development of lung disease in patients with α1AT deficiency is reviewed. In summation, the conclusions remain intriguing but still speculative.

## II. Proteases in Airway Disease

Patients with chronic bronchitis, and especially patients with cystic fibrosis (CF), have large accumulations of inflammatory cells, particularly neutrophils, in both sputum (9–12) and bronchoalveolar lavage (BAL) fluid (13,14). Neutrophil elastase, the protease most frequently implicated in the causation of emphysema with α1AT deficiency, can be detected in active form in chronic bronchitis (14) and particularly in patients with CF (15,16), even without α1AT deficiency. Neutrophil elastase is the predominant protease in the airway in CF (17). In most patients with CF, neutrophil elastase is present but inactivated or inhibited by α1AT. Damage to the airways by neutrophil elastase appears likely in both chronic bronchitis and CF. Instillation of neutrophil elastase into hamsters leads to changes resembling those in chronic bronchitis (18,19).

Neutrophils are increased and there is an antiprotease deficiency as well in the BAL fluid of cigarette smokers (19a). Neutrophils are also increased in BAL fluid during the late-phase response to challenge of both atopic and occupational asthmatics (20,21). Also, peripheral neutrophils are activated after allergen challenge or exercise (22,23). The role of neutrophils in the development of either chronic bronchitis or asthma remains unclear since only a small proportion (20–30%) of smokers who have increased neutrophils in BAL fluid develop obstructive airways disease, and even fewer asthma. Clearly, other factors of host susceptibility are necessary.

In asthma, eosinophils and mast cells are more predominant than neutrophils in the airway (24–26), as well as in BAL fluid (26). Mast cells release a variety of reactive substances, histamine, prostaglandin, leukotrienes, platelet activity factor (PAF), and, perhaps most intriguing, two proteases, tryptase and chymase. PAF recruits and activates eosinophils (27). PAF release is stimulated by proteases and inhibited by α1AT and alpha1–antichymotrypsin (α1ACT) (28). Eosinophils generate similar cytokines and, in addition, a major basic protein (MBP) that is known to be toxic to the bronchial epithelium (26,29). Damage and loss of epithelium by tryptase, chymase, or MBP is hypothesized to lead to BHR through several possible mechanisms: loss of protective effect of the epithelium, exposure of intraepithelial nerves, generation of mediators, or loss of putative relaxant factor (26,30). Analysis of BAL fluid in subjects with mild atopic asthma has shown a correlation between BHR and the percentage of mast cells, eosinophils, and, in particular, the amount of MBP (26).

The potential for the mast-cell proteases tryptase and chymase to play a role in asthma has been emphasized by Nadel and Caughey (31,32). These enzymes constitute more than 20% of the protein in mast cells. Chymase is a chymotrypsin-like proteinase closely related to neutrophil cathepsin G and inhibited by alpha 1–antichymotrypsin (α1ACT) and alpha 2–macroglobulin (α2M), but not α1AT. Chymase is predominantly in the mast cells that are in association with the bronchial submucosal glands. Chymase augments vascular permeability by histamine, stimulates degranulation of serous cells, and inactivates sensory neuropeptides: substance P and vasoactive intestinal peptides (VIP). Tryptase may be a member of a new group of serine proteases not related to trypsin, and is more predominant than chymase in the human airway mast cells. It has been implicated in augmenting bronchoconstriction by inactivating VIP, a bronchodilating neuropeptide, but not substance P, a bronchoconstrictor; this was shown in isolated human airway preparations (33). Tryptase also potentiates histamine; this system has been implicated in aspirin-induced respiratory reactions by the finding of elevation of serum tryptase and histamine in three subjects who demonstrated systemic symptoms in response to aspirin (34).

Yet another source of protease in the airway is the macrophage. These cells are derived from peripheral monocytes and have been found mostly in alveoli and lung interstitium, but some appear to be resident in the airways adhering tightly to the epithelial cells (35). Macrophages are a complex factory for numerous proteins, including antiproteases. Alveolar macrophages (AMs) accumulate in the lungs in response to cigarette smoke in much greater numbers than neutrophils (36), are found in the walls of bronchioles (37,38), and are found in numbers 10 times higher in BAL fluid from cigarette smokers than in that from nonsmokers (39). Elastolytic enzymes found in AMs include cathepsin B and D, as well as neutrophil elastase, which is possibly from phagocytosed neutrophils. Cathepsin B is similar to the plant enzyme papain; both have been used to induce not only emphysema in hamsters (40) but also airway and peribronchial inflammation (41). These enzymes are not inhibited by α1AT but may degrade or inactivate α1AT, which is also found in AMs (35,41).

Thus, there is a wide variety of proteases active in the airway, many, but not all, inhibited by the predominant serum protease inhibitor, α1AT. Clearly other protease inhibitors are in the airway and need to be considered.

## III. Antiproteases in the Airway

Lung secretions contain several elastase inhibitors, but the major ones are α1AT and secretory antileukocytic protease inhibitor (SLPI). In tracheobronchial secretions, SLPI exceeds α1AT by threefold or more (42,43), suggesting that SLPI is the more important protease inhibitor in protecting bronchial epithelium from proteolytic injury. It is a reversible inhibitor of several serine proteinases, including neutrophil elastase and cathepsin G. SLPI is found to vary 10-fold in patients with chronic bronchitis, but is not clearly associated with the severity of this disease (44). Nevertheless, it has been suggested that protease–antiprotease imbalance plays a role in the development of human chronic bronchitis (8,45).

In contrast to tracheobronchial secretions, BAL fluid from the peripheral airspaces shows that α1AT is 10-fold greater than SLPI (46,46a). Despite this molar excess of α1AT SLPI may play a role in the peripheral airways since SLPI is found in association with elastase fibers in the alveolar wall (47). SLPI is currently undergoing trials in a CF population, in which its efficacy in controlling inflammatory airways disease may best be tested.

SLPI has been measured in bronchial secretions in a small group of asthmatic patients, but its levels were not different from those in normal subjects (48). In fact, SLPI levels were lower in asthmatics when normalized for the higher albumin levels. However, these were mild asthmatics, and neutrophils in the BAL samples were not increased. There has been a scarcity of studies of this type in the U.S. literature. Plusa et al. (49) have reported an increase of acid protease, α1AT, and, especially, α2M in 28 asthmatic subjects.

α2M may be yet another major antiprotease in the airway, as reviewed by Wewers (50). α2M enters the lower respiratory tract by diffusion from the blood (51). It is a unique inhibitor that sequesters but does not inactivate elastase, thus allowing small, low-molecular-weight substances to interact and inhibit elastase. α2M increases 100-fold in ARDS (52), and may be a factor in protecting the lung from destruction in ARDS (50).

Lindmark et al. (84,85) have recently emphasized the possible importance of α1ACT. α1ACT is also a serine protease inhibitor of neutrophil elastase and cathepsin G, is in high concentration in plasma, increases several-fold with inflammation, and is found in sputum in higher concentration than expected from diffusion from plasma (53). Moreover, a heterozygous deficiency state for α1ACT has been associated with asthma (84) and abnormal pulmonary function (85).

In summary, although there are multiple lines of evidence implicating many proteases and antiproteases in the development of inflammatory airways disease, there is no clear definition of a protease–antiprotease imbalance in asthma. There is a paucity of studies evaluating the presence (or absence) of protease inhibitors in asthmatic secretions or in pathophysiological studies of patients with RAWD. Epidemiological and clinical evidence for an association between RAWD and protease inhibitors is considered next.

## IV. Epidemiological Associations Between Protease Inhibitors and Reactive Airways Disease

If there were a causative link between α1AT deficiency and RAWD, it should be expected that such an association would be most obvious in the severe deficiency states. Population studies that would provide some insight into the association of asthma to α1AT deficiency have been divided into three types: 1) generally healthy working populations in which predominantly heterozygotes with intermediate deficiency are detected (Table 1), 2) populations of cases of severe deficiency (predominantly ZZ), generally referred to centers for known or suspected OAD, and 3) populations with known or suspected asthma.

### A. Healthy-Population Studies

Studies in the general, nondiseased population that give some information regarding asthma or RAWD are summarized in Table 1. The original study that started the α1AT-deficiency story was reported by Laurell and Eriksson in 1963 (54) from a screen of 7000 subjects in northern Sweden. They found four severely deficient subjects, three of whom had OAD characterized as emphysema. Larger collections of ZZ subjects in Sweden were subsequently reported, as summarized in Table 2. The other random-population studies in the United States (55–57) found only MS and MZ subjects with no difference in the percentage with asthma or wheeze, nor was there any difference in OAD between heterozygotes and MM subjects. Note the high percentage of subjects having wheezing symptoms in some series. Three studies of industrial populations in Canada and Northern Ireland (58,59,59a) likewise failed to show any difference in allergies or OAD between MM and MS and/or MZ subjects.

During the two decades following the discovery of α1AT deficiency, there were many studies that looked for an association of the more common heterozygote states, particularly MZ and OAD. In general, those studies that started with diseased populations tended to find more MZs, while in those studies in which MZs were found from random or general, healthy populations no differences in OAD were found between MM and MZ subjects, as summarized by Morse et al. (72). Perhaps the most definitive was a multicenter study comparing 143 MZs with matched MM controls; there were no symptomatic or physiological differences (73). In a case–control study by Buist et al. (61), there was an increase in asthma in the 34 combined MZ and MS subjects; however, the authors noted that

**Table 1** General Population Survey

| Ref. | Year | Country | *n* | Population | MM | MS | MZ | Comments |
|---|---|---|---|---|---|---|---|---|
| Laurell and Eriksson (54) | 1963 | Sweden | 7000 | | | | | 4 PiZ; 3 OAD |
| Webb et al. (56) | 1973 | U.S. (NY) | 500 | | 395 | 30 | 18 | No increased OAD or RAWD in MS or MZ |
| | | | | % $FEV_1$ | 92 | 101 | 102 | |
| | | | | % Wheeze | 16 | 7 | 11 | |
| Chan-Yeung et al. (58) | 1975 | Canada | 1138 sawmill workers | % | 89 | 8.0 | 2.7 | No significant increases in allergies |
| | | | | % Allergic | 15.1 | 14.3 | 9.7 | |
| Cole et al. (59a) | 1976 | N. Ireland | 1995 working population | % | 86.5 | 8.0 | 3.9 | No significant differences |
| | | | | % Wheeze | 7.1 | 6.3 | 10.8 | |
| | | | | % B or E[a] | 16.4 | 15.2 | 20.3 | |
| | | | | $FEV_1$[b] | 3.58 | 3.86 | 3.71 | |
| Patterson et al. (57) | 1976 | U.S. | 65 matched | *n* | 65 | — | 65 | No significant difference in wheeze or OAD |
| | | | | % Wheeze | 60 | — | 45 | |

| | | | | | | | | |
|---|---|---|---|---|---|---|---|---|
| Buist et al. (61) | 1979 | U.S. | 34 matched | *n* | 68 | | 34 | Asthma significantly higher in MS/MZ, but authors felt asthma misdiagnosed |
| | | | | % Asthma | 2 | | 6 | |
| | | | | % Bronchitis | 14 | | 12 | |
| Morse et al. (55) | 1977 | U.S. | 2944 gen'l population | % Total | 89.5 | 7.1 | 3.0 | No increase in asthma; high % with wheeze |
| | | | | % Asthma | 7.2 | 5.9 | 8.1 | |
| | | | | % Wheeze | 34 | 35 | 37 | |
| Ostrow et al. (59) | 1978 | Canada | 391 (polluted industrial town) | N | 331 | 26 | 3 | No MM–MS difference in lung-disease smokers or nonsmokers; low no. of MZ |
| | | | | % $FEV_1$[c] | 92 | 98 | — | |
| | | | | % Abn $FEV_1$/FVC[c] | 15 | 17 | — | |
| Bruce et al. (73) | 1984 | U.S. | 16,500 gen'l population 143 matched MZ | | | | | MM age stratified; no difference in pulmonary symptoms or function |
| Sveger (63) | 1984 | Sweden | 200,000 newborns | | | | | 13 (8%) of PiZ and SZ had asthma by age 8 |
| Wall et al. (62) | 1990 | U.S. | 107,000 newborns | | | | | 18 PiZ and 4 PiSZ; only 2 siblings with mild asthma by adolescence |

[a]Bronchitis or emphysema.
[b]Age-adjusted, males.
[c]Smokers only.

bronchial infections may have been misdiagnosed as asthma in six of the Pi variants and therefore state that their data do not support an association of asthma with Pi variants.

Perhaps the most important and pertinent studies are those of the large populations of newborns screened in Sweden [200,000 by Sveger (60)] and in Oregon [107,000 by Buist et al. (61) and Wall et al. (62)]. At age 8, 13 or 8% of the ZZ or SZ subjects, respectively, had asthma in the Swedish study (63). This may be high, since only 2.4% of 8-year-old Swedish children were reported to have asthma in a separate study (64). Studied from ages 3 to 7, 19 ZZ and SZ subjects showed no evidence of OAD in the Oregon Group (61). Later the Oregon group reported that of 22 ZZ and SZ subjects studied in adolescence, only two siblings had mild reversible asthma (62).

Except for the possibly high incidence of asthma in severely deficient children reported by Sveger, there is no support from these studies for an association between asthma and $\alpha$1AT deficiency. It may be that the ZZ subjects in the two larger studies are too young to demonstrate RAWD. Older, referred, severely deficient populations are summarized in Table 2.

### B. Populations of Referred ZZ and SZ Subjects

It should be recognized that most of the ZZ subjects [or SZ, for Hutchison et al. (65)] summarized in Table 2 are derived largely from patients referred specifically for OAD. In the two series from England (104,105) and the St. Louis study (108), the index cases were separated from nonindex cases; in each case, there is less OAD in the nonindex cases. In most of these reports, asthma is based on clinical history and ranges from as low as 1% to a high of 34% in the latest and largest series from the NHLBI Registry (109). The 20% incidence in the earlier series by Brantly et al. (107) is based on either a history of asthma or a "significant response in $FEV_1$ to bronchodilators." When the latter criterion was used in the NHLBI Registry series, 27% were found to have a >12% increase in $FEV_1$. As with the population studies in Table 1, wheezing is found in a much larger number of patients, 80% of the 20 patients in the series of Rawlings et al. (101) and 35% in the NHLBI Registry series. In contrast, four studies reported that less than 5% of subjects had respiratory symptoms or asthma before age 20. This is similar to the expected incidences of asthma in a general population, and consistent with the findings of less than 8% asthma in the population studies shown in Table 1.

The question that remains is how many of these 30% or more individuals with a history of asthma or wheezing or response to bronchodilators have RAWD that is not a nonspecific association with narrowed airways and COPD? Is the high percentage with asthma in the last two series an example of this phenomenon as the percentage with OAD is 100% and 85% in these two series? Perhaps the answer may be found by looking at populations with known or presumed asthma.

**Table 2** Referred Populations

| Ref. | Year | Country | *n* | % OAD | % Wheeze | % Asthma | % Asthma or symptoms < age 20 | % Reversible airway obstr.[a] |
|---|---|---|---|---|---|---|---|---|
| Eriksson (99)[b] | 1965 | Sweden | 33 | 70 | | 9 | 1 | — |
| Keuppers and Black (100) | 1974 | U.S. | 76 | | | | | |
| Rawlings et al. (101) | 1976 | U.S. | 20 | 90 | 80 | — | 5 | — |
| Larson (102)[c] | 1978 | Sweden | 246 | 65 | | 4 | 0 | |
| Keuppers and Black (103) | 1978 | U.S. | 22 | 83 | — | — | 0 | — |
| Tobin et al. (104)[d] | 1983 | England | I 126 | 91[e] | — | 11 | — | — |
| | | | NI 40 | 73 | | | | |
| Hutchinson et al. (105)[d] | 1983 | England | I 14 | 11[f] | — | 15 | — | 4 of 6 |
| | | | NI 11 | 1 | — | 9 | — | 1 of 1 |
| Janus et al. (106) | 1985 | N. Zealand | 69 | 50 | — | 1 | — | — |
| Brantly et al. (107) | 1988 | U.S | 120 | 100 | — | 20 | 4 | 20 |
| Silverman et al. (108)[d] | 1989 | U.S. | I 22 | 100 | — | — | — | — |
| | | | NI 30 | 33 | — | — | — | — |
| | | | $FEV_1$ <65 | 100 | 1 | 25 | — | — |
| | | | $FEV_1$ >65 | 0 | 20 | 0 | — | — |
| | | | 20 | | | | | |
| NHLBI Registry (109) | 1992 | U.S. | 773 | 85 | 50 | 34 | — | 27 |

[a]More than 12% increase in $FEV_1$.
[b]30% had peptic ulcers; only 5% in Tobin's series.
[c]37 (15%) had glomerular renal damage (proteinuria or hematuria); 11 (4.5%) had rheumatoid arthritis, 7 other arthritis; 1 ankylosing spondylitis; 2 SLE; 29 (12%) had liver disease (3 with excess alcohol).
[d]Populations divided into index (I) and nonindex (NI).
[e]Based on radiological evidence.
[f]10 of 11 with OAD were smokers; one nonsmoker had asthma.

### C. Asthmatic Population Studies

Table 3 summarizes the studies that focus on subjects with lung disease, asthma, or BHR. The initial report of this type, by Fagerhol and Hauge in 1969 (66) of 503 patients with a variety of lung diseases, found a statistical association between the S allele and asthma. There were six MS and one SS in 39 asthmatics. There was no association of asthma or OAD with MZs. Subsequently, two large surveys of asthmatic children in Poland and the United States (67,68) failed to find an increase in Pi variants. However, Katz et al. (69) did find an increased (although not statistically significant) number of MZ subjects in the steroid-dependent asthmatic children, suggesting that this variant was associated with more severe disease. Similar associations were observed in the smaller selected series of Werner et al. (70) and Hyde et al. (71), who found increased numbers of MS and MZ subjects in adult asthmatics; they also noted that those with $\alpha 1$AT had more persistent and more severe OAD, and OAD was more frequent in the families of Pi variants.

Yet another carefully done comparison of 34 MZ subjects, aged 48 to 52, from a screening of healthy subjects in Malmo, Sweden (74), looked not only at baseline data but also at BHR response to methacholine. They report no difference in OAD or BHR between 34 MZ and 31 MM subjects, but BHR was much greater in smokers and ex-smokers. Among the 21 nonsmokers (11 MZ and 10 MM), only two showed BHR while 21 (10 MZ and 11 MM) of 44 smokers and ex-smokers showed BHR. This study would support the concept of nonspecific airway reactivity occurring in smokers.

In 1990, two studies again raised the question of an association between PiMS and asthma. Colp et al. (76) studied a predominantly Puerto Rican section of New York City and documented what had long been suspected, that asthma was more prevalent among the Puerto Rican population. In a random survey of a general medical clinic, 65% of Puerto Ricans studied had a history of asthma, but only 35% of other ethnic groups. The authors found a high incidence of MS in both asthmatics and controls, but no increase in Pi variants in the asthmatic group. It was noted that more of the MS subjects were nonsmokers, and the authors suggested that the MS gene rather than cigarette smoking was a factor in their asthma. Similarly, Townley et al. (77), in an extensive study of 489 subjects from asthmatic families, found asthma in 13 of 36 MS, 8 of 34 MZ, and 88 of 419 MM, indicating a significant difference between MS and MM but not between MZ and MM. More striking was that MS subjects from both the asthmatic and the nonasthmatic families showed significantly higher BHR than either MZ or MM phenotypes. The most recent study of 90 asthmatics in South Africa (83) shows small but not significant increases in MS and MZ subjects, and a curious significant increase in the $M_2M_2$ phenotype in the asthmatic population. Of most interest in this study was the decrease in elastase inhibitory capacity (EIC) despite a higher α1AT concentration in the plasma of the asthmatics, suggesting dysfunction or complex formation of the α1AT.

From these studies of asthmatic groups, the curious association with the S gene is recurrent while the more deficient Z allele has been less prominent. Lieberman and Colp (78) argue that the lability of the S allele (79,80) is possibly a factor in the reduced protection of the airways in response to an immunological insult. Since α1AT is important in anti-immunological responses (81,82), a labile or reduced α1AT could contribute to a greater protease load, greater damage, and greater airways disease. The finding of Gaillard et al. (83) of reduced EIC in asthmatics supports the idea that asthma somehow alters the protease–antiprotease balance. These and other clinical and pathophysiological speculations are discussed below.

### D. Clinical and Physiological Correlations

Protease–antiprotease balance is clearly related to inflammatory and immunological states. α1AT is a major acute-phase reactant, increasing 2- to 10-fold in response to inflammatory states. Asthma is increasingly recognized as a primary inflammatory disease of the airways, involving multiple cells, cytokines, proteases, and antiproteases, as discussed above. The studies summarized in Table 3 point out the slightly increased α1AT levels in asthmatics [although actually less in those controlled with steroids (68)], but it is not clear if large increases in α1AT occur in response to an acute asthma. More studies are needed like those of Plusa et al. (49) that document the role of protease and antiprotease–Pi complexes in the serum, as well as airway or BAL secretions of acute asthmatics. Is the decreased EIC in stable asthmatics noted by Gaillard et al. (83) amplified in acute asthma, and can free protease or protease–antiprotease complexes be documented in acute asthma?

Immunological response has been shown to be modulated by α1AT (81,82). Other antiproteases are present in the airway, but their role in immunological reactions has not been well studied. α1AT and α1ACT have been implicated in PAF release, which may be critical in asthmatic inflammation (27,28). Heterozygous deficiency of α1ACT has also been associated with asthma (84) and an increased prevalence of high residual volume (85). A variety of immunologically based diseases have been sporadically reported in association with α1AT deficiency, as cited in Table 2 from the studies of Larsson (102). Others have also reported associations of Pi variants with rheumatoid arthritis (87), juvenile polyarthritis (88), and vasculitis (89). However, these associations, as in most of the studies of asthma cited in Table 3, are weak and not borne out in larger series. This suggests that multiple factors need to be satisfied to produce these complex immunological diseases. Antiprotease deficiency alone cannot induce an asthmatic condition.

**Table 3** Asthmatic Populations

| Ref. | Country | Year | Population | Results/comments |
|---|---|---|---|---|
| Fagerhol and Hauge (66) | Norway | 1969 | 503 patients with lung disease | Significant association of asthma with S gene; asthma in 6/13 MS, 1/1 SS, 7/39 asthmatic S variants |
| Szczeklik et al. (67) | Poland | 1974 | 240 with asthma<br>215 normal | No increase in heterozygotes but emphysema found in 6/12 patients with asthma and decreased TIC |
| Werner et al. (70) | U.S. | 1974 | 60 asthmatic children<br>10 Pi variants matched with 16 MMs | Increased heterozygotes (5 MS, 4 MZ); more severe and persistent OAD in heterozygotes |
| Katz et al. (69) | U.S. | 1976 | 152 asthmatic children<br>230 controls | Increased MS in steroid-dependent asthmatics, but not significant |
| Schwartz et al. (68) | U.S. | 1977 | 1054 asthmatics<br>930 controls | No difference in frequency of S and Z variants; steroid-dependent asthmatics had decreased α1AT |
| Hyde et al. (71) | U.S. | 1979 | Selected 46 Caucasians from 57 chronic asthmatics | 5 MS, 6 MZ in 46 Caucasians with asthma; 50% of families of these had COPD |

| | | | | |
|---|---|---|---|---|
| Kabiraj et al. (74) | Sweden | 1982 | 34 MZ men matched for age and smoking<br>31 MM men | No difference in OAD or BHR by methycholine response |
| Townley et al. (77) | U.S. | 1990 | 489 subjects from asthma families; 234 subjects from normal families | Asthma in 13 of 36 MS subjects; increased methylcholine response in MS over MM and MZ |
| Colp et al. (76) | U.S.<br>NYC Puerto Ricans | 1990 | 55 asthmatics<br>61 controls | MM% / MS% / MZ% / MV%<br>74.5 / 16.4 / 5.5 / 3.6<br>80.2 / 14.8 / 5.0 / 0<br>Not significantly different from controls |
| Gaillard et al. (83) | South Africa | 1992 | 90 asthmatics<br>240 gen'l population | MM / MS / MZ / $M_2M_2$ / α1AT mg% / EIC[a]<br>81.2 / 8.9 / 3.3 / 6.6 / 214 / 33<br>91.1 / 6.3 / 1.3 / 1.3 / 195 / 42<br>Significantly higher % $M_2M_2$, but not MS or MZ; significantly lower EIC |

[a]Elastase inhibitory capacity.

If asthma or RAWD were strongly dependent on α1AT deficiency, one should expect to see it most easily in the severely deficient subjects. Yet, as shown in Tables 1 and 2, the incidence of asthma in childhood or pulmonary symptoms before age 20 is no higher than the expected incidence of asthma, and less than 8%. In the asthmatic populations (Table 3), the association is strongest with the least deficient MS variants (and, in one case, even $M_2M_2$). Lieberman's argument that the "lability" of the MS variant causes a functional deficiency of antiprotease should be amplified, and therefore reinforced, in the persistent, severe deficiency found in ZZ subjects. Is the high percentage of reported asthma and wheezing and RAWD in the more recent studies of ZZ subjects cited in Table 2 a confirmation of this? Or are these findings simply nonspecific reflections of the more severe OAD and emphysema in these later series?

Over the past decade, BHR has been considered a possible important determinant of susceptibility to OAD (6,7,90). Clinical studies of patients with COPD have shown a high frequency of BHR; for example, one study of 54% of patients with COPD showed a 20% decrease in $FEV_1$ to 3.9 μmol histamine (91). Similarly, 35% of asymptomatic, nonatopic cigarette smokers with normal pulmonary function had greater than 20% decreases in $FEV_1$ following less than 25 mg/ml of methacholine (92). In another, larger population study, pulmonary symptoms, including asthmatic attacks, were strongly correlated with BHR equal to and independent of smoking history (93). However, it is not clear from these and many other cross-sectional studies if these correlations precede or are a result of airway disease. It has been shown that BHR is related to baseline airway caliber (91). More recent studies of mathematical models based on pathological studies have shown that both airway size and loss of elastic recoil (as would be expected in α1AT-deficient subjects) may account for some of the increase in airway reactivity (94). In view of these findings, it would seem likely that much of the high incidence of wheezing and response to bronchodilators reported in the series cited in Table 2 may be accounted for by the high prevalence of OAD in these populations. The current Lung Health Study (95) is attempting to answer the question of whether BHR is etiologically important in the development of COPD or a nonspecific associated effect of OAD. Baseline studies of 5877 smokers with early COPD showed a very high prevalence of nonspecific BHR; a decrease of greater than 20% in $FEV_1$ with less than 25 ng/ml methacholine was found in 63% of men and 87% of women (95). Longitudinal studies of this large population may clarify the role of RAWD in COPD (95).

Whatever the sequence of pathophysiology, it is clear that the development of OAD in patients with α1AT deficiency is dependent on more than just the deficiency state. Clearly cigarette smoke accelerates the development of OAD, with onset of symptoms in α1AT-deficient smokers occurring in the fourth decade, while not until the fifth or sixth decade in nonsmokers. Similarly, several authors have noted the more severe and persistent OAD noted in Pi-variant asthmatics

(Table 3). Unknown familial factors have been recognized as significant in the development of OAD by several studies in non-α1AT-deficient populations (86,96–98). The St. Louis study of referred ZZ subjects (108,108a) (Table 2) and their families further emphasized not only familial factors but the possible importance of asthma and atopy (IgE) as a contributing factor in the development of OAD. Therefore, although there is not yet a clear causal link between α1AT deficiency and asthma or RAWD, there is strongly suggestive evidence that the two conditions interact to result in more severe and probably accelerated OAD.

Asthma is clearly a complex, multifactional, inflammatory disease. Protease–antiprotease balance must occur, but the precise role of α1AT and other antiproteases in the development of asthma and RAWD is yet to be defined.

## References


1. Corrigan CJ, Kay AB. The roles of inflammatory cells in the pathogenesis of asthma and of chronic obstructive pulmonary disease. Am Rev Respir Dis 1991; 143:1165–1168.
2. Woolcock AJ. Bronchial hyperreactivity in COPD. Chest 1984; 85(suppl:20S–23S).
3. Greenspon LW, Parrish B. Inhibition of methacholine induced bronchoconstriction in patients with chronic obstructive pulmonary disease. Am Rev Respir Dis 1988; 137:281–285.
4. Burrows B, Bloom JW, Traver GA, Cline MG. The course and prognosis of different forms of chronic airways obstruction in a sample from the general population. N Engl J Med 1987; 317:1309–1314.
5. Burrows B, Knudson RJ, Cline MG, Lebowitz MD. A reexamination of risk factors for ventilatory impairment. Am Rev Respir Dis 1988; 138:829–836.
6. Sparrow D, O'Connor G, Weiss ST. The relation of airways responsiveness and atopy to the development of chronic obstructive lung disease. Epidemiol Rev 1988; 10:29–47
7. Sparrow D, O'Connor G, Colton T, Barry CL, Weiss ST. The relationship of nonspecific bronchial responsiveness to the occurrence of respiratory symptoms and decreased levels of pulmonary function: the normative aging study. Am Rev Respir Dis 1987; 135:1255–1260.
8. Snider GL. Chronic obstructive pulmonary disease: Risk factors, pathophysiology, and pathogenesis. Am Rev Respir Dis 1989; 40:411–429.
9. Chodosh S, Medici TC. The bronchial epithelium in chronic bronchitis. I. Exfoliative cytology during stable, acute bacterial infectial and recovery phases. Am Rev Respir Dis 1971; 104:888–898.
10. Carilli AD, Gohd RS, Brown D. A cytologic study of chronic bronchitis. Am Rev Respir Dis 1970; 101:696–699.
11. Ghafouri MA, Patil KD, Kass I. Sputum changes associated with the use of ipratropium bromide. Chest 1984; 86:387–393.
12. Boat TF. Cystic fibrosis. In: Murray JF, Nadel JA, eds. Textbook of Respiratory Medicine. Baltimore: WB Saunders, 1988:1126–1152.

13. Stockley RA. Chronic bronchitis: The antiproteinase/proteinase balance and the effect of infection and corticosteroids. Clin Chest Med 1988; 9:643–656.
14. Fujita J, Nelson N, Daughton D, Dobry C, Spurzem JR, Irino S, Rennard S. Evaluation of elastase and antielastase balance in patients with pulmonary emphysema. Am Rev Respir Dis 1990; 142:471–501.
15. Suter S, Schaad UB, Tegner H, Ohlsson K, Desgrandchamps D, Waldvogel FA. Levels of free granulocyte elastase in bronchial secretions from patients with cystic fibrosis: Effects of antimicrobial treatment against *Pseudomonas aeruginosa.* J Infect Dis 1986; 153:902–909.
16. Goldstein W, Doring G. Lysosomal enzymes from polymorphonuclear leukocytes and proteinase inhibitors in patients with cystic fibrosis. Am Rev Respir Dis 1986; 134:49–56.
17. Berger M, Sorensen RU, Tosi MF, Dearborn DG, Doring G. Complement receptor expression on neutrophils at an inflammatory site, the pseudomonas-infected lung in cystic fibrosis. J Clin Invest 1989; 84:1302–1313.
18. Breuer R, Leucy EC, Stone PJ, Christensen TG, Snider GL. Proteolytic activity of human neutrophil elastase and porcine pancreatic trypsin causes bronchial secretory cell metaplasia in hamsters. Exp Lung Res 1985; 9:167–175.
19. Christensen TG, Korthy AL, Snider GL, Hayes JA. Irreversible bronchial goblet cell metaplasia in hamsters with elastase-induced panacinar emphysema. J Clin Invest 1977; 59:397–404.
19a. Gadek JE, Fells GA, Crystal RG. Cigarette smoking induces functional antiprotease deficiency in the lower respiratory tract of humans. Science 1979; 206(14):1315–1316.
20. Metzger WJ, Zavala D, Richardson HB, et al. Local allergen challenge and bronchoalveolar lavage of allergic asthmatic lungs: Description of the model and local airway inflammation. Am Rev Respir Dis 1987; 135:433–440.
21. Fabbri LM, Boschetto P, Zocca E, et al. Bronchoalveolar neutrophilia during late asthmatic reactions induced by toluene diisocyanate. Am Rev Respir Dis 1987; 136: 36–42.
22. Durham SR, Carroll M, Walsh GM, Kay AB. Leukocyte activation in allergen-induced late-phase asthmatic reactions. N Engl J Med 1984; 311:1398–1402.
23. Moqbel R, Durham SR, Shaw RJ, et al. Enhancement of leukocyte cytotoxicity after exercise-induced asthma. Am Rev Respir Dis 1986; 133:609–613.
24. Reid LM, Gleich GJ, Hogg J, Kleinerman J, Laitinen LA. Pathology. In: Holgate, ed. The roles of Inflammatory Processes in Airway Hyperresponsiveness. London: Blackwell Scientific Publications, 1989:36–79.
25. Laitinen LA, Laitinen A. Mucosal inflammation and bronchial hyperreactivity. Eur Respir J 1988; 5:488–489.
26. Wardlaw AJ, Dunnette S, Gleich GJ, Collins JV, Kay AB. Eosinophils and mast cells in bronchoalveolar lavage in mild asthma: relationship to bronchial hyperreactivity. Am Rev Respir Dis 1988; 137:62–69.
27. Wardlaw AJ, Moqbel R, Cromwell O, Kay AB. Platelet activating factor: a potent chemotactic and chemokinetic factor for human eosinophils. J Clin Invest 1986; 78: 1701–1706.
28. Camussi G, Tatta C, Bussolino F, Baglioni C. Synthesis and release of platelet

activating factor is inhibited by plasma alpha$_1$ proteinase inhibitor or alpha$_1$ antichymotrypsin and is stimulated by proteinases. J Exp Med 1988; 168:1293–1306.
29. Gleich GJ, Frigas E, Loegering DA, Wassom DL, Steinmuller D. Cytotoxic properties of the eosinophil major basic protein. J Immunol 1979; 123:2925–2927.
30. Flavahn NA, Aarhus LL, Rimelle TJ, Van-Houtte PM. Respiratory epithelium inhibits bronchial smooth muscle tone. J Appl Physiol 1985; 58:834–838.
31. Nadel JA, Caughey GH. Roles of mast cell proteases in airways. Chest 1989; 95(6): 1328–1330.
32. Caughey GH. The structure and airway biology of mast cell proteinases. Am J Respir Cell Mol Biol 1991; 4:387–394.
33. Tam EK, Franconi GM, Nadel JA, Caughey GH. Protease inhibitors potentiate smooth muscle relaxation induced by vasoactive intestinal peptide in isolated human bronchi. Am J Respir Cell Mol Biol 1990; 2:449–452.
34. Bosso JV, Schwartz LB, Stevenson DD. Tryptase and histamine release during aspirin induced respiratory reactions. J Allergy Clin Immunol 1991; 88:830–837.
35. Sibille Y, Reynolds HY. Macrophages and polymorphonuclear neutrophiles in lung defense and injury. Am Rev Respir Dis 1990; 141:471–501.
36. Janoff A. Elastases and emphysema: current assessment of the protease-antiprotease hypothesis. Am J Respir Dis 1985; 132:417–433.
37. Niewoehner DE, Kleinerman J, Rice DB. Pathologic changes in the peripheral airways of young cigarette smokers. N Engl J Med 1974; 291:755–758.
38. McLaughlin RF, Tueller EE. Anatomic and histologic changes of early emphysema. Chest 1971; 59:592–599.
39. Chang JC, Lesser M, Yoo OH, Orlowski M. Increased cathepsis B-like activity in alveolar macrophages and bronchoalveolar lavage fluid from smokers. Am Rev Respir Dis 1986; 134:538–541.
40. Gross P, Bubyak M, Tolken E, Kashak M. Enzymatically produced pulmonary emphysema: A preliminary report. J Occup Med 1964; 6:481–484.
41. Lesser M, Padilla ML, Cardozo C. Induction of emphysema in hamsters by intratracheal instillation of cathepsin B. Am Rev Respir Dis 1992; 145:661–668.
42. Tegner H. Quantitation of human granulocyte protease inhibitors in non-purulent bronchial lavage fluids. Acta Otolaryngol 1978; 85:282–289.
43. Morrison HM, Kramps JA, Afford SC, Burnett D, Dukman JH, Stockley RA. Elastase inhibitors in sputum from bronchitic patients with and without alpha$_1$-proteinase inhibitor deficiency: partial characterization of a hitherto unquantified inhibitor of neutrophil elastase. Clin Sci 1987; 73:19–28.
44. Dukman JH, Kramps JA, Franken C. Antileukoprotease in sputum during bronchial infections. Chest 1986; 89:731–736.
45. Snider GL. Experimental studies on emphysema and chronic bronchial injury. Eur J Respir Dis 1986; 69(suppl 146):17–35.
46. Boudier C, Pelletier A, Gast A, Tournier JM, Pauli G, Bieth JG. The elastase inhibitory capacity and the alpha*1*-proteinase inhibitor and bronchial inhibitor content of bronchoalveolar lavage fluids from healthy subjects. Biol Chem Hoppe-Seyler 1987; 981–990.
46a. Kramps JA, Franken C, Dukman JH. Quantity of antileukoprotease relative to

alpha1-proteinase inhibitor in peripheral airspaces of the human lung. Clin Sci 1988; 75:351–353.
47. Kramps JA, TeBoekhorst AHT, Fransen AM, Ginsel LA, Dukman JH. Anti-leukoprotease is associated with elastin fibers in the extracellular matrix of the human lung: An immunoelectromicroscopic study. Am Rev Respir Dis 1989; 140: 471–476.
48. Ochnio JJ, Abboud RT, Lam S, et al. Bronchial leukocyte proteinase inhibitor levels in bronchial washings in asthma patients. Chest 1988; 93(5):1008–1012.
49. Plusa T, Tchorzewski H, Raczka A. Archivum Immunologie et Therapiae Experimentalie 1987; 35:49–55.
50. Wewers M. Pathogenesis of emphysema: Assessment of basic science concepts through clinical investigation. Chest 1989; 95(1):190–195.
51. Taylor AE, Guyton AC, Bishop VS. Permeability of the alveolar membrane to solutes. Circ Res 1965; 16:353–362.
52. Holter JF, Weiland JE, Pacht ER, Gadek JE, Davis WB. Protein permeability in the adult respiratory distress syndrome: loss of size selectivity of the alveolar epithelium. J Clin Invest 1986; 78:1513–1522.
53. Eriksson S, Lindmark B, Lilja H. Familial alpha-1-antichymotrypsin deficiency. Acta Med Scan 1986; 220:447–453.
54. Laurell CB, Eriksson S. The electrophoretic $alpha_1$ globulin pattern of serum in alpha1 antitrypsin deficiency. Scand J Clin Lab Invest 1963; 15:132–140.
55. Morse JO, Jebowitz MD, Knudson RJ, Burrows B. Relation of protease inhibitor phenotypes to obstructive lung disease in a community. N Engl J Med 1977; 296: 1190–1194.
56. Webb DR, Hyde RW, Schwartz RH, et al. Serum $alpha_1$ antitrypsin variants: Prevalence and clinical spirometry. Am Rev Respir Dis 1973; 108:918–925.
57. Patterson CD, Mackenthum A, Hammarsten JF, et al. Pi MZ subjects and pulmonary disease. Am J Respir Dis 1976; 113(suppl):158.
58. Chan-Yeung M, Ashley MJ, Corey P, Maledy H. Pi phenotypes and the prevalence of chest symptoms and lung function abnormalities in workers employed in dusty industries. Am Rev Respir Dis 1978; 117:239–245.
59. Ostrow DN, Manfreda J, Tse KS, Dorman T, Cherniack RM. $Alpha_1$-antitrypsin phenotypes and lung function in a moderately polluted northern Ontario community. CMA J 1978; 18.
59a. Cole RB, Nevin NC, Blundell G, Merrett JD, McDonald JR, Johnston WP. Relation of $alpha_1$-antitrypsin phenotype to the performance of pulmonary function tests and to the prevalence of respiratory illness in a working population. Thorax 1976; 31: 149–157.
60. Sveger T. Liver disease in $alpha_1$-antitrypsin deficiency detected by screening of 200,000 infants. N Engl J Med 1976; 294:1316–1321.
61. Buist AS, Adams BE, Azzam AH, Sexton GJ. Pulmonary function in young children with $alpha_1$-antitrypsin deficiency. Am Rev Respir Dis 1980; 122:817–822.
62. Wall M, Moe E, Eisenberg J, Powers M, Buist N, Buist AS. Long-term follow up of a cohort of children with $alpha_1$-antitrypsin deficiency. J Pediatr 1990; 116:248–251.
63. Sveger T. Prospective study of children with $alpha_1$-antitrypsin deficiency: Eight year old follow up. J Pediatr 1984; 104:91–94.

64. Kjellman M. Immunoglobulin E and atopic allergy in childhood. Thesis, Linkoping University Medical Dissertations 1976; 36:37.
65. Hutchison DCS, Tobin MJ, Cook PJL. Alpha$_1$-antitrypsin deficiency: Clinical features in heterozygotes of Pi type SZ. Br J Dis Chest 1983; 77:28–34.
66. Fagerhol MK, Hauge HE. Serum Pi types in patients with pulmonary diseases. Acta Allergologica 1969; 24:107–114.
67. Szczelik A, Turowska B, Czerniawska-Mysik G, Opolska B, Nizankowska E. Serum alpha$_1$-antitrypsin in bronchial asthma. Am Rev Respir Dis 1974; 109:487–490.
68. Schwartz RH, Van Ess JD, Johnstone DE, Dreyfuss EM, Ali Abrishami M, Chai H. Alpha-1 antitrypsin in childhood asthma. J Allergy Clin Immunol 1977; 59:31–34.
69. Katz RM, Lieberman J, Siegel SC. Alpha$_1$-antitrypsin levels and prevalence of Pi-variant phenotypes in asthmatic children. J Allergy Clin Immunol 1976; 57:41.
70. Werner P, Hyde JS, Lourenco RV, Talamo RC. Alterations in lung function in children with chronic asthma and Pi variants. J Allergy Clin Immunol 1975; 55:128–129.
71. Hyde JS, Werner P, Kumar CM, Moore BS. Protease inhibitor variants in children and young adults with chronic asthma. Ann Allerg 1979; 43:8–13.
72. Morse JO, Lebowitz MD, Knudson RJ, Burrows B. Relation of protease inhibitor phenotypes to obstructive lung diseases in a community. N Engl J Med 1977; 296(21):1190–1194.
73. Bruce RM, Cohen BH, Diamond EL, Fallat RJ, et al. Collaborative study to assess risk of lung disease in Pi MZ phenotype subjects. Am Rev Respir Dis 1984; 130: 386–390.
74. Kabiraj MU, Simonsson G, Groth S, Bjorklund A, Bulow K, Lindell SE. Bronchial reactivity, smoking, and alpha$_1$-antitrypsin: A population-based study of middle-aged men. Am Rev Respir Dis 1982; 126:864–869.
75. Peterson B, Kristenson H, Sternby NH, Trell E, Fex G, Hood B. Alcohol consumption and premature death in middle-aged men. Br Med J 1980; 280:1403–1406.
76. Colp C, Talavera W, Goldman D, Green J, Multz A, Lieberman J. Profile of bronchospastic disease in Puerto Rican patients in New York City. Arch Intern Med 1990; 150:2349.
77. Townley RG, Southard JG, Radford P, Hopp RJ, Bewtra AK, Ford L. Association of MS Pi phenotype with airway hyperresponsiveness. Chest 1990; 98:594–599.
78. Lieberman J, Colp C. A role for intermediate heterozygous alpha$_1$-antitrypsin deficiency in obstructive lung disease. Chest 1990; 93(3):522–523.
79. Lieberman J. Heat lability of alpha$_1$-antitrypsin variants. Chest 1973; 64:579–584.
80. Engh R, Lubermann H, Schneider M, Wiegand G, Huber R, Laurell CB. The S-variant of human alpha$_1$-antitrypsin, structure and implications for function and metabolism. Protein Engineering 1989; 2:407–415.
81. Arora PK, Miller HC. Alpha$_1$-antitrypsin is an effector of immunological stasis. Nature 1978; 274:589–590.
82. Breit SN, Wakefield D, Robinson JP, Luckhurst E, Clark P, Penny R. Review: The role of alpha$_1$-antitrypsin deficiency in the pathogenesis of immune disorders. Clin Immunol Immunopathol 1985; 35:363–380.
83. Gaillard MC, Kilroe-Smith A, Nogueira C, Dunn D, Jenkins T, Fine B, Kallenbach J. Alpha-1-protease inhibitor in bronchial asthma: Phenotypes and biochemical characteristics. Am Rev Respir Dis 1992; 145:1311–1315.

84. Lindmark B. Asthma and heterozygous alpha$_1$-antichymotrypsin deficiency: a possible association. J Intern Med 1990; 227:115–118.
85. Lindmark BE, Arborelius M, Eriksson SG. Pulmonary function in middle-aged women with heterozygous deficiency of the serine protease inhibitor alpha$_1$-antichymotrypsin. Am Rev Respir Dis 1990; 141:884–888.
86. Larson RK, Barman ML, Kueppers F, et al. Genetic and environmental determinants of chronic obstructive pulmonary disease. Ann Intern Med 1970; 72:627–632.
87. Cox DW, Huber O. Rheumatoid arthritis and alpha$_1$-antitrypsin. Lancet 1976; i: 1216–1217.
88. Arnaud P, Galbraith RM, Faulk WP, Ansell BM. Increased frequency of the MZ phenotype of alpha$_1$ protease inhibitor in juvenile chronic polyarthritis. J Clin Invest 1977; 60:1442–1444.
89. Lewis M, Kallenbach J, Zaltzman M, Levy H, Lurie D, Baynes R, King P, Meyers A. Severe deficiency of alpha$_1$-antitrypsin associated with cutaneous vasculitis, rapidly progressive glomerulonephritis, and colitis. Am J Med 1985; 79:489–494.
90. Weiss ST, Speizer FE. Increased levels of airways responsiveness as a risk factor for development of chronic obstructive lung disease. Chest 1984; 86:3–4.
91. Yan K, Salome CM, Woolcock AJ. Prevalence and nature of bronchial hyperresponsiveness in subjects with chronic obstructive pulmonary disease. Am Rev Respir Dis 1985; 132:25–29.
92. Casale TB, Rhodes BJ, Donnelly AL, Weiler JM. Airway responses to methacholine in asymptomatic nonatopic cigarette smokers. J Appl Physiol 1987; 62(5):1888–1892.
93. Rijcken B, Schouten JP, Weiss ST, Speizer FE, Van Der Lende R. The relationship of nonspecific bronchial responsiveness to respiratory symptoms in a random population sample. Am Rev Respir Dis 1987; 136:62–68.
93a. Tashkin DP, Altose MD, Bleecker ER, Connett JE, Kanner RE, Lee WW, Wise R, The Lung Health Study Group. The Lung Health Study: Airway responsiveness to inhaled methacholine in smokers with mild to moderate airflow limitation. Am Rev Respir Dis 1992; 145:301–310.
94. Wiggs BR, Bosken C, Pare PD, James A, Hogg JC. A model of airway narrowing in asthma and in chronic obstructive pulmonary disease. Am Rev Respir Dis 1992; 145:1251–1258.
95. Buist AS, Connett J, et al. Chronic Obstructive Pulmonary Disease Early Intervention Trial (Lung Health Study). Chest 1993; 103(6):1863–1872.
96. Keuppers F, Miller RD, Gordon H, Hepper NG, Offord K. Familial prevalence of chronic obstructive pulmonary disease in a matched pair study. Am J Med 1977; 63: 336–342.
97. Larson RJ, Barman ML. The familial occurrence of chronic obstructive pulmonary disease. Ann Intern Med 1965; 63:1001.
98. Higgins M, Keller J. Familial occurrence of chronic respiratory disease and familial resemblance in ventilatory capacity. J Chron Dis 1975; 28:239.
99. Eriksson S. Studies in alpha$_1$-antitrypsin. Acta Med Scand 1965; 177(suppl 432): 1–85.
100. Keuppers F, Black LF. Alpha$_1$-antitrypsin and its deficiency. Am Rev Respir Dis 1974; 110:176–194.

101. Rawlings W Jr, Kreiss P, Levy D, et al. Clinical, epidemiologic, and pulmonary function studies in alpha-1 antitrypsin-deficient subjects of Pi Z type. Am Rev Respir Dis 1976; 114:945–953.
102. Larsson C. Natural history and life expectancy in severe $alpha_1$ antitrypsin deficiency, PiZ. Acta Med Scand 1978; 204:345–356.
103. Black L, Keuppers F. $Alpha_1$-antitrypsin deficiency in non-smokers. Am Rev Respir Dis 1978; 117:421–428.
104. Tobin MJ, Cook PJL, Hutchison DCS. $Alpha_1$-antitrypsin deficiency: the clinical and physiological features of pulmonary emphysema in subjects homozygous for Pi type Z: a survey by the British Thoracic Society. Br J Dis Chest 1983; 77:14–27.
105. Hutchison DCS, Barter CE, Cook PJL, Laws JW, Martelli NA, Hugh-Jones P. Severe pulmonary emphysema: a comparison of patients with and without $alpha_1$-antitrypsin deficiency. Q J Med 1972; 41:301–315.
106. Janus ED, Phillips NT, Carrell RW. Smoking, lung function and $alpha_1$-antitrypsin deficiency. Am Rev Respir Dis 1974; 110:176–194.
107. Brantly ML, Paul LD, Miller BH, Falk RT, Wu M, Crystal RG. Clinical features and history of the destructive lung disease associated with $alpha_1$-antitrypsin deficiency of adults with pulmonary symptoms. Am Rev Respir Dis 1988; 138:327–336.
108. Silverman EK, Pierce JA, Province MA, Rao DC, Campbell EJ. Variability of pulmonary function in $alpha_1$-antitrypsin deficiency: clinical correlates. Ann Intern Med 1989; 111:982–991.
108a. Silverman EK, Province MA, Rao DC, Pierce JA, Campbell EJ. A family study of the variability of pulmonary function in $alpha_1$-antitrypsin deficiency. Am Rev Respir Dis 1990; 142:1015–1021.
109. NHLBI Registry for Patients with Severe Deficiency of Alpha 1-Antitrypsin. Bethesda, MD: National Institutes of Health, November 1991.

# 18

# Natural History of α1AT Deficiency

**JANET WITTES**

Statistics Collaborative, Inc.
Washington, D.C.

**MARGARET C. WU**

National Heart, Lung, and Blood Institute
National Institutes of Health
Bethesda, Maryland

## I. Introduction

An association between severe alpha 1-antitrypsin (α1AT) deficiency and chronic obstructive pulmonary disease (COPD) was recognized in the early 1960s by Laurell and Eriksson (1). A few years later, reports described associations of the α1AT deficiency state with cirrhosis (2), neonatal liver disease (2,3), and childhood renal disease (4).

The aim of this chapter is to describe the frequency with which α1AT-deficient individuals experience diseases associated with the deficiency. In any study of the association between a state (here, α1AT deficiency) and disease (here, COPD, liver disease, and renal disease), accurate quantification of the degree of that relationship is predicated upon unbiased ascertainment of a representative sample of people with the disease. Although the usual mode of identification of α1AT-deficient individuals is through presentation for medical problems, unbiased identification would be through population screening to determine prevalence of α1AT deficiency and longitudinal follow-up to assess incidence and time course of the associated disease. In genetically determined conditions, another relatively unbiased method of ascertainment is follow-up of siblings of patients who have presented with symptoms. In this chapter, which reviews the literature on the association of $\alpha$1AT deficiency and subsequent disease, we describe the method of ascertainment of cases as well as the reported associations. Unless otherwise stated, the $\alpha$1AT individuals to which this chapter refers are phenotypically PiZZ.

## II. Infancy to Late Adolescence

### A. Available Data

There have been two reported neonatal screenings designed to identify $\alpha$1AT deficiency, one in Sweden in 1972 to 1974 (5) and one in Oregon between 1971 and 1974 (6). The $\alpha$1AT-deficient individuals identified by screening provide the most unbiased data from which to make inferences about the relationship of $\alpha$1AT deficiency and disease in children. Other data come from reports of siblings of affected probands (5) and from case studies (7,8).

### B. Liver Disease

About 20% of infants with $\alpha$1AT deficiency have mildly abnormal liver function during early childhood (6,7). These problems sometimes manifest themselves in severe childhood liver disease leading to death or liver transplantation (7). Most of the abnormalities resolve during adolescence (6). The literature relevant to these findings is described below.

An 8-year follow-up of 122 PiZZ infants identified by screening 200,000 infants in Sweden found that approximately 17% of the PiZZ infants manifested some clinical evidence of liver disease (5). In this cohort, the prevalence of abnormal liver function decreased from infancy through the age of roughly 8 years. Of the 14 children who had neonatal cholestasis, two died of cirrhosis by age 2. A third child died at age 5 in an accident; at the time of death, he had a mild increase in periportal fibrous tissue. No cases of cirrhosis were reported among the children with normal liver function in infancy.

Wall et al. (6) described results of long-term follow-up of a cohort of 29 $\alpha$1AT-deficient individuals identified by screening neonates in Oregon and by identification of siblings of probands. Twenty-two people in the cohort were located and tested as adolescents (mean age, 15.1 years). Of these 22, 18 were type PiZZ and 4 type PiSZ. The adolescents were examined for evidence of liver abnormalities. None had symptoms or physical findings consistent with liver disease. One child, a boy, had high alkaline phosphatase; in his case, the abnormal value was considered to be of bone origin. No member of the cohort had had neonatal hepatitis, but several had had mild abnormal liver function during early childhood. This low prevalence is consistent with previously reported data (5).

Ibarguen et al. (7) reviewed the clinical charts of 98 children with a diagnosis of $\alpha$1AT deficiency at the University of Minnesota between the years 1967 and 1988. Age at diagnosis ranged from 5 days to 16 years (mean, 2.3 years; median, 6 weeks). The 98 children included 85 index cases with evidence of liver disease at presentation; the remaining 13 were siblings identified by screening the families of index cases. Of the 85 index cases, 35 were symptom-free at follow-up (mean, 6.4 years; range, 1–25 years). By the end of follow-up, 18 continued to have serum laboratory abnormalities, but in 15, laboratory values became normal within 1 to 15 years (mean, 5 years). Twenty-six of the 50 index cases who did not remain free of symptoms received a liver transplant. Eight died from postoperative complications. Of the 24 who did not receive a transplant, 17 had died by the time of the report. The wide range of age of presentation, the variable length of follow-up, and the long period of time covered (1967–1988) make it difficult to quantify the frequency of severe liver disease. Certainly, however, the grave sequelae of a large proportion of children who presented with symptoms of liver disease suggest that disease, if present, may be very severe in children with α1AT deficiency.

One source of data on the frequency of liver disease in children with α1AT deficiency is information on liver disease in siblings of index cases. If one α1AT-deficient child has liver disease, a PiZZ sibling will have about a 20% chance of developing severe liver disease (7).

### C. Renal Disease

Some children with α1AT deficiency (3,4,7), especially those with liver disease, have renal complications (3,4,7). Of 85 children presenting with liver disease, 17% had renal complications either at presentation or during follow-up (7). Furthermore, 45% of all patient deaths were attributed to renal complications (7).

### D. Pulmonary Complications

Symptomatic lung disease is associated with α1AT deficiency in childhood (8,9), although the prevalence is low (6). For example, in a cohort of 18 PiZZ adolescents (mean age, 15.1 years; range, 12–18 years), all had normal lung volume, normal carbon monoxide diffusing capacity values, and normal spirometric values after bronchodilator aerosol inhalation. A sibling pair, both PiSZ, with known reactive airways showed reversibility to normal range after inhalation of a β-agonist. The authors conclude that most children with α1AT deficiency reach late adolescence with normal lung function (6).

Children with α1AT deficiency who come to medical attention have a high rate of pulmonary complications. For example, the above case series of 98 α1AT-deficient children reported 18% with pulmonary symptoms (7); the median age of presentation with pulmonary disease was 7 years (range, 7 months to 15 years). Because 85 of these children were identified when they presented with liver disease, the observed 18% is not relevant to an unselected population of α1AT-deficient children. Nonetheless, the high rate of pulmonary complications can be viewed as an indication that children with one abnormality associated with α1AT deficiency are probably at increased risk of other abnormalities, including pulmonary complications. Some PiZZ adults have had childhood histories of respiratory-tract infections, atopy with asthma, recurrent pneumonias, or chronic cough with sputum (10).

### E. Summary of the Natural History of α1AT Deficiency in Children

Table 1 summarizes the data on the prevalence of liver and pulmonary disease in children with PiZZ. Included with the estimated prevalence are calculated confidence intervals. About 80% of people with α1AT deficiency exhibit no manifestation of disease during childhood, while about 20% have abnormal liver function. Some of these children develop severe, perhaps fatal, liver disease. Only a few children have pulmonary problems.

## III. Adult Years

### A. Pulmonary Disease

COPD among α1AT-deficient individuals occurs as early as the age of 25 years and generally between 25 and 40 years (11–13). Silverman et al. (14), in a series of 30 persons of type PiZ identified by family screening, found a high proportion with normal $FEV_1$. Although people of type PiZ have been known to live to their eighth (15) or ninth (13) decade, they are likely to develop obstructive airways disease eventually (16). COPD is the most prevalent disease and most common cause of death reported among PiZZ adults.

Studies of PiZZ adults have reported a strong association of tobacco smoking with the development of, and mortality from, pulmonary disease (11–13,15–17). People who begin smoking in their early teen years often have disabling pulmonary disease in their 30s (10). Larsson (11) estimated that smoking shortens median survival by 23 years. Data show considerable variability among PiZZ

**Table 1** Proportion of Liver and Pulmonary Disease in PiZZ Children Identified on Neonatal Screening or as Siblings of Index Cases

| | | | Liver disease (%) | | Abnormal pulmonary function (%) | |
|---|---|---|---|---|---|---|
| Study | *n* | Age | Rate | 95% Conf. limit | Rate | 95% Conf. limit |
| Sveger (5) | 122 | Infancy | 17 | 11–25 | — | — |
| Wall et al. (6) | 18 | Teenage | 0 | 0–19 | 0 | 0–19 |

individuals with respect to the severity of pulmonary disease and the effect of smoking. In particular, lung function is well preserved in some PiZZ smokers but severely impaired in some nonsmokers (11–13,15–17). The following text presents in more detail several reports related to pulmonary disease in the PiZZ adult.

Larsson (11) studied natural history and life expectancy of 246 Swedish α1AT-deficient PiZZ individuals identified from blood samples. Most of the individuals had diagnoses of COPD. Tobin et al. (12) described clinical and physiological features of COPD in 166 PiZZ individuals identified from a British multicenter study. The cohort included 126 index cases identified through chest clinics and 40 nonindex cases identified through family studies of the index cases. Janus et al. (13) studied the relationship between lung function and smoking in 69 PiZZ adults in New Zealand, while Black and Kueppers (15) reported clinical course and lung function of 22 PiZZ smokers and 36 PiZZ smokers from the midwestern United States. Using data from Larsson (11), Wu and Eriksson (17) studied the relationship between smoking and lung function in the 158 PiZZ adults who had at least one measurement of lung function.

Table 2 presents the frequency of COPD as well as the causes of death for all the above mentioned papers that presented relevant data. COPD was present in 44–74% of the study participants, and pulmonary disease accounted for 62–88% of the reported deaths. To examine the association of smoking with pulmonary disease and death, the mean or median age of onset of dyspnea and the mean age at death are presented in Table 3 by smoking status for three studies with the relevant information. The average age of onset of dyspnea ranged from 32 to 44 years in smokers and 43 to 53 years in nonsmokers, while the age at death ranged from 48 to 52 years for smokers and 60 to 68 years for nonsmokers. Although no significant difference was observed in ages at onset of dyspnea between smokers in the small number of nonindex cases with dyspnea reported by Tobin et al. (12), the mean $FEV_1$ as percent of predicted in smokers was 19% lower than that in the nonsmokers for both the index and nonindex cases (see Table 4). Furthermore, the nonindex cases had significantly higher average lung function than the index cases.

Buist et al. (18) reported data on annual rate of change in $FEV_1$ for PiZ individuals in the United States and Sweden who had $FEV_1$ measured at least twice. The time of follow-up varied considerably (Range, 12–181 months; mean, approximately 70 months). The people included had been identified in a number of ways. Some were patients with lung disease or relatives of such patients; others had been identified by blood-bank screening or population studies. The group studied included a small number of healthy young adults with normal or near-normal $FEV_1$ who experienced only a very slow decline in $FEV_1$ during follow-up. Among those with initial $FEV_1$ below 30% predicted, the morality was very high. Finally, in those with initial $FEV_1$ between 30% and 65% predicted, the average (±SD) annual rate of decline was 111 ± 102 ml, a rate the authors point out

**Table 2** Frequency Distribution of Emphysema, Liver Disease, and Death in Three Studies of $\alpha_1$AT-Deficient Individuals

| Study | Description | Smoker | *n* | Age | Disease | No. with disease | No. deaths |
|---|---|---|---|---|---|---|---|
| Janus et al. (13) | New Zealand | Yes and No | 69 | 0–87 | COPD | 33 | 14 |
| | PiZZ cases 1970–1983 | Yes and No | 246 | >20 | Liver disease | 12 | 4 |
| Larsson (11) | Sweden PiZZ | Yes and No[a] | 246 | >20 | COPD | 184 | 56 |
| | | Yes | 151 | >20 | COPD | 129 | 56 |
| | | No | 95 | >20 | COPD | 55 | 0 |
| | | Yes and No | 246 | >20 | Liver disease | 30 | 12 |
| | | Yes and No | 246 | >20 | Other | — | 23 |
| Black and Kueppers (15) | Midwest U.S. | Yes | 36 | 22–66 | COPD | 33 | 5 |
| | | No | 22 | 18–79 | COPD | 10 | 7 |
| | | | | | Suicide | — | 1 |
| | | | | | Other | 8 | — |

[a]61% were smokers.

**Table 3** Mean Age of Onset of Dyspnea and Mean Age of Death by Smoking Status for Four Studies

| | Onset of Dyspnea | | Death | |
|---|---|---|---|---|
| Study | Mean age ± SD | *n* | Age | *n* |
| Janus et al. (13) | | | | |
| Smokers | 32 ± 9 | 22 | 48 ± 13 | 10 |
| Nonsmokers | 51 ± 10 | 11 | 67 ± 4 | 5 |
| Tobin et al. (12) | | | | |
| Index cases | | | | |
| Smokers | | | | |
| Male | 39 | 69 | 55 | 15 |
| Female | 39 | 30 | 43 | 5 |
| Nonsmokers | | | | |
| Male | 46 | 6 | — | 0 |
| Female | 49 | 8 | 60 | 3 |
| Nonindex cases | | | | |
| Smokers | 44 | 14 | — | 0 |
| Nonsmokers | 43 | 7 | — | 0 |
| Larsson et al. (20) | | | | |
| Smokers | 40[a] | — | — | 0 |
| Nonsmokers | 53[a] | — | | |
| Total | | 169 | | |
| Black and Kueppers (15) | | | | |
| Smokers | 37 ± 10 | 35 | 51 | 5 |
| Nonsmokers | 51 ± 9 | 18 | 68 | 3 |

[a]Median age.

is nearly twice that of decline in ordinary COPD. The authors conclude that "PiZ subjects who develop clinically significant airflow limitation go through a phase of their disease in which there is a relatively high rate of functional decline."

Two studies (13,17) report both cross-sectional and longitudinal analyses of pulmonary function ($FEV_1$) by smoking status (see Table 4). Cross-sectional analysis of the most recent $FEV_1$ measurement (13) indicates that on average smokers had significantly lower lung function than nonsmokers.

Longitudinal analysis of serial measurements also indicates significantly faster $FEV_1$ decline in smokers than in nonsmokers; the rate of decline in ex-smokers is somewhere in between (13). Longitudinal analysis of follow-up $FEV_1$ measurements showed mean $FEV_1$ declines of 60 ml/year, 60 ml/year, and 80 ml/year for smokers, nonsmokers, and ex-smokers, respectively (17). The mean age of the smokers, however, was approximately 9 years lower than that of the non-

**Table 4** $FEV_1$ by Smoking Status: Cross-Sectional and Longitudinal Analyses

| | Cross-sectional analysis of $FEV_1$ | | Longitudinal analysis | | |
|---|---|---|---|---|---|
| Study | $FEV_1$ | *n* | $FEV_1$ slope ± SD (ml/yr) | *n* | Mean age |
| Wu and Eriksson (17) | (Initial $FEV_1$) | | | | |
| Never-smokers | −30 ml/yr | 40 | −60 ± 100 | 10 | 49.8 |
| Ever-smokers | −41 ml/yr | 118 | — | — | — |
| Ex-smokers | — | — | −80 ± 70 | 22 | 48.8 |
| Current smokers | — | — | −60 ± 170 | 40 | 40.1 |
| Janus et al. (13) | (Most recent $FEV_1$ predicted ± SD) | | | | |
| Smokers | 38% ± 37% | 22 | −316 ± 196 | 5 | |
| Nonsmokers | 77% ± 36% | 13 | −80 ± 101 | 2 | |
| Ex-smokers | — | — | −61 ± 122 | 8 | |
| Tobin et al. (12) | | | | | |
| Index cases | | | | | |
| Smokers | 35% | 96 | | | |
| Nonsmokers | 54% | 14 | | | |
| Nonindex cases | | | | | |
| Smokers | 62% | 17 | | | |
| Nonsmokers | 81% | 14 | | | |

and ex-smokers. After adjusting for age and other important covariates, the rates of $FEV_1$ decline did not differ significantly among smokers, nonsmokers, and ex-smokers. This similarity of age-adjusted rates of decline should not be viewed as evidence that the course of disease is the same in smokers as in nonsmokers, because in the same study, the risk of death for smokers was approximately three times the risk for nonsmokers. A reasonable hypothesis is that the higher death rate in smokers censors differentially those with fastest decline in lung function. Thus, the observed similarity in rates of decline by smoking status is likely an artifact of differential mortality. In particular, the period of most rapid decline in $FEV_1$—the months prior to death—is excluded from the comparison of slopes.

### B. Other PiZZ-Associated Disease

After COPD, liver disease has been reported to be the next most common disease associated with type PiZZ in adults (12,13,18), but its frequency is unknown.

Rawlings et al. (19) reported a high rate of miscarriages in women with PiZZ. Among the eight women in the case series who were pregnant at least once, five had at least one miscarriage.

## IV. Other Phenotypes

Some investigators report an increased risk of COPD associated with the PiSZ phenotype (20,21). The phenotype is uncommon; only one of the 124 patients referred to in the study of Brantly et al. (22) with α1AT deficiency and pulmonary symptoms and three of the 98 cases reviewed by Ibarguen et al. (7) were of the PiSZ phenotype. Other phenotypes associated with α1AT deficiency are rare (23,24).

## V. Summary

A child with α1AT deficiency has elevated risk of early liver disease. A small proportion who have severe liver disease do not survive to adulthood. Adults with α1AT deficiency are at high risk for early COPD and death from respiratory failure. Smoking is associated with an accelerated rate of decline in $FEV_1$; it is therefore very important that people with α1AT deficiency do not smoke. In trying to estimate the elevation in risk of severe pulmonary disease and early related mortality, and in trying to elucidate the relationship of smoking with the acceleration of the process of deterioration of the lung, the available data are necessarily limited. The most ill patients are the ones who are seen by medical care facilities; an asymptomatic person, or one whose pulmonary function is not severely affected, may not be identified as a PiZZ individual. In the absence of population follow-up of asymptomatic PiZZ individuals, only a qualitative assessment of the burden of illness is possible. The data surely point to a very high prevalence of COPD in PiZZ individuals. The actual proportion of people who develop COPD and the distribution of age of onset are, however, unknown.

Similarly, the rate of early mortality in PiZZ individuals is certainly very high relative to that in an unaffected population, but the proportion of people who live to at least the sixth decade of life is unknown. Finally, there is ample evidence that smoking is related to an accelerated downward course in PiZZ individuals and suggestive evidence that cessation of smoking reduces the risk of pulmonary disease and early death to somewhere between that of current smokers and those who never smoked. Again, a precise estimate of the rate of decline of pulmonary function in an unselected PiZZ population is not available.

Quantification of the strength of association of risk factors with morbidity and mortality in α1AT-deficient people and more complete delineation of the time course of the disease would require rigorous, large-scale study of asymptomatic individuals with PiZZ, PiSZ, and related phenotypes. Such studies could provide further information about the levels of serum α1AT that portend early COPD.

## References

1. Laurell CB, Eriksson S. The electrophoretic alpha$_1$-globulin pattern of serum in alpha$_1$-antitrypsin deficiency. Scand J Clin Lab Invest 1963; 15:132.
2. Sharp HL, Bridges RA, Krivit W, Freir EF. Cirrhosis associated with alpha-1-antitrypsin deficiency: a previously unrecognized inherited disorder. J Lab Clin Med 1969; 73:934.
3. Moroz SP, Cutz E, Cox DW, Sass-Kortsak A. Liver disease associated with $\alpha_1$-antitrypsin deficiency in childhood. J Pediatr 1976; 88:19–25.
4. Strife CF, Hug G, Chuck G, McAdams AJ, Davis CA, Klein JJ. Membranoproliferative glomerulonephritis and $\alpha_1$-antitrypsin deficiency. Pediatrics 1983; 71:88–92.
5. Sveger T. Prospective study of children with alpha$_1$-antitrypsin deficiency: eight-year-old follow-up. J Pediatr 1984; 104:91–94.
6. Wall M, Moe E, Eisenberg J, Powers M, Buist N, Buist AS. Long-term follow-up of a cohort of children with alpha-1-antitrypsin deficiency. J Pediatr 1990; 116:248–251.
7. Ibarguen E, Gross CR, Savik K, Sharp HL. Liver disease in alpha-1-antitrypsin deficiency: Prognostic indicators. J Pediatr 1990; 117:864–870.
8. Hustek J, Copora M, Zapetal A, Tomasova H, Hamenek M, Alpha$_1$-antitrypsin deficiency in a child with chronic lung disease. Chest 1975; 64:773.
9. Talamo RC, Levison H, Lynch MJ, Herez A, Hyslop NE, Bain HW. Symptomatic pulmonary emphysema in childhood associated with hereditary $\alpha_1$-antitrypsin and elastase inhibitor deficiency. J Pediatr 1971; 79:20.
10. Pierce JA. Antitrypsin and emphysema. JAMA 1988; 259:2890–2895.
11. Larsson C. Natural history and life expectancy in severe alpha$_1$-antitrypsin deficiency, PiZ. Acta Med Scand 1978; 204:345–351.
12. Tobin MJ, Cook PJL, Hutchison DCS. Alpha$_1$-antitrypsin deficiency: the clinical and physiological features of pulmonary emphysema in subjects homozygous for Pi type Z. Br J Dis Chest 1983; 77:12–27.
13. Janus ED, Phillips NT, Carrell RW. Smoking, lung function and $\alpha_1$-antitrypsin deficiency. Lancet 1985; 1:152–154.
14. Silverman EK, Pierce JA, Province MA, Roa DC, Campbell EJ. Variability of pulmonary function in alpha-1-antitrypsin deficiency: clinical correlates. Ann Intern Med 1989; 111:982– 986.
15. Black LF, Kueppers F. Alpha$_1$-antitrypsin deficiency in nonsmokers. Am Rev Respir Dis 1978; 117:421–428.
16. Snider GL. Pulmonary disease in alpha-1-antitrypsin deficiency. Ann Intern Med 1989; 111:957–959.
17. Wu MC, Eriksson S. Lung function, smoking and survival in severe alpha$_1$-antitrypsin deficiency, PiZZ. J Clin Epidemiol 1988; 41:1157–1165.
18. Buist AS, Burrows B, Eriksson S, Mittman C, Wu M. The natural history of air-flow obstruction in PiZ emphysema. Report of an NHLBI Workshop. Am Rev Respir Dis 1983; 127(suppl):43–45.
19. Rawlings W, Kreiss P, Levy D, Cohen B, Menkes H, Brashears S, Permutt S. Clinical, epidemiologic, and pulmonary function studies in alpha$_1$-antitrypsin-deficient subjects of PiZ type. Am Rev Respir Dis 1976; 114:945–953.

20. Larsson C, Dirksen H, Sundstromg, Eriksson S. Lung function studies in asymptomatic individuals with moderately (PiSZ) and severely (PiZ) reduced levels of $\alpha_1$-antitrypsin. Scand J Respir Dis 1976; 57:207–280.
21. Gadek JE, Crystal RG. $\alpha_1$-antitrypsin deficiency. In: Stansbury JB, Wyngaardon JB, Frederikson DS, Goldstein JI, Brown MS, eds. The Metabolic Basis of Inherited Disease. 5th ed. New York: McGraw-Hill, 1982:450–467.
22. Brantly ML, Paul LD, Miller BH, Falk RT, Wu M, Crystal RG. Clinical features and history of the destructive lung disease associated with $\alpha_1$-antitrypsin deficiency of adults with pulmonary symptoms. Am Rev Respir Dis 1988; 138:327–336.
23. Fagerhol MK, Hauge HE. Serum Pi type in patients with pulmonary disease. Acta Allergol 1969; 24:107–114.
24. Cox DW, Billingsley GD, Smyth S. Rare types of $\alpha_1$-antitrypsin associated with deficiency. In: Allen RC, Arnaud P, eds. Electrophoresis '81. Berlin: Walter de Gruyter, 1981:505–510.

# 19

# The Prevalence of α1AT Deficiency Outside the United States and Europe

**TOSHIHIRO NUKIWA**

Tohoku University
Sendai, Japan

**KUNIAKI SEYAMA and SHIRO KIRA**

Juntendo University School of Medicine
Tokyo, Japan

## I. Introduction

### A. Prevalence of α1AT Deficiency in Orientals

Whereas the gene frequency for the Z-type alpha 1–antitrypsin (α1AT)-deficient variant is relatively high (0.01–0.02) among Caucasians, deficient variants outside the United States and Europe—for example, among Orientals—have been recognized to be very rare (1,2). Obviously one reason would be the lack of sufficient laboratory examination systems in countries outside the United States and Europe. However, some countries, including Singapore, Korea, Japan, and Taiwan, have equally sophisticated laboratory examination systems. Nonetheless, only a few cases have been reported except among those of Caucasian descent with the Z deficient variant. For example, only 12 cases with deficient α1AT serum levels have been reported in Japan, as described in detail later. More than 2 million Orientals from China, Korea, and Japan—immigrants or their descendants—live in North America; again, there are only a few reports of α1AT deficiency among these U.S. Orientals despite the fact that they receive high-quality medical examinations. One null variant, $Null_{hongkong}$ [two nucleotides' deletion at residue 318 causing premature termination at residue 334 (3)] was reported as a variant in a family from China (4). α1AT deficiency is also rare in American Indians.

### B. Prevalence in Blacks and Other Races

Although a few cases with the Z-deficient α1AT variant among American blacks have been reported (5), the gene frequency of the Z-type variant among 204 American black subjects in one study was only 0.005 (two subjects with the Z variant) (6) and zero in 186 American blacks in another study (7). Although several normal variants with different isoelectrofocusing (IEF) mobility have been reported (8), no new deficient variant analyzed at the gene level is known to occur in blacks. Furthermore, according to studies with African blacks, no subject with a Z variant was observed among blacks from Mozanbique and Bantu (9,10). As for other races, studies of more than 5000 native people, including those of the Pacific islands, Papua New Guinea, and central Australia in addition to China, Japan, and India, revealed no cases with the Z-type deficient variant (2).

Taking these reports together, it can be concluded that α1AT deficiency in non-Caucasians is extremely rare in both the Z-type deficient variant and other deficient variants. In other words, the clinically significant and highly prevalent Z-type deficient variant appears to be limited to Caucasians, although it is expected that intermarriage between Caucasians and other races will eventually increase the prevalence of the Z-type variant.

## II. α1AT Deficiency in Japan

### A. Evaluation of the Incidence of Unique Allelic Marker $Ala^{213}$(GCG) to $Val^{213}$(GTG) Mutation in Japanese

The Ala(GCG) to Val(GTG) substitution at residue 213 was first described as a second mutation in addition to Glu(GAG) to Lys(AAG) at residue 342 in the Z-type deficient variant (11). It turned out that the root of this substitution is found in a normal variant, M1, as phenotyped by IEF (12). Because alanine and valine are both nonpolar amino acids, the substitution of these residues does not affect the mobility on isoelectrofocusing. However, GCG to GTG mutation corresponding to these 213 residues could be distinguished by restriction endonucleases, BstEII (11), MaeIII (13), and BstPI. This enables the discrimination of two normal α1AT variants, M1($Ala^{213}$) and M1($Val^{213}$), that are otherwise identical on isoelectrofocusing. In those of North America Caucasian descent, about one-third of electrophoretically designated M1 variants are M1($Ala^{213}$) and two-thirds are M1($Val^{213}$) (Table 1) (12,13). As the Z-type α1AT-deficient variant has alanine on the 213 residue and no other substitution of residue except for residue 342 (Glu-

**Table 1** Incidence of Unique Allelic Marker of Residue 213 (Ala/Val Substitution) in α1AT Gene in a Japanese Population and in U.S. Whites

| | | | U.S. white population (phenotype M1)[b] | |
|---|---|---|---|---|
| Amino acid on residue 213 | Main variant included | Japanese population[a] | Nukiwa et al. (12) | Cox et al. (13) |
| Ala213 | M1(Ala213) | 0 | 0.32 | 0.34 |
| | Z | (0/312) | (25/78) | (13/38) |
| Val213 | M1(Val213) | 1.0 | 0.68 | 0.66 |
| | M2 | (312/312) | (53/78) | (25/38) |
| | M3 | | | |
| | M4 | | | |

[a]The Japanese population was studied based on the DNA analysis in exon III of the α1AT gene, not on serum protein phenotype.
[b]Analysis of RFLP was performed in a U.S. white population with phenotype M1 on IEF.

Lys), it is likely that this highly prevalent deficient variant might be derived from M1($Ala^{213}$), although a precise haplotype study would be necessary to prove it.

Because the Z-type deficient variant is so rare in Japan and the Z-type variant is characterized by residue 213 as Ala, we attempted to examine which amino acid substitution (Ala or Val) is found at α1AT residue 213 in Japanese (14). In this context, a DNA fragment in exon III of α1AT was amplified by PCR and subsequently digested with BstPI. All 312 alleles from 156 genomic DNA samples from a Japanese population revealed that they have valine on residue 213 of α1AT (Table 1), indicating that, in contrast to U.S. whites, most α1AT genes in Japanese are likely derived from M1($Val^{213}$) including the major normal variants M2, M3, and M4. This result is consistent with the fact that in Japanese and other Orientals, the Z-type α1AT-deficient variant (with alanine at the 213 residue) is extremely rare. It is highly probable that with more detailed studies in nonexonic regions of the α1AT gene in addition to the exonic region sequence as the above Ala213–Val substitution, the α1AT genes in Japanese or other Orientals will be proved to be quite different from those in Caucasians, accounting for the rarity of the Z-type α1AT deficiency in these countries. Although some exceptions such as $Z_{augusburg}$ (15), which has $Glu^{342} \rightarrow$ Lys mutation on M2 background and not on the usual M1($Ala^{213}$) background, might be found in the future, the vast majority of the deficient variants in Oriental populations would not be related to the Z-type deficient variant.

### B. Three α1AT Deficient Variants in Japan Analyzed at the Gene Level

Three deficient variants in Japan have been analyzed at the gene level: $M_{nichinan}$ [del $Phe^{52}$, $Gly^{148}$(GGG) to $Arg^{148}$(AGG)] (16), $S_{iiyama}$[$Ser^{53}$(TCC) to $Phe^{53}$(TTC)] (26), and $M_{malton}$ (del $Phe^{52}$) (17).

$M_{nichinan}$ was found in a 42-year-old woman with bronchitis (18). Although the proband was a light smoker, her pulmonary function did not meet the criteria for emphysema. Consistent with Z-type α1AT deficiency, the aggregation of α1AT molecules was demonstrated histologically in hepatocytes. The genomic DNA of the α1AT gene of the proband was cloned and sequenced along with the entire 10627 bp. Within the coding exons, the TTC trinucleotide deletion and a G substitution were identified that corresponded to the deletion $Phe^{52}$ and substitution of $Gly^{148}$(GGG) to Arg(AGG). Deletion of $Phe^{52}$—identical to the defect with the $M_{malton}$-type deficient variant (19)—is likely to accumulate within the cell and be deficient in serum. Although not confirmed by expression, the second $Gly^{148} \rightarrow$ Arg mutation is assumed not to be the cause of deficiency in both the amount in the serum and the function because this position is not in a highly conserved part of the serpin backbone. In addition, one serpin, protein C inhibitor, has Arg on the corresponding residue 148 of protein C inhibitor structure when amino acid sequences were aligned with those of α1AT.

The analysis of $M_{nichinan}$ has been unique in that investigators have sequenced the whole 10627 bp of both $M_{nichinan}$ and M1($Val^{213}$), a normal variant. This information made it possible for the first time to compare the entire genomic α1AT nucleotide sequences of the reported S variant (20) to those of M1($Val^{213}$) from a Japanese normal individual and of $M_{nichinan}$. In other words, the entire nonexonic α1AT genomic nucleotide sequence from a Caucasoid individual can be compared with those from Mongoloid individuals. In this context, apart from the coding exons as described above, Matsunaga et al. (16) reported that the sequences of the 5′ flanking regions, of four introns, and of 3′ flanking regions revealed 58 bp differences between the $M_{nichinan}$ and S genes, 47 bp between the M1($Val^{213}$) and S genes, and only 15 bp between the M1($Val^{213}$) and $M_{nichinan}$. Thus, more than twice as many nucleotides were detected in the haplotype genes of Caucasoids as in those of Mongoloids, probably because of the historical and geographical differences between the races.

The $S_{iiyama}$ variant was found in a 38-year-old man from the central area of Japan with pulmonary emphysema. The accumulation of the α1AT proteins was detected in a liver-biopsy specimen. On isoelectrofocusing, a very faint banding around the S region was finally confirmed on crossed immunoelectrophoresis, and the phenotype was designated $S_{iiyama}$ after the birthplace of the proband. When coding regions were amplified and sequenced, the amino acid substitution, $Ser^{53}$(TCC) to Phe(TTC), occurred on the conserved residue of the serpin backbone. This was the first case fitted to the theoretical interpretation and prediction of the three-dimensional crystallographic structure of the α1AT molecule. In this context, the amino acid substitution found in α1AT $S_{iiyama}$ ($Ser^{53}$–Phe) occurred on one of 51 residues noted by Huber and Carrell (21) as being conserved. Mutation at $Ser^{53}$ has a profound effect on the three-dimensional structure of the α1AT molecule because Oγ of $Ser^{53}$ initiates helix B, hydrogen-bonded to N of $Ser^{56}$, and stabilizes a portion of sheet 5B by bonding to O of $Leu^{383}$. It also participates in the folding of the internal core, which consists mainly of the most conserved secondary structural elements (helix B and sheets 3A, 4B, and 5B). It can be assumed that the changes in properties resulting from the replacement of hydrophilic $Ser^{53}$ with hydrophobic $Phe^{53}$ may influence the integrity and organization of the α1AT molecule. This would be related to the marked cathodal shift to S on IEF and the existence of immunoreactive aggregates in hepatocytes from the proband. The intracellular events caused by altered protein structure eventually result in the reduction in the serum level of α1AT.

$M_{malton}$ in Japan was identified in 49-year-old woman with dyspnea and wheeze (22). Although her serum α1AT level was 70 mg/dl and she was a nonsmoker, she suffered from mild hypoxemia and showed a pattern of obstructive pulmonary function. Her phenotype was initially determined as $PiM_{null}$. Nucleotide sequencing of the coding exons by PCR revealed the heterozygous deletion of three-nucleotide TTC, which corresponds to deletion of $Phe^{52}$, known as the $M_{malton}$ deficient variant (17). At least four independent $M_{malton}$ cases have been reported (17,19,23,24) and the M2 α1AT structure was found in two Caucasoid cases (19,23); i.e., allelic markers on the coding sequence were $His^{101}$, $Val^{213}$, and $Asp^{376}$ (27). In this context, it is of interest that $M_{nichinan}$ has the identical defect of deletion $Phe^{52}$ on M1($Val^{213}$) structure; i.e., allelic markers are $Arg^{101}$, $Val^{213}$, and $Glu^{376}$, indicating that the pathological defect occurs independently at a "hot spot." This is caused either by intrachromosomal recombination between directly repeated sequences or by so-called frameshift mutagenesis, because of the presence of ATC–TTC–TTC–TCC in codons 51–54 (16,19). In this sense, $\Delta Phe^{52}$-type deficient variants might be found more frequently outside the United States and Europe.

## III. α1AT $S_{iiyama}$ Deficient Variant Is Prevalent in Japan

Although α1AT deficiency is rare in Japan, 12 unrelated families including the above three deficient variants have been reported (Table 2). We attempted to examine whether five other known cases have independent genetic defects on the α1AT gene or share the identical mutations. For screening we used allele-specific polymerase chain reaction (PCR) by preparing a pair of oligonucleotides with mutated bases in exon 2 of the α1AT $S_{iiyama}$ gene at the 3′ end. Interestingly, all

**Table 2** Reported Cases with α1AT Deficiency in Japan: Prevalence of $S_{iiyama}$ Deficient Variant

| No. | Proband (age and sex) | Phenotype originally reported | Serum level (mg/dl) | Allele of deficient variant by gene analysis | Authors |
|---|---|---|---|---|---|
| 1 | 33F, 33M | Pizz | 18 | NA[a] | Kozuru et al., 1975 |
| 2 | 27M, 33F, 37M | $Pi_{nullnull}$ | >10 | $Pi*S_{iiyama}$ | Ohashi et al., 1978 |
| 3 | 49F | $PiM_{null}$ | 70 | $Pi*M_{malton}$ | Kitada et al., 1978 |
| 4 | 42F, ?F | $PiM_{nichinan}M_{nichinan}$ | 17.9 | $Pi*M_{nichinan}$ | Nakamura et al., 1980 |
| 5 | 56M | $PiM_{numazu}M_{numazu}$ | 10 | $Pi*S_{iiyama}$ | Otani et al., 1980 |
| 6 | 52M | PiSS | 19 | NA[a] | Tsuda et al., 1983 |
| 7 | 1M | $PiM1_{null}$ | 104 | del 14q (q24.3 to q32.1)[b] | Yamamoto et al., 1986 |
| 8 | 38M | $PiS_{iiyama}S_{iiyama}$ | 14 | $Pi*S_{iiyama}$ | Takabe et al., 1989 |
| 9 | 33M | $Pi_{nullnull}$ | 12 | $Pi*S_{iiyama}$ | Sugimoto et al., 1990 |
| 10 | 40M | ? | 25 | $Pi*S_{iiyama}$ | Sato et al., 1990 |
| 11 | 50F, 53F | $PiM_{numazu}2M_{numazu}2$ | 22, 11 | $Pi*S_{iiyama}$ | Fujita et al., 1990 |
| 12 | 35F | ? | 40 | $Pi*S_{iiyama}$ | Konishi et al., 1991 |

[a]Samples from proband or family members are not available.
[b]A sporadic case, not familial; del 14q syndrome was confirmed by chromosomal analysis.

five cases were identified as carrying the $S_{iiyama}$ deficient variant in a homozygous fashion. Additionally, one family was independently identified as carrying the $S_{iiyama}$ deficient variant. Thus, seven families (70%) of 10 examined cases with α1AT deficiency in Japan are carrying the $S_{iiyama}$ α1AT deficient variant (25). All cases showed consanguinity in family pedigrees; parents of all seven probands were cousins. Seven families are distributed widely on the central island (Honshu) of Japan. To date no other deficient variant analyzed at the gene level was reported with an accumulation like that of $S_{iiyama}$ except for Z and S. Although there is no report of α1AT-deficient variants from other Asian countries, it will be of interest to explore whether the $S_{iiyama}$ variant is common to Orientals because of the relatively high accumulation in Japan and the migration of people from the Asian continent in both the prehistoric and historic past.

Through this attempt to search for identical deficient variants in Japan, we realized the necessity of direct examination at the nucleotide level. Because of difficulties in determining a deficient phenotype on a faint isoelectrofocusing band, these families with the identical genetic defect were misnamed at the serum protein level (Table 2), hence misrepresenting the incidence of deficient variants.

## IV. Summary

Z-type α1AT deficiency is one of the most common genetic disorders in Caucasians, but it is extremely rare outside the United States and Europe, even though medical-examination systems are less sophisticated in many of these areas. Only a few cases of deficient variants in non-Caucasians have been reported. In addition, the Z-type deficient variant itself appears to be limited to Caucasians: no deficient variant was reported in African blacks; no Z type was found in more than 5000 natives of China, Japan, Thailand, India, Indonesia, Pacific Islanders, Papua New Guinea, and Central Australia. The Z-type deficient variant is characterized by its two amino acid residues (Ala at residue 213 as a marker for an older variant in the phylogenetic tree and Lys at residue 342 as a pathological substitution in terms of the protein structure). When 312 α1AT alleles in Japanese were examined to determine which amino acid—Ala(GCG) or Val(GTG)—is coded for at residue 213 using PCR-RFLP, all were found to have Val at residue 213, characteristic of newer variants and different from the Z-type variant. This partly explains the rarity of the Z-type deficient variant in Japan. Only 12 cases with deficient α1AT in serum have been reported in Japan. Three were analyzed at the gene level and identified as $M_{nichinan}$, $S_{iiyama}$, and $M_{malton}$. When six other cases were examined using allele-specific PCR or direct sequencing, all were identified as $S_{iiyama}$. Thus, $S_{iiyama}$ is the most common deficient α1AT variant in Japan. It will be of interest to learn whether the $S_{iiyama}$ deficient variant is common in other Oriental populations.

## References


1. Miyake K, Suzuki H, Oka H, Oda T, Harada S. Distribution of $\alpha$1-antitrypsin phenotypes in Japanese: Description of Pi M subtypes by isoelectric focusing. Jap J Human Genet 1979; 24:55–62.
2. Kamboh MI, Kirk RL, Clark P. Alpha-1-antitrypsin (PI) types in Asian, Pacific and Aboriginal Australian populations. Disease Markers 1983; 1:33–42.
3. Sifers RN, Brashears-Macatee S, Kidd VJ, Muensch H, Woo SLC. A frameshift mutation results in a truncated $\alpha$1-antitrypsin that is retained within the rough endoplasmic reticulum. J Biol Chem 1988; 263:7330–7335.
4. Muensch H, Gaidulis L, Kuppers F, So SY, Escano G, Kidd VJ, Woo SLC. Complete abscence of serum alpha-1-antitrypsin in conjunction with an apparently normal gene structure. Am J Hum Genet 1986; 38:898–907.
5. Mostafavi S, Lieberman J. Intermediate alpha 1-antitrypsin deficiency with apical lung bullae and spontaneous pneumothorax. Chest 1991; 99:1545–1546.
6. Pierce JA, Eradio B, Dew TA. Antitrypsin phenotypes in St. Louis. JAMA 1975; 231: 609–612.
7. Lieberman J, Gaidulis L, Roberts L. Racial distribution of alpha 1-antitrypsin variants among junior high school students. Am Rev Respir Dis 1976; 114:1194–1198.
8. Hug G, Chuck G, McGill M. $PiW_{finneytown}$: a new alpha-1-antitrypsin allele in an American Negro family. Hum Heredity 1982; 32:280–284.
9. Kellermann G, Walter H. Investigations on the population genetics of the alpha-1-antitrypsin polymorphism. Humangenetik 1970; 10:145–150.
10. Welch SG, McGregor IA, Williams K. Alpha-1-antitrypsin (Pi) phenotypes in a village population from the Gambia, West Africa. Hum Genet 1980; 53:223–235.
11. Nukiwa T, Satoh K, Brantly ML, Ogushi F, Fells GA, Courtney M, Crystal RG. Identification of a second mutation in the protein-coding sequence of the Z type alpha 1-antitrypsin gene. J Biol Chem 1986; 261:15989–15994.
12. Nukiwa T, Brantly M, Ogushi F, Fells G, Satoh K, Stier L, Courtney M, Crystal RG. Characterization of the M(ala213) type of $\alpha$1-antitrypsin, a newly recognized, common "normal" $\alpha$1-antitrypsin haplotype. Biochemistry 1987; 26:5259–5267.
13. Cox DW, Billingsley GD. Restriction enzyme MaeIII for prenatal diagnosis of alpha 1-antitrypsin deficiency. Lancet 1986; ii(8509), 741–742.
14. Nukiwa T, Seyama K, Takahashi H, Takahashi K, Ohwada A, Matsuda K, Kira S. Why is Z type $\alpha$1-antitrypsin deficiency not found in Japan? Jap J Thoracic Soc 1991; 29(suppl):371.
15. Faber J-P, Weidinger S, Olek K. Sequence data of the rare deficient alpha1-antitrypsin variant PI Zaugusburg. Am J Hum Genet 1990; 46:1158–1162.
16. Matsunaga E, Shiokawa S, Nakamura H, Maruyama T, Tsuda K, Fukumaki Y. Molecular analysis of the gene of the $\alpha$1-antitrypsin deficiency variant, Mnichinan. Am J Hum Genet 1990; 46:602–612.
17. Sakai T, Satoh K, Narumi A, Nagai H, Motomiya M. A case of deficient $\alpha$1-antitrypsin Mmalton analyzed at the gene level. Jap J Thoracic Soc 1991; 29(suppl):386.
18. Nakamura H, Ogawa A, Hisano S, Fukuma M, Tachibana N, Tsuda K. A family with a new deficient variant of alpha 1-antitrypsin $PiM_{nichinan}$—with special reference to

diastase-resistant, periodic acid-Schiff positive globules in the liver cells. J Jap Soc Int Med 1980; 69:967–974.

19. Curiel DT, Holmes MD, Okayama H, Brantly ML, Vogelmeier C, Travis WD, Stier LE, Perks WH, Crystal RG. Molecular basis of the liver and lung disease associated with the α1-antitrypsin deficiency allele $M_{malton}$. J Biol Chem 1989; 264:13938–13945.
20. Long GL, Chandra T, Woo SLC, Davie EW, Kurachi K. Complete sequence of the cDNA for human α1-antitrypsin and the gene for the S variant. Biochemistry 1984; 23:4828–2837.
21. Huber R, Carrell RW. Implications of the three-dimensional structure of α1-antitrypsin for structure and function of serpins. Biochemistry 1989; 28:8951–8966.
22. Kitada O, Sugita M, Kikuchi H, Hourai Z, Inokuma S. Study on a case with pulmonary emphysema combined with alpha 1-antitrypsin deficiency and its family. J Jap Soc Int Med 1978; 67:295–300.
23. Fraizer GC, Harrold TR, Hofker MH, Cox DW. In-frame single codon deletion in the $M_{malton}$ deficiency allele of α1-antitrypsin. Am J Hum Genet 1989; 44:894–902.
24. Graham A, Kalsheker NA, Newton CR, Bamforth FJ, Powell SJ, Markham AF. Molecular characterization of three alpha-1-antitrypsin deficiency variants: proteinase inhibitor (Pi) $null_{cardif}$ ($Asp^{256}$–Val); $PiM_{malton}$ ($Phe^{51}$-deletion) and PiI ($Arg^{39}$–Cys). Hum Genet 1989; 84:55–58.
25. Seyama K, Nukiwa T, Aiba M, Kira S. Seven independent families in Japan are carrying α1-antitrypsin deficient variant Siiyama ($Ser^{53}$(TCC) to $Phe^{53}$(TTC)): Is it local accumulation or common to Orientals? Am Rev Respir Dis 1992; 145(suppl).
26. Seyama K, Nukiwa T, Takabe K, Takahashi H, Miyake K, Kira S. Siiyama (serine 53 (TCC) to phenylalanine 53 (TTC)): a new α1-antitrypsin deficient variant with mutation on a predicted conserved residue of the serpin backbone. J Biol Chem 1991; 266:12627–12632.
27. Nukiwa T, Brantry ML, Ogushi F, Fells GA, Crystal RG. Characterization of the gene and protein of the common alpha 1–antitrypsin normal M2 allele. Am J Hum Genet 1988; 43:322–330.

# 20

# The National Institutes of Health/National Heart, Lung, and Blood Institute Registry for Patients with Severe Deficiency of Alpha 1–Antitrypsin

**JAMES K. STOLLER**

Cleveland Clinic Foundation
Cleveland, Ohio

## I. Introduction

Since the first description of alpha 1–antitrypsin (α1AT) deficiency by Laurell and Eriksson in 1963 (1), major advances have been made in understanding the basic scientific aspects of this disorder. As discussed in another chapter, the structures of the protein and the gene for α1AT have been elucidated, the gene has been cloned, and transfer of the gene to animal host cells has been accomplished both in vitro and in vivo (2,3). Although these strides are especially impressive for having occurred in the short span of 32 years, they highlight a paradox that the basic scientific understanding of α1AT deficiency far outstrips clinical understanding. Specifically, basic clinical questions about clinical features of affected individuals, risk factors for airflow obstruction, and the natural history of α1AT deficiency remain unanswered, largely because of the difficulty of assembling a large cohort for study. Indeed, estimates of the rate of decline of $FEV_1$ in affected individuals vary greatly in available series (i.e., from as low as 42 ml/year to as high as 317 ml/year) (4–9). Furthermore, until the recent publication of experience from the Danish Registry (10) (with $n = 565$ participants) and from the NIH-sponsored Registry of Patients with Severe Deficiency of Alpha 1–Antitrypsin

(11) (with $n = 1129$ participants)—the subject of this chapter—the largest available series consisted of 264 enrollees (12).

The need to better characterize the natural history of α1AT deficiency has fostered this multicenter Registry to assemble and follow a large cohort of affected individuals. Another factor promoting the Registry was the conclusion rendered by an expert panel that a randomized trial of intravenous augmentation therapy would be unlikely because the statistical and financial requirements of a successful trial were deemed unachievable (13,14). Thus, in 1989, the Registry for Patients with Severe Deficiency of Alpha 1–Antitrypsin was sponsored by the National Institutes of Health/National Heart, Lung, and Blood Institute to characterize the laboratory and clinical course of individuals with severe deficiency of α1AT, whether or not they were receiving intravenous augmentation therapy (11). This Registry is reviewed in this chapter. Specifically, the goals and design of the Registry are described, followed by a brief review of features of the baseline cohort that have been published to date.

## II. Goals and Structure of the Registry

The main purpose of the Registry is to characterize the natural history of severe deficiency of α1AT in affected individuals, whether or not they are receiving augmentation therapy. It bears emphasis that the Registry is not a randomized clinical trial of augmentation therapy, because decisions about participants' treatment (e.g., whether to use intravenous augmentation) remain with their managing physicians, not with the Registry. To achieve the Registry's goals of characterizing the clinical and laboratory course of affected individuals, the primary outcome measures include change in lung function (especially $FEV_1$) and survival. Secondary outcome measures include laboratory test results (e.g., chest-radiograph features and liver-function tests), enrollees' functional status (using the Modified Dyspnea Index) (15), and health status. Table 1 lists the data elements that are recorded at baseline and yearly thereafter for the duration of follow-up in the Registry.

Figure 1 presents the structural elements of the Registry, which consists of:

1. Thirty-seven participating Clinical Centers in 25 states and one Canadian province (Appendix).
2. A Steering Committee composed of experts in the field, some of whom are principal investigators at participating Clinical Centers.
3. A Central Phenotyping Laboratory, at which blood specimens from participants are tested to confirm serum α1AT levels and phenotypes. Because serum levels and phenotypes could be confounded by exogenous α1AT infusions in prospective participants committed to continuing intravenous augmentation therapy at the time of Registry enroll-

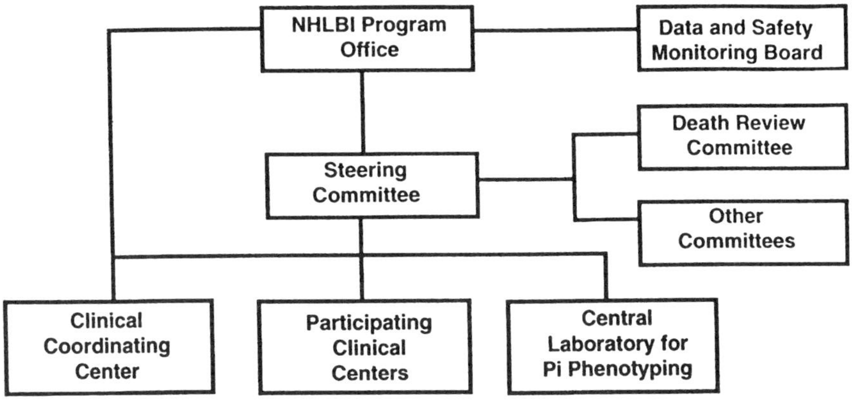


**Figure 1** Organization of the Registry for Patients with Severe Deficiency of Alpha 1–Antitrypsin.

ment, their eligibility was determined by gene-probe analysis (GeneScreen, Dallas, Texas).

4. A Data and Safety Monitoring Committee to oversee data quality and identify any hazardous circumstances associated with the Registry.
5. A Death Review Committee, whose purpose is to ascertain the cause of death in deceased participants and to review findings from postmortem examinations whenever possible.
6. A Clinical Coordinating Center, which is responsible for Registry design and for data collection, editing, storage, and analysis.

Eligibility criteria for the Registry include: 1) age $\geqslant$18 years, 2) a serum $\alpha$1AT level $\leqslant$11 $\mu$M or a high-risk phenotype (e.g., PI*ZZ, Null Z, or Null variants) based on molecular probe testing, and 3) completion of baseline spirometry testing. Eligible subjects underwent baseline testing during which data were collected regarding demographic features, pulmonary symptoms (using the ATS-DLD 78 questionnaire) (16), functional status (based on the Modified Dyspnea Index) (15), available laboratory testing, and chest-radiographic features (Table 1). Thereafter, participants were encouraged to return to one of the 37 participating Clinical Centers once every 6 months until November 1, 1993, and once yearly thereafter until the end of longitudinal follow-up in the Registry (April 30, 1996).

Because spirometry measurements were a primary outcome measure and were essential to characterize the natural history of participants' lung function, great attention was given to aquiring high-quality spirometry measurements, viewing and rating submitted spirograms, and providing feedback on spirometry

**Table 1** Data Collection Schedule

| | Screening | Baseline | Follow-up |
|---|---|---|---|
| Demographics | | | |
| Age, gender, race | × | | |
| Education, employment | | × | |
| Marital status, occupation history | | × | × |
| Method of ascertainment | × | | |
| Initial serum α1AT level, phenotype | × | | |
| Augmentation therapy history[a] | × | × | × |
| Adverse reactions | | × | × |
| Smoking history, alcohol use | | × | × |
| Symptom history[b] | | × | × |
| Self-reported medical history of patient, family | | | |
| Diagnoses, hospitalizations, surgeries | | × | × |
| Current medications | | × | × |
| Modified Dyspnea Index | | × | × |
| Pulmonary function tests | | | |
| $FEV_1$ and FVC, pre- and postbronchodilator | | × | × |
| Total lung capacity | | × | × |
| Residual volume | | × | × |
| Diffusing lung capacity | | × | × |
| Alveolar volume | | × | × |
| Slow vital capacity | | × | × |
| Chest roentgenogram, posteroanterior and lateral | | × | × |
| Blood and urine laboratory studies[c] | | × | × |

[a]Augmentation therapy history includes current status, method of treatment, frequency of infusion, changes in treatment (frequency, dose).

[b]Symptom history includes standard ATS questions (ATS-DLD 78) on cough, phlegm, wheezing, breathlessness, and chest colds.

[c]Blood studies include: white blood count, hemoglobin, hematocrit, serum glutamic oxaloacetic transaminase (SGOT), total bilirubin, serum glutamic pyruvate transaminase (SGPT), blood urea nitrogen, creatinine, alkaline phosphatase, arterial oxygen tension ($PaO_2$), pH, arterial carbon dioxide tension ($PaCO_2$), serum bicarbonate ($HCO_3$), hemoglobin oxygen saturation ($SaO_2$), and carboxyhemoglobin level. Urine studies reported include: pH, specific gravity, ketones, total protein, and glucose.

*Source*: Ref. 11.

quality to participating Clinical Centers. Before beginning data collection, pulmonary function technicians from each of the Clinical Centers participated in a $1\frac{1}{2}$-day central training session conducted at the Clinical Coordinating Center. The training session reviewed American Thoracic Society standards for spirometers (17), spirometric criteria for acceptability and reproducibility, and recommended expiratory techniques for spirometry. Protocols for patient recruitment, baseline testing, and follow-up were reviewed, with emphasis on study questionnaires and evaluation instruments and their completion.

During Registry follow-up, the protocol called for mandatory spirometry (both before and after an inhaled bronchodilator) and submission to the Clinical Coordinating Center of hard copies of three acceptable and reproducible spirograms from each session. All baseline spirograms were reviewed and rated for acceptability and reproducibility by two experienced pulmonary function technicians. Although uncommon (1.5% of submitted spirograms), discordant ratings by the two reviewers were adjudicated by a third reviewer (J.K.S.).

## III. Recruitment and Baseline Characteristics of Participants

Recruitment to the Registry extended from March 1, 1989, to October 31, 1992. Over this time, 1384 serum specimens were submitted, of which 1161 were found eligible (84%) based on serum level and/or phenotype (Fig. 2). Of the 1161 eligible subjects, 32 were not enrolled [due to failure to consent or dropout before enrollment (n = 29), age <18 years (*n* = 2), or death prior to enrollment (*n* = 1)], leaving 1129 enrollees. On this basis, actual enrollment exceeded the initial target of 1000 and this Registry represents the largest single cohort of individuals with α1AT deficiency (Fig. 3).

Table 2 presents selected baseline features of Registry participants. A slight

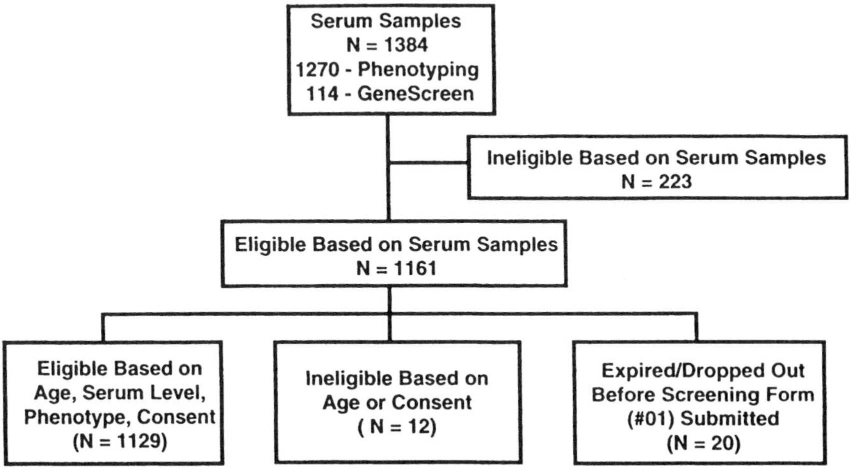


**Figure 2** Assembly of the cohort in the Registry, including eligible patients who were not included. Overall, 84% of eligible subjects participated.

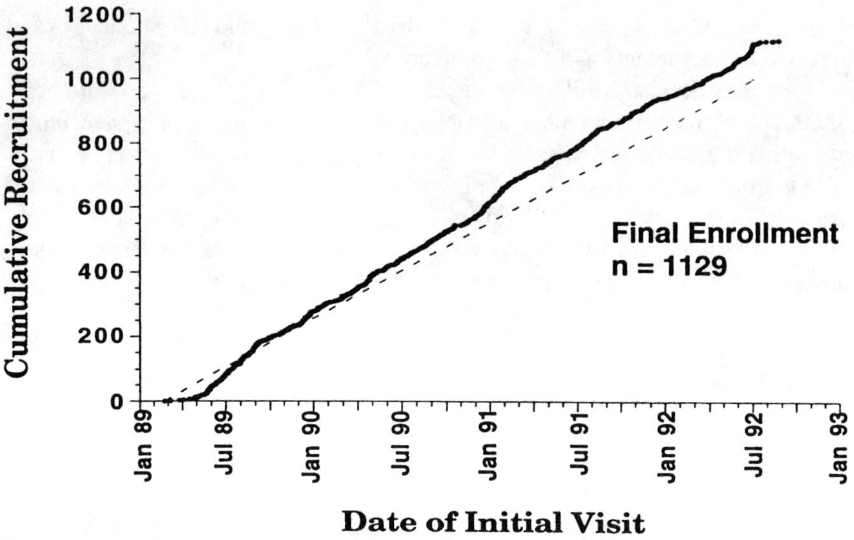


**Figure 3** (Dotted line) Registry recruitment projections and (solid line) actual recruitment. Recruitment was completed as of October 31, 1992, and exceeded the 1000-enrollee target by 11% ($n$ = 1129 final cohort).

**Table 2** Selected Baseline Features of Participants (data as of 10/31/94, $n$ = 1129 enrollees)

| | Mean ± SD | Range |
|---|---|---|
| I. Demographic features | | |
| 1. Age | 46 ± 11 yr | (18–82) |
| 2. % Male | 56% | — |
| 3. Cigarette smoking status | | |
| a. Never-smoker | 20% | — |
| b. Ex-smoker | 72% | — |
| c. Current smoker | 8% | — |
| II. Method of ascertainment | | |
| 1. Symptoms present | 72% | — |
| 2. Family screening | 20% | — |
| 3. Abnormal pulmonary function test or chest radiograph | 3% | — |
| 4. Liver disease | 2% | — |
| 6. Other/unknown | 3% | — |
| IV. Pulmonary function | | |
| 1. $FEV_1$ % predicted (prebronchodilator) | 43% | (7–135%) |

*Source*: Ref. 11.

male predominance was observed (56%), and the mean age (±SD) was 46 ± 11 years. Most participants were ex-smokers (72%), but 8% were current smokers and 20% had never smoked. The baseline mean $FEV_1$ % predicted was 43% ± 30% (SD), indicating a moderate degree of airflow obstruction with a wide range of baseline values among Registry subjects (7–135% predicted).

In keeping with several reports that emphasize the importance of ascertainment method, the Registry has recorded how patients came to attention for enrollment. Most subjects (72%) were ascertained because they had pulmonary symptoms (so-called "index" cases), but 20% were ascertained because a family member was known to have α1AT deficiency ("nonindex" cases). As previously reported by Silverman et al., (18) nonindex individuals have better-preserved lung function (mean $FEV_1$ % predicted 76% ± 33%) than index subjects, whose mean $FEV_1$ % predicted is 32% ± 19%.

As longitudinal follow-up of the cohort continues, the Registry is expected to yield important insight into the clinical and pulmonary function course of patients with severe α1AT deficiency.

## Appendix: Organizational Elements and Participating Investigators

*National Heart, Lung, and Blood Institute*

Zakir Bengali, Ph.D. (through June 1989); Carol E. Vreim, Ph.D. (Program Director); Ann Rothgeb; Margaret Wu, Ph.D.

*Data and Safety Monitoring Board*

Gordon L. Snider, M.D. (Chairman); Katherine Detre, M.D., Dr.P.H.; Herbert Y. Reynolds, M.D.; Melvyn S. Tockman, M.D., Ph.D. and Janet Wittes, Ph.D.

*Steering Committee*

Members: Ronald G. Crystal, M.D. (Chairman); A. Sonia Buist, M.D.; Benjamin Burrows, M.D.; Allen Cohen, M.D.; Robert J. Fallat, M.D.; James E. Gadek, M.D.; Ralph Rousell, M.D.; Mark D. Schluchter, Ph.D.; Richard S. Schwartz, M.D. (through October 1992); Gerard M. Turino, M.D.; Carol E. Vreim, Ph.D.; *Ex officio members*: Mark L. Brantly, M.D.; James K. Stoller, M.D.; Margaret Wu, Ph.D.

*Death Review Committee*

Herbert P. Wiedemann, M.D. (Chairman); Thomas L. Petty, M.D.; James K. Stoller, M.D.; Joseph F. Tomashefski, Jr., M.D.

*Clinical Coordinating Center*

The Cleveland Clinic Foundation, Cleveland, OH, Biostatistics Section:

George W. Williams (through June 1991) (Co-Director); Mark D. Schluchter, Ph.D. (Co-Director); Raghid Ajamoughli, B.S.; Gerald J. Beck, Ph.D.; Richard P. Connelly, M.S.; Beth Dobish; Marlene Goormastic, M.P.H.; Judith Leatherman, B.S.; June McMahan; Betty Moore, Susan G. Sherer, B.S.; DeAnn Swinderman; Michael Tuason, B.S.; Pulmonary Section: James K. Stoller, M.D. (Co-Director); Kevin McCarthy, R.C.P.T.; Herbert P. Wiedemann, M.D.; Consultant: Thomas L. Petty, M.D.

*Central Phenotyping Laboratory*

National Institutes of Health, NICHD, Human Genetics Branch, Bethesda, MD, Mark L. Brantly, M.D.; Jeffrey Hildesheim, B.A.; Jeffrey Redwine, B.A.; Barbara Rundquist, B.S.

*Clinical Centers*

**Arapahoe Pulmonary Consultants, Denver, CO**

Robert A. Sandhaus, M.D., Ph.D. (Principal Investigator); C. William Bell, M.D.; Janis Berend, M.S.N., C.N.P.; C. Allen Burry, C.R.T.T.; Kathleen Irvine, B.S.; Dixie Krantz, R.R.T., C.P.F.T.; Susan Lewis, volunteers.

**William Beaumont Hospital, Royal Oak, MI**

K. P. Ravikrishnan, M.D. (Principal Investigator); Robert Begle, M.D.; Karen Burgess, M.A.; Barbara Cameron, R.N.; Shirley Cotton, C.P.F.T.; David Erb, M.D.; Chet Jaworsky, R.R.T., C.P.F.T.; Joel Seidman, M.D.; Stanley Sherman, M.D.; Mercedes True, B.S., R.P.F.T.

**Beth Israel Hospital, Boston, MA**

Steven Wienberger, M.D. (Principal Investigator); Kristen Armstrong, B.A., Richard Johnston, C.P.F.T.; Carol Murree; Mitchell Rosenberg, M.D.; Jeanne B. La Rock, B.S.; Alison Vargas, B.A.

**California Pacific Medical Center, San Francisco, CA**

Robert J. Fallat, M.D. (Principal Investigator); Leonard Moriyama, R.R.T., R.C.P.T.; Keith Willard, R.C.P.T.

**The Cleveland Clinic Foundation, Cleveland, OH**

Alejandor Arroliga, M.D. (Principal Investigator); David P. Meeker, M.D. (through September 1994) (Principal Investigator); Eugene Cassidy, C.P.F.T.; Joseph A. Golish, M.D.; Daniel Laskowski, R.P.F.T.; Atul Mehta, M.D. Lynn Pagliaccio, P.A.-C.; Richard Pillar, R.C.P.T.; Gloria Rhodes, R.C.P.T.; Jenera Scott, R.C.P.T., Linda Hutchins, R.N.

**Dallas Pulmonary Associates, Dallas, TX**

W. John Ryan, M.D. (Principal Investigator); Kathy Johnson, P.A.-C.; James P. Loftin, M.D.

**Danbury Hospital, Danbury, CT**
Arthur Kotch, M.D. (Principal Investigator); Trudy Clark, R.N., R.C.P.T.

**Graduate Hospital, Philadelphia, PA**
Paul E. Epstein, M.D. (Principal Investigator); Pam Del Buono, R.C.P.T.

**Group Health Cooperative Puget Sound, Redmond, WA**
Robert E. Sandblom, M.D. (Principal Investigator); Loretta Collar, B.S.N., R.N.; Mary Curtis, M.D.; James B. DeMaine, M.D.; Richard C. Hert, M.D.; Brenda Melson, C.R.T.T., C.P.F.T.

**Henry Ford Hospital, Detroit, MI**
Michael S. Eichenhorn, M.D. (Principal Investigator); Richard Beauchamp, R.C.P.T., R.P.F.T.; Susan Hupfer, C.C.P.T.; Charisse Lukaszek, Richard Mackewich, R.P.F.T., R.C.P.T., C.R.T.T.; Christine Wilson, C.P.T.

**Indiana University Medical Center, Indianapolis, IN**
W. Mark Breite, M.D. (through August 1994) (Principal Investigator); Joseph P. McMahan, M.D. (Principal Investigator); Robert DeAtley, M.S.; Deb Mylet, R.N.; Kari Surr; Tina Williams

**Lahey Clinic Medical Center, Burlington, MA**
David Webb-Johnson, M.D. (Principal Investgator); Dana Boiszert; Joyce Corbett, C.R.T.T.; Lissa Judd, C.R.T.T.; Deborah McManus, R.N.; Judith Pierce, C.R.T.T.

**Mayo Clinic Jacksonville, Jacksonville, FL**
Michael J. Krowka, M.D. (Principal Investigator); Jean Adams; Zafar Awan, R.R.T.; Rebecca Fehrenkamp, R.R.T.; Madeleine Madden, R.R.T., C.P.F.T.; Kathy Schultz, R.R.T.; Nancy Wheatley, R.R.T., R.P.F.T.

**Mayo Clinic Rochester, Rochester, MN**
Udaya B. S. Prakash, M.D. (Principal Investigator); Deb Nesler, C.P.F.T.; Lin Scott, C.P.F.T.; Paul Scanlon, M.D.; Bruce Staats, M.D., Robert Viggiano, M.D.

**Medical University of South Carolina, Charleston, SC**
Charlie Strange, M.D. (Principal Investigator); Michael Baumann, M.D.; Barbara Burns; Ruth Oser, R.N., M.S.; Margaret Youmans, B.S., R.P.F.T.; Marc Judson, M.D.

**Mercy Hospital, Portland, ME**
Dermot N. Killian, M.D. (Principal Investigator); Brenda Bell; Terry Clark, R.C.P.T.; William Demicco, M.D.; Lewis Golden, M.D.; Steven A. Hess, M.D.; Rebecca Hitchcock, R.N., C.R.N.P.; Gilman Raymond, C.P.F.T.

**National Heart, Lung, and Blood Institute, Bethesda, MD**
Ronald G. Crystal, M.D. (through August 1993) (Principal Investigator);

Joel Moss, M.D., Ph.D. (Principal Investigator); Pauline Barnes, R.N.; Dotty Czerski, R.N.; Jane Healy, R.N.; Clara Jolley; N. Gerard McElvaney, M.D.; Renee Lay; Woodrow Robinson III, B.S.; Gregory Taylor, C.R.T.T.

**National Naval Medical Center, Bethesda, MD**

Bruce M. Meth, M.D. (through August 1992) (Principal Investigator); David Holden, M.D. (Principal Investigator); Richard W. Ashburn, M.D.; Gil Crowder, C.R.T.T.; Robert Dolensky, R.C.T.; Joseph Forrester, M.D.; Christel Hamilton, C.R.T.T.; Carol Harkness, C.R.T.T.; Sheila Jones, R.N.; Rose Pereria; Robert F. Sarlin, M.D.; Ronald P. Sen, M.D.; Bruce Shelton, C.R.T.T.; Barbara Schuler, R.N.; Mona Tyler, C.R.T.T.; Thomas E. Walsh, M.D.; Julio Zarate, C.R.T.T.

**Ohio State University, Columbus, OH**

Mark Wewers, M.D. (Principal Investigator); Janice Drake, R.R.T.; James E. Gadek, M.D.; Betsy James, R.R.T.; Brenda Swank

**Oregon Health Sciences University, Portland, OR**

Alan F. Barker, M.D. (Principal Investigator); A. Sonia Buist, M.D.; Ray D'Silva, R.P.F.T.; Lynn Oveson, R.N.; Laura Winther, R.N.

**Pulmonary Care, P.C., Fall River, MA**

William C. Sheehan, M.D. (Principal Investgator); Robert M. Aisenberg, M.D.; Len Chadbourne, R.R.T., B.A.; Patricia Demers, R.N.; Perry Little, R.R.T., R.N.; Nick Mucciardi, M.D.; Doreen Olivera-Williams, C.P.F.T., R.R.T.; Ann Sheehan, B.S.

**St. Luke's/Roosevelt Hospital, New York, NY**

Gerard M. Turino, M.D. (Principal Investigator); Edward Eden, M.D.; Thomas Lugh, R.P.F.T., R.R.T.; Sharad I. Parmar, B.S., C.P.F.T.; M. Lynn Middleton, L.P.N.; David Montague, B.S.; Patricia Murphy, R.R.T., C.P.F.T.

**University of Arizona, Tucson, AZ**

Mary Klink, M.D. (through September 1991); Benjamin Burrows, M.D. (Principal Investigator); Barbara Albright; E. P. Beeler, B. A., C.P.T., Barbara Boyer, R.N.; Martha Cline, M.S.; Russell R. Dodge, M.D.; Darlene Gordon, R.N.; Nancy Poiner, R.N.

**University of California, Davis Medical Center, Sacramento, CA**

Carroll E. Cross, M.D. (Principal Investigator); Jo Ann Booth, R.N., M.A.; Andrew Chan, M.D.; Richard Fekete, R.P.F.T.; Heino Kemnitz, R.P.F.T.; Ben Studebaker; William Volz, R.N., R.P.F.T.

**University of California, Los Angeles, CA**

Donald F. Tierney, M.D. (Principal Investigator); Linda Ezell, R.C.P.; John Haugh, R.C.P.; Bertrand Shaprio, M.D.

**University of California, San Diego Medical Center, San Diego, CA**
Jack L. Clausen, M.D. (Principal Investigator); JoAnna Borders, M.S., Charlene Dent, R.P.F.T.; Donna Elliott; Catherine Fonzi, R.P.F.T., R.C.P.; Robert Ford, R.P.F.T.s, B.S.; Angela Kimbrough, M.S.; Sheila J. King, R.P.F.T.; Carlos Lopez, R.P.F.T.

**University of Iowa, Iowa City, IA**
Jeff Wilson, M.D. (Principal Investigator); Marsha Anderson, R.R.T., R.P.F.T.; Jan Buchmayer, R.N.; Jeneva Ford; Angie Kemp, C.R.T.T.

**University of Minnesota Hospital and Clinic, Minneapolis, MN**
Peter Bitterman, M.D. (Principal Investgator); Beth Dosland, R.N.; Cheryl Edin, R.N.; Keith Harmon, M.D.; Marshall Hertz, M.D.; Shelly Krause, B.S.; Pat Lindquist, M.T.; Marnie Loven-Bell, M.T.; Kathy Plooster, R.N.

**University of Nebraska Medical Center, Omaha, NE**
Stephen I. Rennard, M.D. (Principal Investigator); Ron Cheney, P.A.-C.; Deb Cirian, R.R.T.; Jane Diamond, R.R.T.; Kevin Epperson, R.R.T.; Richard Fogleman, R.R.T.; John Houchins, R.R.T.; Jen Jones, R.N., M.S.N.; Sandy McGranaghan, C.P.F.T.; Theresa Pignotti, R.R.T.; Tom Pursel, R.C.P.T.; Richard A. Robbins, M.D.

**University of North Carolina, Chapel Hill, NC**
James F. Donohue, M.D. (Principal Investigator); Lyn Davis, R.N.; Katherine W. Hohneker, R.N.; Betty Hornaday, C.P.T.; Jeanine Mascrella, M.S., R.N.; Lynne Sobol, B.S., R.N.; Steven Turpin, M.D.

**University of Rochester Medical Center, Rochester, NY**
Richard W. Hyde, M.D. (Principal Investigator); Richard Lynch, R.R.T.; Barbara Spohn, R.N.

**University of Tennessee/Memphis Clinical Center, Memphis, TN**
Norman T. Soskel, M.D. (Principal Investigator); Charyl Grisham, C.R.T.T.; Carol Jones, R.N., B.S.N.; Tosha Patrick; Vicki Smith

**University of Texas Health Center, Tyler, TX**
James M. Stocks, M.D. (Principal Investigator); Willie J. Blevins, B.S., R.P.F.T.; Allen Cohen, M.D.; Sam Fields, R.P.F.T.; Janet Hinojosa, C.R.T.T.; Debbie Waldrop, R.N., B.S.N.; Edith Wilson, C.R.T.T.

**University of Utah Health Sciences Center, Salt Lake City, UT**
Richard E. Kanner, M.D. (through June 1990) (Principal Investigator); Edward J. Campbell, M.D., (Principal Investigator); James Behnke, M.S., R.P.F.T.; Steven Blaine, C.P.F.T.; Brad Gwyher, B.S.; Linn Hyer, C.P.F.T.; Phaedra McPherson, B.S.; Cynthia Moore, B.S., R.P.F.T.; Cathy Pope, R.N.; Darin Ryujin, M.S., R.P.F.T.; Kathy Sherwood, B.S., C.P.F.T.; Connie Thelander, M.A.; Mark Weight, B.S., R.F.T.; Kay Willden

**Veterans Administration Hospital, Hines, IL**
Nicholas Gross, M.D., Ph.D. (Principal Investigator); Frank King, B.S.

**Victoria General Hospital, Victoria, British Columbia, Canada**
Ian Waters, M.D. (Principal Investigator); Les MacNeill, R.R.T.

**Washington University Medical Center, St. Louis, MO**
Patricia Nelson, M.D. (Principal Investigator); Beverly Franklin, C.P.F.T., C.R.T.; Michelle Jenkerson, C.R.T.; Jack A. Pierce, M.D.; Edward Silverman, M.D.; Nichola Story, R.P.F.T., R.R.T.; Margie Wade, R.P.F.T.; Pamela Wilson

## References

1. Laurell CB, Eriksson S. The electrophoretic $alpha_1$-globulin pattern of serum in $alpha_1$-antitrypsin deficiency. Scand J Clin Lab Invest 1963; 15:132–140.
2. Canonico AE, Conary JT, Meyrick BO, Brigham KL. Aerosol and intravenous transfection of human alpha 1-antitrypsin gene to lungs of rabbits. Am J Respir Crit Care Med 1994; 10:24–29.
3. Rosenfeld MA, Siegfried W, Yoshimura K, Yonegama K, et al. Adenovirus-mediated transfer of a recombinant alpha 1-antitrypsin gene to the lung epithelium in vivo. Science 1991; 252:431–434.
4. Janus ED, Phillips NT, Carrell RW. Smoking, lung function and $alpha_1$-antitrypsin deficiency. Lancet 1985; i:152–154.
5. Hutchison DCS, Tobin MJ, Cooper D, Lowe D. Longitudinal studies in alpha 1-antitrypsin deficiency: A survey by the British Thoracic Society. In: Taylor JC, Mittman C, eds. Pulmonary Emphysema and Proteolysis. New York: Academic Press, 1987:7–15.
6. Wu MC, Eriksson S. Lung function, smoking, and survival in severe alpha 1-antitrypsin deficiency, PI*ZZ. J Clin Epidemiol 1988; 41:1157–1165.
7. Brantly ML, Paul LD, Miller BH, Falk BH, Wu M, Crystal RG. Clinical features and history of the destructive lung disease associated with alpha 1-antitrypsin deficiency of adults with pulmonary symptoms. Am Rev Respir Dis 1988; 138:327–336.
8. Workshop on the Natural History of PI*ZZ Emphysema. Am Rev Respir Dis 1983; 127(suppl):543–545.
9. Viskum K, Kok-Jensen A. Criteria for alpha 1-antitrypsin substitution. Lung 1990; 1(suppl):586–591.
10. Seersholm N, Kok-Jensen A, Dirksen A. Survival of patients with severe alpha 1-antitrypsin deficiency with special reference to non-index cases. Thorax 1994; 94:695–698.
11. The Alpha 1-Antitrypsin Deficiency Registry Study Group. Prepared by: Schluchter MD, Barker AF, Crystal RG, Robbins RA, Stocks JM, Stoller JK, Wu MC. A registry of patients with severe deficiency of alpha 1-antitrypsin: design and methods. Chest 1994; 106:1223–1233.
12. Larsson C. Natural history and life expectancy in severe $alpha_1$-antitrypsin deficiency, PI*Z. Acta Med Scand 1978; 204:345–351.

13. Burrows B. A clinical trial of efficacy of antiproteolytic therapy: Can it be done? Am Rev Respir Dis 1983; 127(suppl):S42–S43.
14. Idell S, Cohen AB. Alpha$_1$-antitrypsin deficiency. Clin Chest Med 1983; 4:359–375.
15. Stoller JK, Ferranti R, Feinstein AR. Further specification and evaluation of a new clinical index for dyspnea. Am Rev Respir Dis 1986; 134:1129–1134.
16. Ferris BG (Principal Investigator). Epidemiology standardization project. Am Rev Respir Dis 1978; 118(part 2):55–88.
17. American Thoracic Society. Standardization of spirometry—1987 update. Am Rev Respir Dis 1987; 136:1285–1298.
18. Silverman EK, Pierce JA, Province MA, Rao DC, Campbell EJ. Variability of pulmonary function in alpha 1-antitrypsin deficiciency: Clinical correlates. Ann Intern Med 1989; 111:982–991.

# Part Four

## TREATMENT

# 21

# Therapy of α1AT Deficiency

**NOEL G. McELVANEY**

Pulmonary and Critical Care Medicine Branch
National Heart, Lung, and Blood Institute
National Institutes of Health
Bethesda, Maryland

**RONALD G. CRYSTAL**

The New York Hospital–Cornell Medical Center
New York, New York

## I. Introduction

There are marked differences in the pathogenesis of the lung and liver disorders in alpha 1–antitrypsin (α1AT) deficiency. In this regard, it is not surprising that the therapeutic strategies for these different manifestations of α1AT deficiency should also differ markedly.

## II. Liver Disease

Other than transplantation, there is no available therapy for the liver disease associated with α1AT deficiency (1–3). Liver transplantation has been used successfully to treat the liver disease in α1AT-deficient children and, indeed, α1AT deficiency is the second most common indication for liver transplantation in childhood, with 5-year survival rates exceeding 70% (1,2). The long-term survival for liver transplantation in adults with α1AT deficiency and liver disease is somewhat lower, at 60% (3). However, despite being the definitive therapy for α1AT deficiency, liver transplantation has a number of important drawbacks, including scarcity of donors, lifelong immunosuppressive therapy, and a significant mortality rate.

As for other therapeutic modalities, intravenous augmentation therapy with plasma-purified α1AT has no proven effect on the liver disease associated with α1AT deficiency, consistent with the concept that the liver disease in α1AT deficiency is not due to lack of antiprotease protection. The mild liver-function-test abnormalities seen in some α1AT-deficient adults with emphysema are not affected by intravenous α1AT augmentation therapy (4). Other therapeutic options are mainly theoretical, such as efforts directed toward reducing α1AT synthesis and/or increasing the rate of its translocation from the rough endoplasmic reticulum (4,5). Another potential strategy is gene therapy. Since Z homozygote individuals are at risk for developing clinically significant liver disease but MZ heterozygotes are not (6), this strategy would involve inserting the normal α1AT cDNA into hepatocytes, thereby converting them into the equivalent of MZ heterozygote cells. The possibilities of achieving this in humans with currently available gene-therapy vectors is not known. Thus, at present, the therapy for the liver manifestations of α1AT deficiency is that for any chronic liver disease.

## III. Lung Disease

### A. Augmentation of Liver Synthesis and/or Secretion of α1AT

As the liver is the major site of α1AT production, one possible approach to augmenting the lung antiprotease protective screen in α1AT deficiency would be to increase the amount of α1AT secreted by the liver. This is possible through liver transplantation, which theoretically would "cure" both the lung and liver manifestations of this disorder. In this regard, following liver transplantation in Z homozygotes there is conversion of serum α1AT to the α1AT phenotype of the transplanted liver, together with normalization of serum α1AT levels (1). However, while liver transplantation may be acceptable in children or adults with progressive severe liver disease, the morbidity and mortality associated with liver transplantation are not as acceptable in adults with lung disease, in which the process being treated is slowly progressive and potentially amenable to other therapies.

Various attempts have been made to increase the endogenous production and/or release of α1AT by the liver in α1AT deficiency. With the knowledge that plasma α1AT levels are elevated in fever, trauma, shock, and pregnancy, patients with α1AT deficiency have been treated in a number of short-term studies with typhoid vaccine and estrogen–progesterone combinations (7,8) but with no significant increases in serum α1AT levels. Other strategies have included the use of danazol, a derivative of the synthetic steroid 17 α-ethinyl testosterone that has properties similar to those of testosterone but does not have its androgenic effects

(9). Danazol has been shown to increase serum concentrations of C1-esterase in hereditary angioedema, a disorder that, like α1AT, is characterized by serum deficiency of a hepatocyte-produced antiprotease. However, while danazol causes a modest increase in α1AT serum levels in some α1AT-deficient individuals (9,10), the increases are insufficient to provide an adequate protective screen in serum and respiratory epithelial lining fluid (ELF).

Another medication that has been tried in the therapy of α1AT deficiency is tamoxifen, an agent that binds to intracytoplasmic estrogen receptors and thus may mimic the increases in α1AT serum levels normally associated with pregnancy. However, while trials with tamoxifen have shown increases in serum α1AT above the protective levels in SZ and PZ individuals, administration to Z homozygous individuals does not result in α1AT levels sufficient to re-establish the normal anti–neutrophil elastase (NE) protection of the lung (11,12).

### B. Intravenous Augmentation Therapy with Plasma-Purified α1AT

The most direct approach to augmenting anti-NE protection in the lungs of individuals with α1AT deficiency is to administer exogenous α1AT, either systemically or directly to the lung. The amount of exogenous α1AT required to provide adequate anti-NE protection for the lungs of individuals with α1AT deficiency can be inferred from animal studies and from studies in normals and in individuals with α1AT deficiency. It is known that serum levels of α1AT >11 μM are usually not associated with α1AT-deficiency-related emphysema. Put together with bronchoalveolar-lavage studies to evaluate lung ELF α1AT levels, it can be inferred that for the epithelial surface of the lung the minimum protective level is between 1 and 2 μM, while for the interstitium the threshold protective levels are between 5 and 7 μM.

With this as background, Gadek et al. (13) demonstrated that it was feasible to augment serum and lung α1AT levels in six individuals with α1AT deficiency by administering a partially purified preparation of human α1AT prepared from human plasma. This was given intravenously once weekly for 4 weeks. This strategy resulted in significant increases in ELF α1AT with no significant adverse effects. Following this study, methods were developed to purify α1AT from pooled plasma of human donors. The plasma-purified product prepared in this manner was heat-treated to lower the risk of plasma-borne pathogens and was 80% pure, the remainder being composed of various plasma proteins. The α1AT in the preparation was approximately 75% active, the active α1AT having a normal association rate for NE. Studies with this preparation showed that once-weekly intravenous infusions with 60 mg/kg α1AT were sufficient to maintain serum levels of α1AT >11 μM throughout the course of the study period (14). Not only were the serum levels of α1AT increased, but so also were the α1AT levels in respiratory ELF 6 days after infusion. Importantly, there was a concomitant increase in anti-NE capacity in serum and ELF, demonstrating the biochemical efficacy of this therapeutic approach. This preparation was thereafter approved by the Food and Drug Administration for use in the treatment of α1AT deficiency and is now administered to over 2000 individuals with α1AT deficiency worldwide.

The regimen of once-weekly infusions, while widely accepted by individuals with α1AT deficiency, still presented a not inconsiderable intrusion into their daily lives, being time-consuming and requiring frequent venous access and supervision by medical personnel. With this in mind, studies were initiated to determine whether a larger dose, 250 mg/kg, could be given less frequently (once every 4 weeks) and still achieve similar biochemically efficacious results. These infusions took longer (5–7 hours compared to approximately 30 minutes for the 60 mg/kg infusions) but the results were equally efficacious (15). Subsequent attempts to further prolong the interval between infusions have been made using plasma exchange, in which large amounts of α1AT were exchanged for other plasma proteins. Interestingly, although extremely high levels of α1AT were achieved in plasma in the initial days after exchange, the levels did not remain above the protective threshold level much beyond the timepoints achieved by the 250 mg/kg infusions, and this approach has been abandoned. The plasma-exchange approach did show, however, that administration of up to 40 g of α1AT could be tolerated without adverse effects (16).

Today, intravenous augmentation therapy with plasma-purified α1AT, given once weekly at a dose of 60 mg/kg, remains the only therapy for this disorder approved by the Food and Drug Administration. Despite this, a significant number of individuals with α1AT deficiency are on a once-monthly regimen that, while shown to have biochemical efficacy, is not FDA-approved. Further, many patients are treated with biweekly regimens that have been neither approved by the FDA nor demonstrated to have biochemical efficacy.

Because the α1AT preparation is purified from human plasma, there are theoretical concerns about its use, including the possibility of the development of anti-α1AT antibodies or immune-complex disease. Data from the large number of individuals receiving the therapy worldwide have allayed this concern. Infection with human immunodeficiency virus (HIV) or a hepatitis virus is also a theoretical cause for concern. However, the final therapeutic product undergoes a rigorous heat treatment to diminish the possibility of transmission of plasma-borne viruses, and so far no individuals have contracted either HIV infection or hepatitis from this product.

A number of groups have developed recombinant forms of α1AT that, while retaining anti-NE properties, would not have the added problems associated with blood-derived products. Recombinant α1AT has been produced in *E. coli* and yeast directed by the cDNA of the normal M1 form of human α1AT. The recombinant form is identical to the naturally occurring α1AT, but it is not glycosylated and has an additional $NH_2$-terminal methionine. This molecule functions as well in vitro as normal human α1AT does as an inhibitor of NE. However, its plasma half-life is markedly reduced by virtue of its lack of carbohydrate side chains (this results, in part, from the recombinant molecule being excreted in urine), which renders it unsuitable for intravenous administration (17).

### C. Aerosol Augmentation Therapy for α1AT Deficiency

One other possible problem with using plasma-purified α1AT as a therapy for the emphysema associated with α1AT deficiency relates not to the product itself but to the large quantities of α1AT needed for this therapeutic approach. It is estimated that there are in excess of 40,000 Z homozygote individuals in the United States alone. If all these individuals were to require α1AT augmentation therapy, they would require at least 8000 kg of purified plasma α1AT yearly (17). Because other manifestations of α1AT deficiency, such as the liver disease, are not ameliorated by augmentation therapy, a more efficient and cost-effective approach might be to target the lungs directly by aerosolization of α1AT.

The feasibility of aerosolized delivery of α1AT as a therapy for the emphysema associated with α1AT deficiency rests on an important assumption. Whereas proteins normally diffuse from plasma through the interstitium of the lung onto the alveolar epithelial surface (19–21), the aerosolization approach assumes that this process can also work in reverse, i.e., that α1AT aerosolized onto the epithelial surface of the lung not only increases the anti-NE protection but, by diffusing into the interstitum, also provides anti-NE protection for the lung parenchyma, the site of destruction in individuals with α1AT deficiency. Relevant to these questions, studies have demonstrated that plasma-purified α1AT can be aerosolized, without adverse effects, to the lungs of individuals with α1AT deficiency (22). Following aerosolization, plasma-purified α1AT can be recovered in its intact functional form from the respiratory epithelial surface where it re-establishes the normal anti-NE protective screen. Interestingly, intact plasma α1AT of the normal M type can be detected in the plasma of Z individuals following aerosolization, showing that aerosolized α1AT can diffuse from the epithelial surface into plasma. In doing so, it likely increases the anti-NE protection of the interstitium. This finding is corroborated by studies in experimental animals that show that, following aerosolization of plasma α1AT, both the α1AT levels and the anti-NE protection are increased in lung lymph, indicative of an increase in α1AT levels and anti-NE augmentation in the alveolar interstitial fluid (22,23).

The potential for aerosol delivery of α1AT rekindled interest in the use of recombinant α1AT. Following aerosolization, recombinant α1AT effectively augments the anti-NE defenses on the respiratory epithelial surface and also diffuses through the interstitium into plasma (24), indicating some increased protection in the interstitium. Despite these encouraging results, there are several hurdles to overcome before aerosolized α1AT can be used as a therapy for α1AT deficiency. First, the interstitial levels of α1AT predicted from the initial studies are low (22–24). Second, there are difficulties in measuring the lung interstitial levels following aerosol therapy, and thus in determining if the protective threshold for the lung interstitium can be determined for individuals on chronic aerosol therapy.

Another candidate as an anti-NE molecule is recombinant secretory leukoprotease inhibitor (SLPI), a 12 kDa nonglycosylated single-chain polypeptide, identical to the naturally occurring SLPI, which functions as the major anti-NE molecule of the upper respiratory tract (25–28). rSLPI is a potent inhibitor of human NE with concentration- and time-dependent kinetics similar to those of α1AT (29). SLPI has some properties that distinguish it from α1AT. It is acid-stable and thus may remain functional in the decreased pH associated with the metabolic burst (30,31). It has a pI >9, similar to that of NE, and may track and bind to tissue sites favored by NE, such as elastin, where it can inhibit elastin-bound NE (25,31,32). Finally, studies in animals have demonstrated that aerosolization of rSLPI augments, not only the anti-NE defenses of the respiratory epithelial surface, but also the antioxidant defenses by increasing the glutathione levels in the local milieu (33). Despite these properties, the use of aerosolized rSLPI as a therapy for α1AT deficiency is not without obstacles. Although rSLPI has a molecular mass <30% that of recombinant α1AT, simultaneous aerosolization of both molecules to animals shows that, on a mole-for-mole basis, significantly more α1AT than rSLPI molecules is detected in lung lymph (29). The reasons for this are unclear; it may be due to compartmentalization of SLPI to the epithelial surface, adsorption of rSLPI onto epithelial cells, and/or binding of rSLPI to molecules in the interstitium after passing through the epithelium (29,34). Whatever the reasons, these results suggest that aerosolized rSLPI, while potentially useful for inflammatory disorders affecting the epithelial surface of the lung, may not reach the interstitial tissues and therefore has limited value as a therapy for α1AT deficiency. As an alternative approach, studies have been attempted with intravenous administration of rSLPI (34). Unfortunately, rapid intravenous infusion results in presentation of an unacceptably high protein load of rSLPI to the kidneys, obviating this as a strategy. By slowing the rate of infusion, the plasma and lung SLPI levels can be significantly increased while reducing urinary excretion of SLPI to negligible levels, thus presenting a potential alternative to intravenous administration of α1AT as therapy for this disorder (34).

### D. Low-Molecular-Weight Inhibitors of NE

Apart from α1AT and SLPI, normally found in the respiratory tract, a number of synthetic NE inhibitors have been synthesized as potential therapeutic agents for α1AT deficiency. These include irreversible inhibitors such as the peptide chloromethylketones (35) and reversible inhibitors such as peptide boronic acids (36), peptide aldehydes (37), substituted tripeptide ketones (38), or β-lactams that have been modified to inhibit NE (39). These compounds have potent anti-NE activity in vitro and have been evaluated in vivo in experimental animals. The in vivo studies have shown attenuation of lung injury associated with intratracheal administration of NE or porcine pancreatic elastase (PPE) following pretreatment of study animals with these NE inhibitors (35,37,38). Usually, the degree of inflammation induced by either NE or PPE is decreased. However, these experimental models are very unlike the clinical scenario that occurs in the lungs of individuals with α1AT deficiency, and thus human studies are necessary to show that these synthetic molecules can restore the lung anti-NE protective screen as effectively as the plasma-purified α1AT or genetically engineered recombinant α1AT or SLPI.

### E. Gene Therapy

α1AT deficiency theoretically is a relatively easy target for gene therapy because the α1AT molecule functions extracellularly and has a broad safety margin, as evidenced by the therapeutic trials involving plasma exchange. The phenotypical abnormality in this disorder—the deficiency of α1AT—could theoretically be corrected by transferring the normal human α1AT cDNA to the cells of deficient individuals. The cells to which the α1AT cDNA are be transferred could be anywhere in the body, as long as sufficient amounts of α1AT are able to reach the lower respiratory tract. The major problem for gene therapy for α1AT deficiency, however, relates to the ability to stimulate the production of enough α1AT to protect the lung on a persistent basis. It is calculated that 10–20 mg of α1AT must be delivered daily to the alveolar structures for the therapy to be effective (41). In this regard, any gene-therapy strategy purported to treat this disorder must result in the production of this large amount of protein.

Several strategies have been devised to accomplish this, using such vectors as retroviruses, adenoviruses, and liposomes to deliver the α1AT cDNA, and such cell types as fibroblasts, lymphocytes, hepatocytes, and respiratory epithelial cells as the targets for these vectors. The first in vivo studies for α1AT deficiency in experimental animals used fibroblasts as the source of α1AT (41). The genome of murine fibroblasts was modified in vitro with a retrovirus vector containing a fusion gene that consisted of a constituitive promoter from the SV40 virus followed by a cDNA encoding the sequences for the normal human α1AT protein. This produced a clonal population of mouse fibroblasts secreting human α1AT that was glycosylated and inhibited NE in a normal fashion. The clone of fibroblasts was then transplanted into the peritoneal cavities of nude mice. On evaluation, 1 month later, human α1AT was present in both serum and lung ELF of the mice. This study showed that gene therapy of α1AT deficiency was feasible and could be targeted to cells that do not normally produce the protein. However, the theoretical risks associated with transplanting fibroblasts to the peritoneum (with the possible risk of uncontrolled fibroblast growth leading to fibrosis of the peritoneum) obviated this as an in vivo approach in humans.

Other studies have used retroviral vectors to transfer the α1AT cDNA to hepatocytes (42–44). In general, this involves the isolation of primary hepatocytes from a resected liver lobe and transduction with the α1AT gene in vitro followed by autologous intraportal injection. In some studies, as many as 10–15% of hepatocytes have been successfully infected in this manner, with increased α1AT levels sustained for up to 1 year (43,44). However, despite such high in vivo transduction efficiencies, gene expression at the mRNA level is often quite low compared to results in vitro, and the α1AT levels seen are nowhere near the necessary protective levels required. Perhaps the major problem with this strategy as a therapeutic modality is that at present the technique requires hepatectomy and reinfusion of the modified hepatocytes. While allogeneic hepatocyte transplantation may circumvent this problem, it carries the severe drawbacks associated with rejection and immunosuppression and is not generally considered an option (42). Thus, while the hepatocyte seems an obvious cell target for gene therapy for α1AT deficiency, the approach is severely hampered by the difficulty in transferring genes directly to these cells in vivo. Furthermore, in Z homozygotes, the Z gene product aggregates in the rough endoplasmic reticulum of the hepatocytes, and thus it is not clear if these cells are capable of synthesizing and secreting α1AT as directed by a newly transferred normal α1AT gene. Other cells used as targets for the α1AT gene include T lymphocytes—the retrovirus-modified cells are transplanted directly into the lung, thus permitting local production of α1AT (45). Unfortunately, the amounts of α1AT produced in this way are far from the therapeutic levels necessary to protect the lung.

Adenovirus vectors containing the α1AT cDNA have been targeted at various cell types in attempts to develop a therapy for α1AT deficiency. The first site targeted was the lung, based on the knowledge that adenoviruses are tropic for respiratory epithelium (46). The construct was made safer by deleting the part of the adenovirus responsible for replication of the virus, following which a fusion gene of a constituitive promoter and α1AT cDNA were inserted (47). This vector was used to infect the respiratory epithelial cells of cotton rats in vitro and in vivo. After in vivo tracheal administration, human α1AT mRNA was detected in the respiratory epithelium and α1AT protein was synthesized and secreted by lung tissue, with levels detectable in ELF for up to 1 week (47). Despite these encouraging results, potential problems are associated with adenovirus-mediated gene therapy targeted at the lung. These include the propensity of adenovirus to cause inflammation (this may be mitigated by manipulating the viral genome to delete proinflammatory genes or add inflammatory suppressing genes) and the development of a humoral immune response to the adenovirus, thus limiting the effectiveness following repeat administrations (48). There are also the problems of producing the large amounts of α1AT necessary to protect the lungs of α1AT-deficient individuals and the difficulties of proving that such an approach is effective.

Despite these caveats, adenovirus is still the vector of preference for most of the gene-therapy approaches to the lung because of its ability to efficiently transfer genetic material to lung cells, the large fund of knowledge concerning wild-type adenoviral infection, and the steadily growing experience with its in vivo use in humans (49,50). Other organs targeted with adenovirus as potential therapies for α1AT deficiency include the liver (52), peritoneum (53), and endothelium (54). In vivo intraportal administration of a replication-deficient adenovirus vector containing the α1AT cDNA resulted in production of human α1AT, albeit in amounts lower than needed to effectively treat α1AT deficiency, but without the need for the high-morbidity procedures such as hepetectomy associated with retroviral gene-transfer strategies (52). Intraperitoneal injection of an adenovirus vector containing the human α1AT cDNA to cotton rats resulted in human α1AT levels detectable in serum for up to 24 days, with a maximal level of 3.4 μg/ml at 4 days. Interestingly, repeat administrations of this vector to the peritoneum at 1 week and at 1 month failed to show any gene expression but repeat administration at 3 months demonstrated measurable gene transfer and expression, suggesting that immunity against adenovirus may limit frequent repetitive dosing but wears off over time (53). Finally, human endothelial cells can produce α1AT following infection with the appropriate adenoviral vector, opening the possibility of gene transfer in the pulmonary arteries and capillaries (54).

One other method of delivering α1AT genetic material to the tissues is by using cationic liposomes (55). This system is viral-free, and therefore cotransfer of elements of the parent virus genome does not occur. Furthermore, there is no risk of viral recombination or host genome incorporation. Unfortunately, despite these advantages, the use of cationic liposomes is handicapped by the inefficiency of DNA transfer and the necessity of using large amounts of DNA.

Thus, gene-therapy strategies may have a future role in the therapy of α1AT deficiency. However, the necessity of producing large amounts of α1AT, together with the difficulties in monitoring efficacy and the current availability of replacement therapy, present significant hurdles before these strategies can be used effectively to treat this disorder.

## References

1. Esquivel CO, Vicente E, Van Thiel D, Gordon R, Marsh W, Makowka L, Koneru B, Iwatsuki S, Madrigal M, Delgado Milan MA, Todo S, Tzakis A, Starzl TE. Orthoptic liver transplantation for alpha-1-antitrypsin deficiency: an experience in 29 children and 10 adults. Transplant Proc 1987; 19:3798–3802.
2. Esquivel CO, Marino IR, Fioravanti V, Van Thiel DH. Liver transplantation for metabolic disease of the liver. Gastroenterol Clin N Am 1988; 17:167–177.

3. Esquivel CO, Mash JW, Van Thiel DH. Liver transplantation for chronic cholestatic liver disease in adults and children. Gastroenterol Clin N Am 1988; 17:145–155.
4. Crystal RG. α1-antitrypsin deficiency, emphysema, and liver disease: genetic basis and strategies for therapy. J Clin Invest 1990; 85:1343–1352.
5. Birrer P, McElvaney NG, Chang-Stroman LM, Crystal RG. $\alpha_1$-antitrypsin deficiency and liver disease. J Inher Metab Dis 1991; 14:512–525.
6. Eriksson S, Carlson J, Velez R. Risk of cirrhosis and primary liver cancer in alpha$_1$-antitrypsin deficiency. N Engl J Med 1986; 314:736–739.
7. Kueppers F. Genetically determined differences in the response of alpha 1-antitrypsin levels in human serum to typhoid vaccine. Humangenetik 1968; 6:207–214.
8. Laurell CB, Kullander S, Thorell J. Effect of administration of a combined estrogen-progestin contraceptive on the level of individual plasma proteins. Scand J Clin Lab Invest 1967; 21:337–343.
9. Gadek JE, Fulmer JD, Gelfand JA, Frank MM, Petty TL, Crystal RG. Danazol-induced augmentation of serum α-1-antitrypsin levels in individuals with marked deficiency of this antiprotease. J Clin Invest 1980; 66:82–87.
10. Wewers M, Gadek JE, Keogh BA, Fells GA, Crystal RG. Evaluation of danazol therapy for patients with PiZZ alpha-1-antitrypsin deficiency. Am Rev Respir Dis 1986; 134:476–480.
11. Eriksson S. The effect of tamoxifen in intermediate alpha-1-antitrypsin deficiency associated with phenotype PiSZ. Ann Clin Res 1983; 15:95–98.
12. Wewers MD, Brantly ML, Casolaro MA, Crystal RG. Evaluation of tamoxifen as a therapy to augment alpha-1-antitrypsin concentrations in Z homozygous alpha-1-antitrypsin deficient subjects. Am Rev Respir Dis 1987; 135:401–402.
13. Gadek JE, Klein HG, Holland PV, Crystal RG. Replacement therapy of α1-antitrypsin deficiency: reversal of protease-antiprotease imbalance within the alveolar structures of PiZZ subjects. J Clin Invest 1981; 68:1158–1165.
14. Wewers MD, Casalaro MA, Sellers S, Swayze SC, McPhaul KM, Crystal RG. Replacement therapy for alpha 1-antitrypsin deficiency associated with emphysema. N Engl J Med 1987; 316:1055–1062.
15. Hubbard RC, Sellers S, Czerski D, Stephens L, Crystal RG. Biochemical efficacy and safety of monthly augmentation therapy for α1-antitrypsin deficiency. JAMA 1988; 260:1259–1264.
16. Curiel D, Leitmean SF, Hubbard RC, Stier L, Sellers S, Plunkett A, Crystal RG. Plasma exchange/α1-antitrypsin infusion augmentation for treatment of α1-antitrypsin deficiency. Am Rev Respir Dis 1989; 139:A122.
17. Casolaro MA, Fells G, Wewers M, Pierce JE, Ogushi F, Hubbard R, Sellers S, Forstrom J, Lyons D, Kawasaki G, Crystal RG. Augmentation of lung antineutrophil elastase capacity with recombinant human α-1-antitrypsin. J Appl Physiol 1987; 63:2015–2023.
18. Hubbard RC, Casalaro MA, Mitchell M, Sellers SE, Arabia F, Matthay MA, Crystal RG. Fate of aerosolized recombinant DNA-produced α1-antitrypsin: use of the epithelial surface of the lower respiratory tract to administer proteins of therapeutic importance. Proc Natl Acad Sci USA 1988; 86:680–684.

19. Reynolds HY, Newball HH. Analysis of proteins and respiratory cells obtained from human lungs by bronchial lavage. J Lab Clin Med 1974; 84:559–573.
20. Warr GA, Martin RR, Sharp PM, Rossen RD. Normal human bronchial immunoglobulins and proteins: effects of cigarette smoking. Am Rev Respir Dis 1977; 116:25–30.
21. Delacroix DL, Marchandise FX, Francis C, Sibile Y. Alpha-2-macroglobulin, monomeric and polymeric immunoglobulin A, and immunoglobulin M in bronchoalveolar lavage fluid. Am Rev Respir Dis 1985; 132:829–835.
22. Hubbard RC, Brantly ML, Sellers SE, Mitchell ME, Crystal RG. Anti-neutrophil elastase defenses of the lower respiratory tract in α1-antitrypsin deficiency directly augmented with an aerosol of α1-antitrypsin. Ann Intern Med 1989; 111:206–212.
23. Smith RM, Traber LD, Traber DL, Spragg RG. Pulmonary deposition and clearance of aerosolized alpha-1-antitrypsin inhibitor administered to dogs and sheep. J Clin Invest 1989; 84:1145–1154.
24. Hubbard RC, McElvaney NG, Sellers SE, Healy JT, Czerski DB, Crystal RG. Recombinant DNA-produced α1-antitrypsin administered by aerosol augments lower respiratory tract antineutrophil elastase defenses in individuals with α1-antitrypsin deficiency. J Clin Invest 1989; 84:1349–1354.
25. Vogelmeier C, Hubbard RC, Fells GA, Schneble H-P, Thompson RC, Fritz H, Crystal RG. Antineutrophil elastase defense of the normal human respiratory epithelial surface provided by the secretory leukoprotease inhibitor. J Clin Invest 1991; 87: 442–448.
26. Boudier C, Pelletier A, Gast A, Tournier J-M, Pauli G, Bieth JG. The elastase inhibitory capacity and the $\alpha_1$-proteinase inhibitor and bronchial inhibitor content of bronchoalveolar lavage fluids from healthy subjects. Biol Chem Hoppe-Seyler 1987; 368:981–990.
27. Kramps JA, Franken C, Dijkman JH. Quantity of antileucoprotease relative to $\alpha_1$-proteinase inhibitor in peripheral airspaces of the human lung. Clin Sci 1988; 75:351–353.
28. Morrison HM, Kramps JA, Dijkman JH, Stockley RA. Comparison of concentrations of two proteinase inhibitors, porcine pancreatic elastase inhibitory capacity, and cell profiles in sequential bronchoalveolar lavage samples. Thorax 1986; 41:435–441.
29. Vogelmeier C, Buhl R, Hoyt RF, Wilson E, Fells GA, Hubbard RC, Schnebli H-P, Thompson RC, Crystal RG. Aerosolization of recombinant SLPI to augment antineutrophil elastase protection of pulmonary epithelium. J Appl Physiol 1990; 69: 1843–1848.
30. Hochstraser K, Reichert R, Schwartz S, Werle E. Isolierung und charakterisierung eines proteaseninhibitors ausmenschlichem bronchialsekret. Hoppe-Seyler's Z Physiol Chem 1972; 353:221–226.
31. Rice WG, Weiss SJ. Regulation of proteolysis at the neutrophil-substrate interface by secretory leukoprotease inhibitor. Science (Washington, DC) 1990; 249:178–181.
32. Hubbard RC, Crystal RG. Antiproteases. In: Crystal RG, West JB, eds-in-chief; Barnes P, Weibel ER, Cherniak NS, assoc eds. The Lung. Vol 2. Sci Found. New York: Raven Press, 1991:1775–1788.
33. Gillissen A, Birrer P, McElvaney NG, Buhl R, Vogelmeier C, Hoyt RF, Hubbard RC,

Crystal RG. Recombinant secretory leukoprotease inhibitor augments glutathione levels in lung epithelial lining fluid. J Appl Physiol 1993; 75:825–832.
34. Birrer P, McElvaney NG, Gillissen A, Hoyt RF, Bloedow DC, Hubbard RC, Crystal RG. Intravenous recombinant secretory leukoprotease inhibitor augments antineutrophil elastase defense. J Appl Physiol 1992; 73:317–323.
35. Powers JC, Gupton BF, Harley AD, Nishino N, Whitley RJ. Specificity of porcine pancreatic elastase, human leukocyte elastase and cathepsin G: Inhibition with peptide chloromethyl ketones. Biochim Biophys Acta 1977; 484:156–166.
36. Kettner C, Shenvi A, Watanabe S, Soskel N. A peptide boronic acid inhibitor of elastase In: Taylor JC, Mittman C, eds. Pulmonary Emphysema and Proteolysis: 1986. New York: Academic Press, 1987:65–72.
37. Kennedy AJ, Cline A, Ney UM, Johnson WH, Roberts NA. The effect of a peptide aldehyde reversible inhibitor of elastase on a human leukocyte induced model of emphysema in the hamster. Eur J Respir Dis 1987; 71:472–478.
38. Williams JC, Falcone RC, Knee C, Stein RL, Strimpler AM, Reaves B, Giles RE, Krell RD. Biologic characterization of ICI 200,880 and ICI 200,355, novel inhibitors of human neutrophil elastase. Am Rev Respir Dis 1991; 144:875–883.
39. Doherty JB, Ashe BM, Argenbright LW, Barker PL, Bonney RJ, Chandler GO, Dahlgren ME, Dorn CP, Finke PE, Firestone RA, Fletcher D, Hagmann WK, Mumford R, O'Grady L, Maycock AL, Pisano JM, Shah SK, Thompson KR, Zimmerman M. Cephalosporin antibiotics can be modified to inhibit human leukocyte elastase. Nature 1986; 322:192–194.
40. Crystal RG. $\alpha_1$-antitrypsin deficiency. In: Fishman AP, ed. Update: Pulmonary Diseases and Disorders. New York: McGraw-Hill, 1992:19–35.
41. Garver RI, Chytil A, Courtney M, Crystal RG. Clonal gene therapy: transplanted mouse fibroblastclones express human α1-antitrypsin gene in vivo. Science 1987; 237:762–764.
42. Raper SE, Wilson JM. Cell transplantation in liver-directed gene therapy. Cell Transplant 1993; 2:381–400.
43. Kolodka TM, Finegold M, Kay MA, Woo SL. Hepatic gene therapy: efficient retroviral-mediated gene transfer into rat hepatocytes in vivo. Somat Cell Mol Genet 1993; 19:491–497.
44. Hafenrichter DG, Wu X, Rettinger SD, Kennedy SC, Flye MW, Ponder KP. Quantitative evaluation of liver-specific promoters from retroviral vectors after in vivo transduction of hepatocytes. Blood 1994; 84:3394–3404.
45. Curiel D, Stier L, Crystal RG. Gene therapy for α1-antitrypsin deficiency using lymphocytes as vehicles for α1-antitrypsin delivery. Clin Res 1989; 37:578A.
46. Strauss SE. In: Ginsberg HS, ed. The Adenoviruses. New York: Plenum Press, 1984: 451–496.
47. Rosenfeld MA, Siegfried W, Yoshimura K, Yoneyama K, Fukayama M, Stier LE, Paako PK, Gilardi P, Stratford-Perricaudet LD, Stratford-Perricaudet M, Jallat S, Pavirani A, Lecocq J-P, Crystal RG. Adenovirus-mediated transfer of a recombinant α1-antitrypsin gene to the lung epithelium in vivo. Science 1991; 252:431–434.
48. Crystal RG. Protocol for gene therapy of the respiratory manifestations of cystic fibrosis using a replication deficient recombinant adenovirus to transfer the normal

cystic fibrosis transmembrane conductance regulator cDNA to the airway epithelium. Fed Register 1992; 58:21737–21738.
49. Crystal RG, McElvaney NG, Rosenfeld MA. Chu C-S, Mastrangeli A, Hay JG, Brody SL, Jaffe HA, Eissa NT, Danel C. Administration of an adenovirus containing the human CFTR cDNA to the respiratory tract of individuals with cystic fibrosis. Nature Genet 1994; 8:42–51.
50. Zabner J, Couture LA, Gregory RJ, Graham SM, Smith AE, Welsh MJ. Adenovirus-mediated gene transfer transiently corrects the chloride transport defect in nasal epithelium of patients with cystic fibrosis. Cell 1993; 75:207–216.
52. Jaffe HA, Danel C, Longenecker G, Metzger M, Setoguchi Y, Rosenfeld MA, Gant TW, Thorgeirsson SS, Stratford-Perricaudet LD, Perricaudet M, Pavirani A, Lecocq J-P, Crystal RG. Adenovirus-mediated *in vivo* gene transfer and expression in normal rat liver. Nature Genet 1992; 1:368–371.
53. Setoguchi Y, Jaffe HA, Chu CS, Crystal RG. Intraperitoneal in vivo gene therapy to deliver alpha-1-antitrypsin to the systemic circulation. Am J Respir Cell Mol Biol 1994; 10:369–377.
54. Lemarchand P, Jaffe HA, Cid MC, Kleinman HK, Stratford-Perricaudet LD, Stratford-Perricaudet M, Pavirani A, Lecocq J-P, Crystal RG. Adenovirus-mediated transfer of a recombinant human α1-antitrypsin cDNA to human endothelial cells. Proc Natl Acad Sci USA 1992; 89:6482–6486.
55. Canonico AE, Conary JT, Meyrick BO, Brigham KL. Aerosol and intravenous transfection of human α1-antitrypsin gene to lungs of rabbits. Am J Respir Cell Mol Biol 1994; 10:24–29.

# 22

# Augmentation of Liver Production

**MARK D. WEWERS**

The Ohio State University
Columbus, Ohio

## I. Introduction

The primary defect in alpha 1–antitrypsin ($\alpha$1AT) deficiency resides with the hepatocyte. Current concepts suggest that a single amino acid substitution in the PiZ allele (Glu 342 to Lys 342) produces structural changes that impair posttranslational processing of the nascent $\alpha$1AT protein. One hypothesis is that the loss of an internal salt bridge (1) or simply the addition of positive charge itself (2) leads to disturbed protein-folding, which further impairs posttranslational processing and subsequent secretion of the protein. The net result is a slowing of the release of the molecule such that in PiZ deficiency only about 10–15% of the normal amount is released. Importantly, the protein that does get released has a normal half-life and is functional as an antiprotease (3,4). Therefore, a logical approach to therapy for $\alpha$1AT deficiency is to correct the primary defect, i.e., the impaired hepatocyte release. In principle, correcting this defect could both alleviate the risk of hepatocellular injury (which is likely related to the "storage disorder" itself) and provide protection against accelerated emphysema.

## II. α1AT Production

### A. Liver Primary Producer

Based on rates of catabolism, α1AT is produced at a rate of about 17 mg/kg/day (3). The liver is the primary production site, as exemplified by the fact that individuals with PiZ deficiency have normal α1AT levels after liver transplantation (5). Although mononuclear phagocytes and other cells produce small amounts of α1AT (6–8), these sources are of unknown physiological significance. Histological studies have documented that PiZ α1AT is present in abundance in hepatocytes and can be localized to the rough endoplasmic reticulum (9). However, some PiZ protein is glycosylated and secreted. Of note, the half-life of secreted PiZ protein is similar to that of PiM α1AT (3) and PiZ individuals catabolize PiM protein normally (10–12). Taken together, these observations document that the deficiency in the PiZ form is due to a production defect.

Purified, secreted PiZ protein has antitryptic activity similar to that of PiM protein (4,13). Although a subtle defect in the rate of association with neutrophil elastase for PiZ vs. PiM protein (14) has been demonstrated, therapy directed at enhancing hepatocyte release of native PiZ protein could potentially provide sufficient antiprotease protection for the lung.

### B. α1AT Levels Fluctuate

α1AT is an acute-phase reactant; its responsive serum levels suggest the feasibility of pharmacologically augmenting liver production. For example, it has long been recognized that inflammation, pregnancy, and tumors can elevate the antitrypsin capacity of serum (15–17). One of the first demonstrations that α1AT levels could be pharmacologically manipulated appeared with studies using typhoid vaccine (15). However, the magnitude of the response was closely associated with the phenotype of α1AT. Homozygotes for the normal α1AT gene raised their resting trypsin inhibitory capacity twofold; heterozygotes for the deficiency allele raised their levels significantly as well, but homozygotes for the PiZ deficiency allele did not respond significantly.

A major clue to regulatory events was provided by the observation that α1AT levels were increased in pregnancy (18) in association with increased glucocorticoid release. In this regard, exogenous estrogen compounds were demonstrated to be effective augmentors of α1AT levels. Diethylstibesterol was shown to elevate heterozygote levels of α1AT in PiMZ individuals; however, little to no effect on PiZ levels was noted (19). Oral contraceptive steroids (20) were also found to increase various liver-produced proteins, including α1AT. Thus, the possibility that α1AT hepatocyte release could be augmented pharmacologically seemed feasible.

## III. Augmentation of Liver Protein Production

### A. Danazol Affects Protein Production

Other deficiencies of liver-produced plasma proteins have been documented such as those of antithrombin III and C1 esterase. Relevant to possible therapy for α1AT deficiency, these deficiency states have been demonstrated to respond to pharmacological therapy aimed at enhancing hepatocyte release of the deficient protein. As a pertinent example, clinical improvement in C1 esterase deficiency has been documented with danazol therapy which correlates with the enhanced release of C1 esterase (21,22).

### B. Danazol in α1AT Deficiency

In the context of the success seen with the angioneurotic edema of C1 esterase deficiency, the effect of danazol on α1AT levels in PiZ α1AT deficiency was studied. In a trial of six PiZ individuals, danazol raised serum α1AT levels an average of 37% during a 1-month trial. Larger increases were seen with intermediate deficiency states (23). A more extensive trial with danazol showed similar findings (24). However, the response was relatively modest: half of study patients responded (⩾20% increase in α1AT), and of the responders hepatic enzyme elevations were seen in 20% (Fig. 1). These increases were well below the theoretical "threshold" level of α1AT presumed to be needed for protease protection (12).

### C. Tamoxifen as α1AT Inducer

The use of tamoxifen, an antiestrogen compound, suggested promise as an α1AT inducer in a report of its use in PiSZ individuals with liver disease (25). Significant elevations in serum α1AT levels were recorded (25). A potential advantage of tamoxifen is that it would avoid masculinizing side effects in female patients. A trial of tamoxifen in PiZ individuals revealed that side effect were minimal, but only a small percentage of individuals responded and, as with danazol therapy, the increases were modest (26).

In summary, attempts at augmenting α1AT release from the liver are profoundly affected by the underlying phenotype (Table 1). The trials with danazol and tamoxifen closely parallel the prior results with typhoid vaccine and diethylstibesterol. That is, individuals with a deficiency due to the Z mutation exhibit a blunted response to direct stimulation of hepatocytes. It is therefore likely that attempts to enhance endogenous PiZ protein release from affected individuals will need to address the specific protein defect that has impaired export of the aberrant molecule.

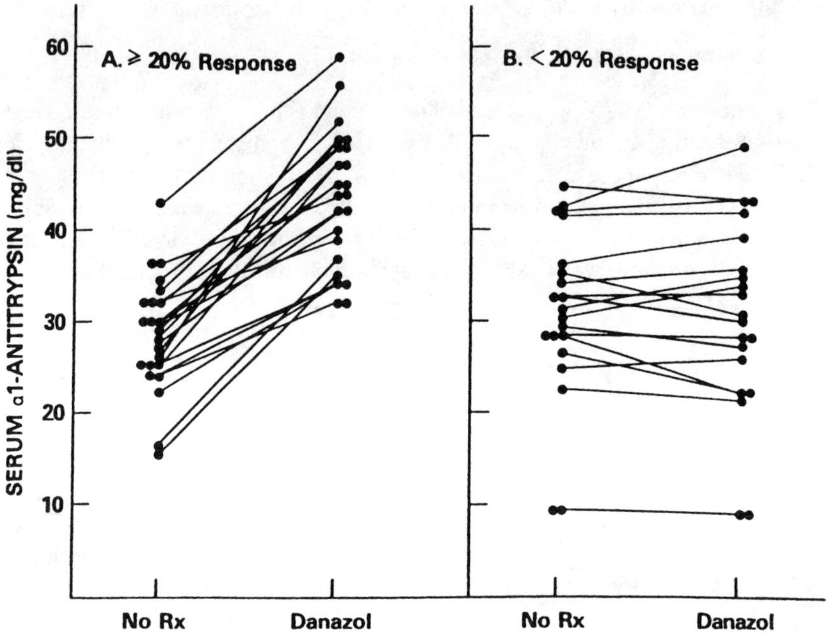


**Figure 1** Effect of 30 days of danazol therapy on serum α1AT-deficient subjects. (A) Pretreatment (No Rx) and treatment (Danazol) values in subjects who had ≥20% increase in serum α1AT with treatment. (B) Pretreatment and treatment values in those who responded with <20% increase in serum α1AT. All subjects received the same therapy (200 mg given orally three times a day). (From Ref. 24.)

## IV. Potential Effect of Intracellular α1AT on Hepatocytes

Recent data suggest that the PiZ form of α1AT accumulates in hepatocytes in an insoluble form that may promote hepatocyte injury (27). The association between liver disease and α1AT deficiency was first made in infants (28). The injury generally occurs within the first 3 months of life (29), but adults who survive past age 50 have an increased risk as well (30). Although the exact mechanism responsible for hepatocellular damage in PiZ α1AT deficiency is still unclear, there is increasing evidence that it is intracellular accumulation of the mutated protein that causes the injury. Indirect support of this hypothesis comes from the observation that, of the PiNull phenotypes identified, none has been associated with either intracellular accumulation of α1AT or premature hepatocellular injury despite a more severe defect in antiprotease screen than is present with the PiZ homozygous state (31–34). In contrast, all individuals with PiZ deficiency allele,

**Table 1** Responsiveness of α1AT Phenotypes to Attempts at Augmenting Hepatic Release

| | Increase in α1AT above baseline[a] | | | | |
|---|---|---|---|---|---|
| Agent (ref.) | PiMM | PiMZ | PiSZ | PiZZ | (units) |
| Typhoid vaccine (15) | 170 | 85 | ND[c] | 10 | (mg/dl) |
| Diethylstibesterol (19) | 0.54 | 0.33 | 0.11 | 0.03 | (units) |
| Danazol (23) | ND | ND | 75 | 12 | (mg/dl) |

ND: group was not studied.
[a]Values displayed represent the average increase in either α1AT concentrations (mg/ml) or in serum trypsin inhibitory capacity (units), a functional index of α1AT concentrations.

including PiZ, PiMZ, and PiSZ, have the intracellular accumulation of insoluble α1AT, and PiZ and PiSZ phenotypes have a predisposition to liver injury (28, 33–35) (Table 2). This relationship implies that there is a divergence between the presence of a defect in circulating levels of α1AT and the development of liver disease, but a convergence between the presence of intrahepatic α1AT accumulation and liver damage.

As previously mentioned, it is believed that the substitution of a positively charged Lys 342 for Glu 342 in the PiZ allele affects proper folding of the nascent protein in the rough endoplasmic reticulum, and that it is the improper folding that promotes aggregation and the insolubility of the protein (1,2). In keeping with this hypothesis, human PiZ α1AT-induced transgenic mice accumulate α1AT in their hepatocytes and also develop liver damage despite adequate circulating levels of normal α1AT (27).

## V. Future Directions

The concept that intracellular accumulation of PiZ α1AT promotes liver injury suggests that future attempts at augmenting liver production of α1AT will need to address this concern. Consistent with this observation is the relatively high frequency of transaminase elevations in individuals treated with androgen or tamoxifen (24–26). Nonspecific stimulators of protein production will likely enhance the net release of α1AT but will do so at considerable risk of increasing the insoluble, intrahepatic fraction of α1AT as well. Thus, all such approaches may increase the risk of hepatic injury. Future approaches will undoubtedly focus on more specific modalities, e.g., gene therapy utilizing genetically modified hepatocytes. These therapies may promote physiologically significant increases in

**Table 2** Relationship Between Hepatocyte α1AT Accumulation and Risk for Cirrhosis

| Phenotype (α1AT % normal)[a] | α1AT accumulation in hepatocytes | Risk[b] for | |
|---|---|---|---|
| | | Emphysema | Cirrhosis |
| MM (100%) | 0 | Normal | Normal |
| MZ (60%) | + | Normal | ?[c] |
| SZ (35%) | ++ | Moderate | Moderate |
| SS (60%) | 0 | Normal | Normal |
| ZZ (10%) | +++ | High | High |
| Null (0%) | 0 | High | Normal[d] |

[a]Approximate serum α1AT concentration expressed as percent of normal levels.
[b]Risk as compared to that of the normal population for either emphysema or cirrhosis.
[c]There is some evidence that individuals with MZ phenotype have increased risk for liver injury but it is largely anecdotal (36).
[d]Because of the rarity of this phenotype, only a few have had histological studies done but none has demonstrated liver injury (25).
*Source*: Adapted from Ref. 33.

α1AT release and are clearly feasible from a technological perspective. More long-range and comprehensive objectives, however, may include approaches that can address both the defect in release and the defect in protein-folding. Correcting the protein-folding problem could provide protection from premature emphysema by boosting the antiprotease screen as well as prevent the potentially harmful accumulation of insoluble α1AT in producer hepatocytes. Thus, more specific therapies may incorporate strategies to either "knock out" the translation of the abnormal PiZ protein or enhance the ability of this protein to fold normally. These are long-range goals and more difficult to achieve.

In summary, pharmacological augmentation of hepatocyte α1AT release can be achieved with various oral agents. However, because the response is modest and side effects are frequent, this approach is currently impractical as a clinically useful approach to treatment of this disorder.

## References

1. Brantly M, Courtney M, Crystal RG. Repair of the secretion defect in the Z form of alpha-1-antitrypsin by addition of a second mutation. Science 1989; 242:1700.
2. Sifers RN, Hardick CP, Woo SLC. Disruption of the 290–342 salt bridge is not responsible for the secretory defect of PiZ alpha-1-antitrypsin variant. J Biol Chem 1989; 264:2997.

3. Laurell C-B, Nosslin B, Jeppson J-O. Catabolic rate of alpha-1-antitrypsin of Pi type M and Z in man. Clin Sci Mol Med 1977; 52:457.
4. Miller RR, Kuhlenschmidt MS, Coffee CJ, Kuo I, Glew RH. Comparison of the chemical, physical, and survival properties of normal and Z-variant alpha-1-antitrypsins. J Biol Chem 1976; 251:4751.
5. Putnam CW, Porter KA, Peters RL, Ashcaval M, Redeker AG, Starzl TE. Liver replacement for alpha-1-antitrypsin. Surgery 1977; 81:258.
6. Takemura S, Rossing TH, Perlmutter DH. A lymphokine regulates expression of alpha-1-proteinase inhibitor in human monocytes and macrophages. J Clin Invest 1986; 77:1207.
7. Mornex J-F, Chytil-Weir A, Martinet Y, Courtney M, Lecocq J-P, Crystal RG. Expression of the alpha-1-antitrypsin gene in mononuclear phagocytes of normal and alpha-1-antitrypsin-deficient individuals. J Clin Invest 1986; 77:1952.
8. Carlson JA, Rogers BB, Sifers RN, Hawkins HK, Finegold MJ, Woo SLC. Multiple tissues express alpha-1-antitrypsin in transgenic mice and man. J Clin Invest 1988; 82:26.
9. Callea F, Fevery J, Massi G, Leivens C, De Groote J, Desmet VJ. Alpha-1-antitrypsin (AAT) and its stimulation in the liver of PiMZ phenotype individuals: A "recruitment-secretory block" ("R-SB") phenomenon. Liver 1984; 4:325.
10. Makino S, Reed CE. Distribution and elimination of exogenous alpha-1-antitrypsin. J Lab Clin Med 1969; 75:742.
11. Gadek JE, Klein HG, Holland PV, Crystal RG. J Clin Invest 1981; 68:1158.
12. Wewers MD, Casolaro MA, Sellers SE, Swayze SC, McPhaul KM, Wittes JT, Crystal RG. Replacement therapy for alpha 1-antitrypsin deficiency associated with emphysema. N Engl J Med 1987; 316:1055.
13. Yoshida A, Lieberman J, Gaidulis L, Ewing C. Molecular abnormality of human alpha-1-antitrypsin variant (Pi-ZZ) associated with plasma activity deficiency. Proc Nat Acad Sci USA 1976; 73:1324.
14. Ogushi F, Fells GA, Hubbard RC, Straus SD, Crystal RG. Z-type alpha 1-antitrypsin is less competent than M1-type alpha 1-antitrypsin as an inhibitor of neutrophil elastase. J Clin Invest 1987; 80:1366.
15. Kueppers F. Genetically determined differences in the response of alpha-1-antitrypsin levels in human serum to typhoid vaccine. Humangenetik 1968; 6:207.
16. Ascoli M, Bezzola UC. Das Verhalten des antitryptischen Vermoegens des Blutserums bei der croupoesen Pneumonie. Berl Klin Wschr 1903; 40:391.
17. Jacobsson K. Studies on the trypsin and plasmin inhibitors in human blood serum. Scand J Clin Lab Invest 1955; 7(suppl 14):83.
18. Faarvang HJ, Lauritsen OS. Increase of trypsin inhibitor in serum during pregnancy. Nature 1963; 199:290.
19. Lieberman J, Mittman C. Dynamic response of alpha-1-antitrypsin variants to diethylstibestrol. Am J Hum Genet 1973; 25:610.
20. Laurell C-B, Kullander S, Thorell J. Effect of administration of a combined estrogen-progestin contraceptive on the level of individual proteins. Scand J Clin Lab Invest 1967; 21:33.
21. Gelfand JA, Sherins RJ, Alling DW, Frank MM. Treatment of hereditary angioedema with danazol: reversal of clinical and biochemical abnormalities. N Engl J Med 1976; 295:1444.

22. Gadek JE, Hosea SW, Gelfand JA, Frank MM. Response of variant hereditary angioedema phenotypes to danazol therapy: Genetic implications. J Clin Invest 1979; 64:280.
23. Gadek JE, Fulmer JD, Gelfand JA, Frank MM, Petty TL, Crystal RG. Danazol-induced augmentation of serum alpha-1-antitrypsin levels in individuals with marked deficiency of this antiprotease. J Clin Invest 1980; 66:82.
24. Wewers MD, Gadek JE, Keogh BA, Fells GA, Crystal RG. Evaluation of danazol therapy for patients with PiZZ alpha-1-antitrypsin deficiency. Am Rev Resp Dis 1986; 134:476.
25. Eriksson S. The effect of tamoxifen in intermediate alpha-1-antitrypsin deficiency associated with the phenotype PiSZ. Ann Clin Res 1983; 15:95.
26. Wewers MD, Brantly ML, Casolaro MA, Crystal RG. Evaluation of tamoxifen as a therapy to augment alpha-1-antitrypsin concentrations in Z homozygous alpha-1-antitrypsin deficient individuals. Am Rev Resp Dis 1987; 135:401.
27. Carlson JA, Rogers BB, Sifers RN, et al. The accumulation of PiZ alpha-1-antitrypsin causes liver damage in transgenic mice. J Clin Invest 1989; 83:1183.
28. Sharp HL, Bridges RA, Krivit W, Freier EF. Cirrhosis is associated with alpha-1-antitrypsin deficiency: a previously unrecognized inherited disorder. J Lab Clin Med 1969; 73:934.
29. Sveger T. Liver disease in alpha-1-antitrypsin deficiency detected by screening of 200,000 infants. N Engl J Med 1976; 294:1316.
30. Cox DW, Smyth S. Risk for liver disease in adults with alpha-1-antitrypsin deficiency. Am J Med 1983; 74:221.
31. Garver RI, Mornex J-F, Nukiwa T, Brantly M, Courtney J-P, Crystal RG. Alpha-1-antitrypsin deficiency and emphysema caused by homozygous inheritance of non-expressing alpha-1-antitrypsin genes. N Engl J Med 1986; 314:762.
32. Nukiwa T, Takahashi H, Brantly M, Courtney M, Crystal RG. Alpha-1-antitrypsin null (granite falls), a nonexpressing alpha-1-antitrypsin gene associated with a frame-shift to stop mutation in a coding exon. J Biol Chem 1987; 262:11999.
33. Crystal RG. Alpha 1-antitrypsin deficiency, emphysema, and liver disease: genetic basis and strategies for therapy. J Clin Invest 1990; 85:1343.
34. Birrer P, McElvaney NG, Chang-Stroman LM, Crystal RG. $\alpha_1$-Antitrypsin deficiency and liver disease. J Inherited Metab Dis 1991; 14:512.
35. Bhan AK, Grand RJ, Colten HR, Alper CA. Liver in alpha-1-antitrypsin deficiency: morphologic observations and in vitro synthesis of alpha-1-antitrysin. Ped Res 1976; 10:35.
36. Carrell RW, Owen MC. Alpha-1-antitrypsin: structure, variation and disease. Essays Med Biochem 1979; 4:83.

# 23

# Low-Molecular-Weight Inhibitors of Neutrophil Elastase

**JAMES C. POWERS, R. RICHARD PLASKON, and CHIH-MIN KAM**

Georgia Institute of Technology
Atlanta, Georgia

## I. Introduction

Human leukocyte elastase (HLE), also known as human neutrophil elastase (HNE), is a serine protease that is responsible for the abnormal turnover of connective-tissue proteins associated with the development of pulmonary emphysema, rheumatoid arthritis, and several inflammatory diseases such as acute respiratory distress syndrome (ARDS) and septicemia (1). HLE is found in the azurophilic granules of polymorphonuclear leukocytes (neutrophils) and has important roles in phagocytosis. Extracellular HLE released from neutrophils is controlled by plasma protease inhibitors, primarily the serpin alpha 1–proteinase inhibitor (α1PI). Conditions leading to a decrease in active α1PI concentration, such as a genetic defect or oxidative destruction of α1PI by cigarette smoking, can result in a protease–protease inhibitor imbalance, which is believed to be responsible for pulmonary emphysema. One approach to the treatment of emphysema is the use of low-molecular-weight elastase inhibitors. Synthetic inhibitors have several advantages over natural protein protease inhibitors: they can be produced

---

Abbreviations are defined following the text.

in large quantities by chemical synthesis or fermentation, they are not likely to be antigenic, and they can be used orally or in aerosol. Various types of synthetic elastase inhibitors, including reversible and irreversible peptide inhibitors, and heterocyclic compounds have been reported. Several inhibitors have been tested in vivo and have the potential for use as therapeutic agents.

## II. Human Leukocyte Elastase

HLE is a glycoprotein with a single peptide chain of 218 amino acid residues and four disulfide bonds. HLE and the related porcine pancreatic elastase (PPE) are the two major serine proteases that cleave the important connective-tissue protein elastin. Both elastases cleave substrates at peptide bonds where the P1 residue* (2) is an amino acid residue with a small alkyl side chain such as Ala or Val. The primary structures of HLE (3) and PPE have been determined and the two enzymes have a sequence homology of approximately 40%. At present, the structures of 21 PPE–inhibitor and three HLE–inhibitor complexes have been determined at atomic resolution by X-ray crystallography. The tertiary structures of these two enzymes are surprisingly alike, especially in the active-site regions, in addition to their sequence homology and similarities in substrate specificity of these two elastases (4). Therefore, information obtained from crystal structures of PPE–inhibitor complexes can be used for elucidating the mechanism of inhibition of HLE by various inhibitors. The catalytic triad (Ser-195, His-57, and Asp-102) and the residues around the binding site (peptide segments 189–195, 213–216, 226–228, and residue 41) are structurally similar in these two enzymes. However, there are important structural differences between these two elastases. For example, HLE has 10 deletions and two insertions in its amino acid sequence compared to PPE, and HLE is more hydrophobic and more basic than PPE.

The first reported crystal structure of HLE is a complex of the enzyme with the third domain of the turkey ovomucoid inhibitor (TOM, 3). TOM forms a tight complex with HLE with an association constant of $6.2 \times 10^9\ M^{-1}$. The active site of HLE makes direct contact with eight residues of the primary binding segment of TOM (P5 Pro-14I to P3′ Arg-21I) and with three to five other residues (Gly-32I, Asn-33I, and Asn-36I) of a secondary binding segment. The majority of the intermolecular contacts occur in the primary binding loop, which mimics a bound substrate in the active site of HLE. Seven hydrogen bonds are formed between the peptide backbone of the inhibitor and HLE. The P3, P2, and P1 residues of TOM form an antiparallel β-sheet structure with the peptide backbone of Ser-214–

*The nomenclature of Schechter and Berger (2) is used to designate the individual amino acid residues (P2, P1, P1′, P2′, etc.) of a peptide substrate and the corresponding subsites (S2, S1, S1′, S2′, etc.) of the enzyme. The scissle bond is the P1–P1′ peptide bond.

Val-216 of HLE. The carbonyl group of Leu-18I (P1 residue) is located in the oxyanion hole (Gly-193N, Ser-195N). The crystal structures of complexes of HLE with MeO-Suc-Ala-Ala-Pro-Val-$CH_2Cl$ and MeO-Suc-Ala-Ala-Pro-Ala-$CH_2Cl$ have also been determined (5,6). The peptide chain of both chloromethyl ketone inhibitors bind to the HLE active site in a manner similar to that of the corresponding P4–P1 residues of TOM.

## III. Synthetic Inhibitors

Various types of synthetic inhibitors for serine proteases have been reported, and this research has been reviewed recently (7). Inhibitors include simple substrate analogs, transition-state analogs, alkylating agents that react with the active-site histidine, acylating agents that react with the active-site serine to form stable acyl enzymes, and mechanism-based (or suicide) inhibitors. The first two classes of compounds are reversible inhibitors, and the last three are irreversible inhibitors.

Reversible inhibitors usually contain substrate-like features, and their potency depends on binding interactions with the enzyme. Since the enzyme–inhibitor complex formed with reversible inhibitors can dissociate, restoration of enzymatic activity may occur as the inhibitor is destroyed or cleared from the system. The strength of the binding is reflected in $K_I$, the dissociation constant for the enzyme–inhibitor complex E·I. Medicinal chemists often report inhibitor potency with $IC_{50}$ ($I_{50}$) values, which are easier to determine than $K_I$ values. Irreversible inhibitors usually inactivate serine proteases by first forming a reversible E·I complex followed by covalent bond formation. The potency of the inhibitor depends on the strength of reversible binding to the enzyme ($K_I$), the rate of the inactivation step ($k_2$), or both ($k_2/K_I$). The most suitable parameter for comparing irreversible inhibitors is $k_2/K_I$, which is equal to $k_{obsd}/[I]$ when $K_I$ is larger than [I]. The more potent reversible and irreversible peptide inhibitors for elastase contain the amino acid sequence Ala-Ala-Pro-Val derived from substrate mapping studies. Several reviews on synthetic elastase inhibitors have appeared (8–11).

### A. Reversible Peptide Inhibitors

Reversible peptide inhibitors can be either simple competitive or slow binding inhibitors. Many of these compounds, including peptidyl aldehydes, boronic acids, α-keto esters, and trifluoromethyl ketones, are transition-state analogs, and show reversible slow tight binding inhibition. The inhibition can be analyzed according to the models proposed by Morrison (12). One model describes the rapid formation of a weak enzyme–inhibitor complex (EI) prior to slow formation of another tight enzyme–inhibitor complex (EI*), where EI* is more stable than EI (Scheme 1).

$$E + I \underset{k_2}{\overset{k_1}{\rightleftharpoons}} EI \underset{k_4}{\overset{k_3}{\rightleftharpoons}} EI^*$$ Scheme 1

$$K_I\ (\text{initial}) = \frac{k_2}{k_1} \qquad \frac{K_I\ (\text{initial})}{K_I\ (\text{final})} - 1 = \frac{k_3}{k_4}$$

The other model has only a single, slowly formed enzyme–inhibitor complex (Scheme 2).

$$E + I \underset{k_{off}}{\overset{k_{on}}{\rightleftharpoons}} EI^* \quad K_I = k_{off} / k_{on}$$ Scheme 2

Kinetic constants such as $K_I$ (initial), $K_I$ (final), or $K_I$, $k_{on}$, and $k_{off}$ are used to measure the potency of these inhibitors. Structures and inhibition constants of several of the most potent reversible inhibitors of HLE are shown in Figure 1.

### *Peptide Aldehydes*

Synthetic peptide aldehydes such as $AdSO_2$-$N^{\varepsilon}$-(4-carboxybenzoyl)-Lys-Ala-Val-H (Ro 31-3537, Fig. 1) and $AdSO_2$-$N^{\varepsilon}$-(succinyl)-Lys-Ala-Val-H inhibit HLE quite potently with $K_I$ values of 0.06 and 0.11 μM, respectively (13). These two aldehydes also inhibit elastase in human bronchial lavage and the complex of HLE with alpha 2–macroglobulin, but they are inactive at 100 μM against other serine proteases such as chymotrypsin and cathepsin G. Another peptide aldehyde, ICI 186,756 (Fig. 1), is also a potent, selective inhibitor of HLE (14).

### *Peptide Boronic Acids*

MeO-Suc-Ala-Ala-Pro-boro-Val-OH (Fig. 1) is a potent and specific transition-state inhibitor of HLE with $K_I$ (initial) and $K_I$ (final) values of 15 and 0.57 nM, respectively (15). This compound also inhibits PPE with a comparable $K_I$, but its inhibition against chymotrypsin and cathepsin G is rather weak. MeO-Suc-Ala-Ala-Pro-boro-Ala-OH inhibits HLE competitively with a $K_I$ (initial) value about fivefold higher than the corresponding boro-Val derivative. The mode of inhibition involves the formation of a hemiacetal-like intermediate with the Oγ of the active site Ser-195 of the enzyme. The complex resembles the tetrahedral intermediate formed during substrate hydrolysis (Fig. 2). In the crystal structure of PPE complexed to Z-Ala-boro-Ile-OH, a covalent bond (1.5 Å) is formed between the boron atom of the inhibitor and the Oγ of Ser-195 of the enzyme. There is also a close direct contact (2.2 Å) between the boron atom and $N^{\varepsilon}$ of His-57 (16). Studies

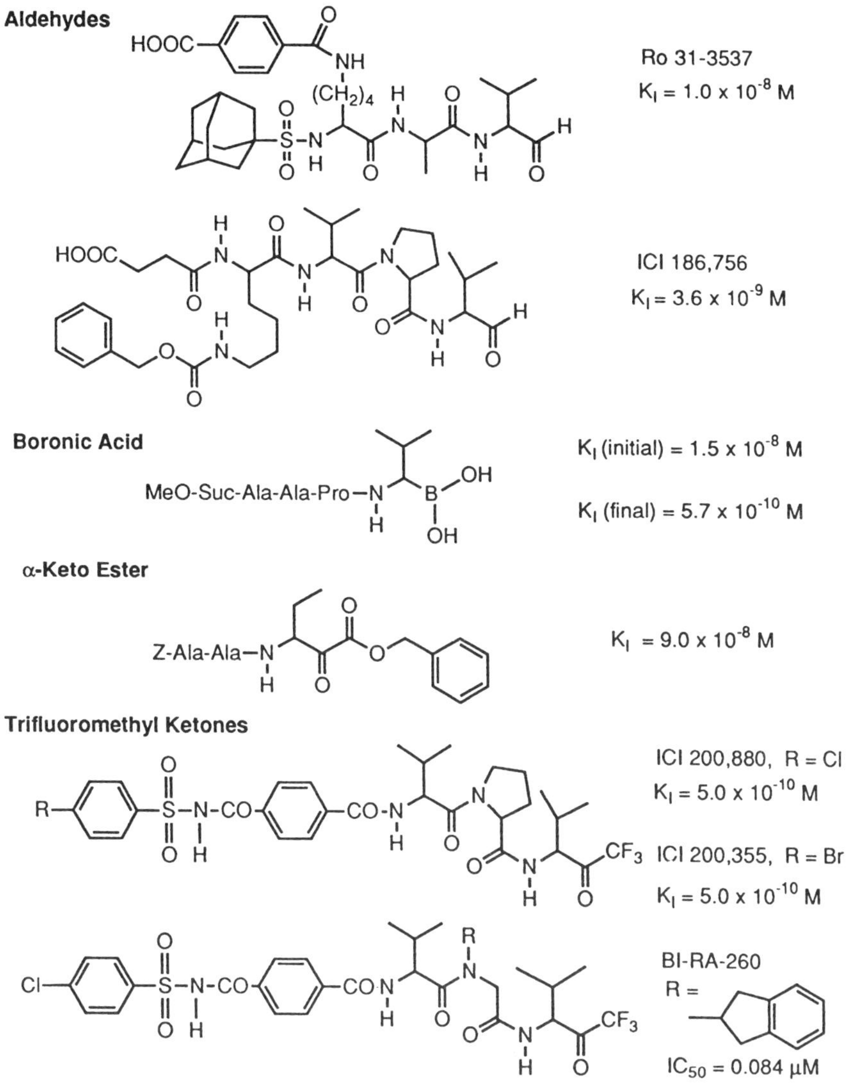


**Figure 1** Structures and inhibition constants of several reversible peptide inhibitors of human leukocyte elastase.

on the inhibition of chymotrypsin by MeO-Suc-Ala-Ala-Pro-boro-Phe-OH using $^{11}B$ NMR have also provided additional evidence of a tetrahedral geometry around boron (17).

### Peptide α-Diketones and α-Ketoesters

Peptide α-ketoesters such as RCO-Abu-COOEt, RCO-Ala-Ala-COOEt, and RCO-Abu-COOBzl (RCO = Z-Ala-Ala, Fig. 1) are potent inhibitors of HLE with $K_I$ values of 0.09–0.3 μM (18). Bz-Ala-COOEt is a much poorer inhibitor than Z-Ala-Ala-Ala-Ala-COOEt by 2000-fold due to lack of subsite interactions at P2–P5. The fact that Bz-Ala-COOEt inhibits HLE more potently than the corresponding acid indicates that the ester alkyl group can make additional interactions with the S1′ subsite of the enzyme. Two α-ketoesters, Ac-Pro-Ala-Pro-Ala-COOMe and MeO-Ala-Ala-Pro-Val-COOMe, show slow binding inhibition toward HLE with $K_I$ (final) values of 0.85 and 0.20 μM, respectively (19). However, RCO-Val-COMe and RCO-Val-COOMe (RCO = N-(4-[(4-chlorophenyl)sulfonylamino-carbonyl]phenylcarbonyl)-Val-Pro) are simple potent, competitive inhibitors of HLE (20). The mechanism of inhibition of elastase by α-ketoesters most likely involves the interaction of Ser-195 with the ketone carbonyl group of the inhibitor to form a hemiketal structure. This model is based on crystal structure of the complex of bovine trypsin and 4-amidinophenylpyruvic acid (APPA) (21), where the amidinophenyl group is located in the primary specificity pocket (S1) of trypsin and the active-site serine has added to the α-carbonyl group of APPA to give a tetrahedral structure.

Two peptidyl α-ketobenzoxazoles, Z-Val-Pro-Val-Box and Ac-Ala-Pro-Val-Box (Box = benzoxazole), are potent, competitive, reversible inhibitors of HLE, with $K_I$ values of 3 and 73 nM, respectively (22). Ac-Ala-Pro-Val-Box also inhibited PPE reversibly with a $K_I$ value of 280 nM. The X-ray crystal structure of the complex of Ac-Ala-Pro-Val-Box with PPE demonstrated that a covalent bond was formed between the S1 carbonyl group of the inhibitor and the hydroxyl group of Ser-195. The nitrogen atom of the benzoxazole ring forms a hydrogen bond with His-57. The benzoxazole functional group is related in structure to both the ester and amide groups of α-ketoesters and α-ketoamides.

### Peptide Fluoroalkyl Ketones

Peptidyl trifluoromethyl ketones containing Val or Ala at the P1 site are potent and selective inhibitors of HLE (19, 23–27). Most of these compounds are slow binding inhibitors. Among the trifluoromethyl ketones, Z-Lys(Z)-Val-Pro-Val-$CF_3$ is the most potent inhibitor, with $K_I < 0.1$ nM (23). The inhibitory potency of these compounds is largely dependent on peptide-chain length; i.e., the $K_I$ values of Val and Pro-Val derivatives are four to five orders of magnitude poorer than those of Lys(Z)-Val-Pro-Val trifluoromethyl ketones. Other potent inhibitors are

ICI 200,880, ICI 200,355 (Fig. 1) (27), Z-Ala-Ala-Pro-Val-$CF_3$ (24), and $N^{\alpha}$-(Ad-$SO_2$)-$N^{\varepsilon}$-(MeO-Suc)Lys-Pro-Val-$CF_3$ (19), with $K_I$ values in the range of 0.5–1 nM. Z-Ala-Ala-Pro-Ala-$CF_3$ and its difluoroketone derivatives have also been tested as inhibitors of HLE (25). Removal of one fluorine atom from a trifluoroketone increases the $K_I$ about 15–30-fold. Replacement of one fluorine atom of Z-Ala-Ala-Pro-Ala-$CF_3$ by a residue (–$CH_2CH_2CO$–Leu-OMe) that can interact with the S1′ and S2′ subsites decreases the $K_I$ by 30-fold when compared to Z-Ala-Ala-Pro-Ala-$CF_2H$. Upon binding to HLE, these compounds undergo addition of the hydroxyl group of Ser-195 on the ketone carbonyl group to form a hemiketal intermediate that is stabilized by the fluoromethyl group (Fig. 2). This mechanism of inhibition is supported by kinetic studies (23), NMR studies (28), and crystal structure of PPE complexed with a peptidyl α,α-difluoro-β-keto amide (29).

Several tripeptide trifluoromethyl ketones containing nonnatural N-substituted glycine residues at the P2 site are effective inhibitors of HLE and have $IC_{50}$ values in the submicromolar range (30). BI-RA-260 (Fig. 1) is one of the most potent inhibitors in the series. Sterically demanding substituents on the P2 nitrogen do not have a large effect on their inhibitory potency. Val is the preferred residue at the P1 position, and the corresponding Gly, Ala, α,α-dimethyl-Gly and Phe analogs are inactive. Deletion of the amino acid at P3 position results in inactive compounds. These compounds are highly selective toward HLE, and they do not inhibit several cysteine, aspartic, metallo, and other serine proteases. Replacement of one fluorine atom of these tripeptide trifluoromethyl ketones that contain Val at the P1 subsite by a residue (–COR, where R is OH, OEt, or linked via the $N^{\varepsilon}$ of L-Lys derivative) results in α,α-difluorostatone-containing peptides that can interact with the S′ subsites of HLE (31). The most potent derivative extends the binding interactions from P3 to P3′ subsite and has an $IC_{50}$ value of 0.057 μM.

An N-protected peptidyl pentafluoroethyl ketone (MDL 101,146) (Fig. 3) is a potent reversible inhibitor of HLE with a $K_I$ of 25 nM and an orally active compound that can inhibit HLE-induced pulmonary hemorrhage (32). Nonpeptidic trifluoromethyl ketones that contain arylpyridone and arylpyrimidone have been designed as reversible inhibitors of HLE based on the molecular model of a tripeptidic trifluoromethyl ketone bound to HLE (33–36). The most potent ones contain a central structure of 3-amino-6-phenylpyridone (Fig. 3) and have $K_I$ values in the range of $10^{-8}$–$10^{-9}$ M (36). These compounds are orally active. Variation of the N-3 substituent in the pyridone derivatives has little effect on in vitro potency. However, it has a dramatic effect on activity after oral administration. The X-ray structure of the complex of one derivative with PPE confirmed the proposed binding interactions, which include the isopropyl group of the inhibitor in the S1 subsite of the enzyme, 6-phenyl substituent in the S2 subsite, and a pair of hydrogen bonds formed between the pyridone and Val-216.

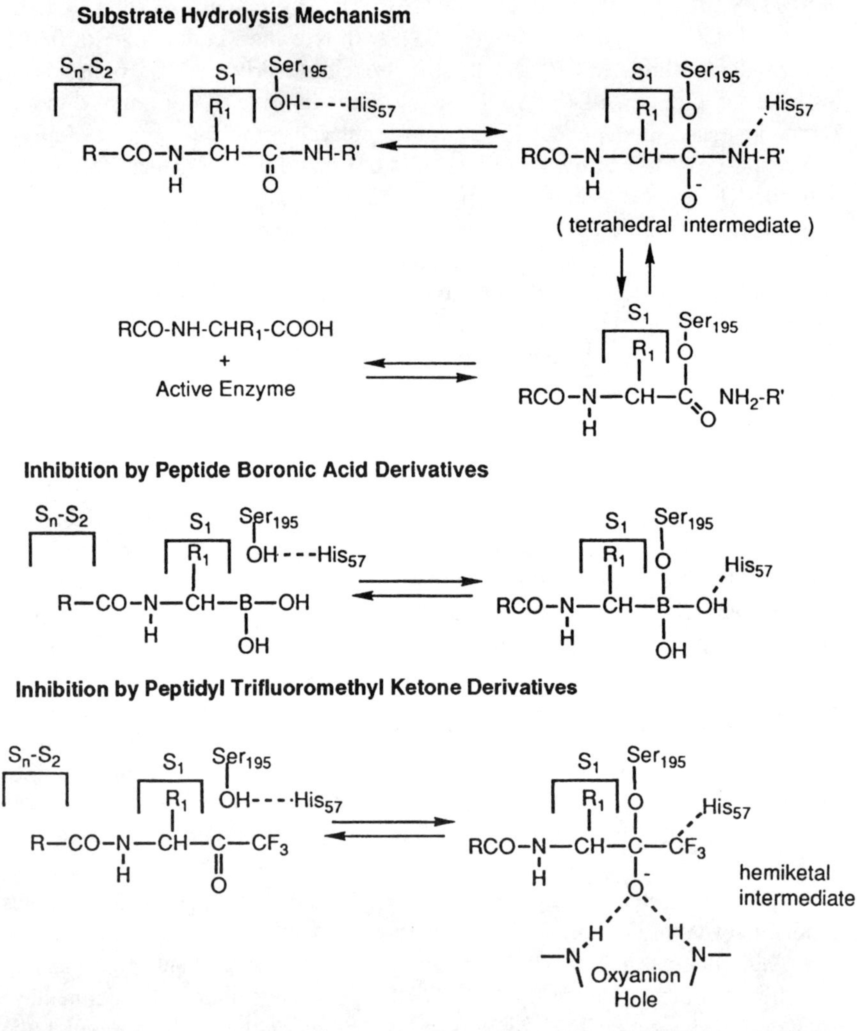


**Figure 2** Mechanism of enzymatic hydrolysis of peptide substrates by neutrophil elastase. Inhibition mechanism of neutrophil elastase by two transition-state analog inhibitors: peptide boronic acid derivatives and peptidyl trifluoromethyl ketone derivatives.

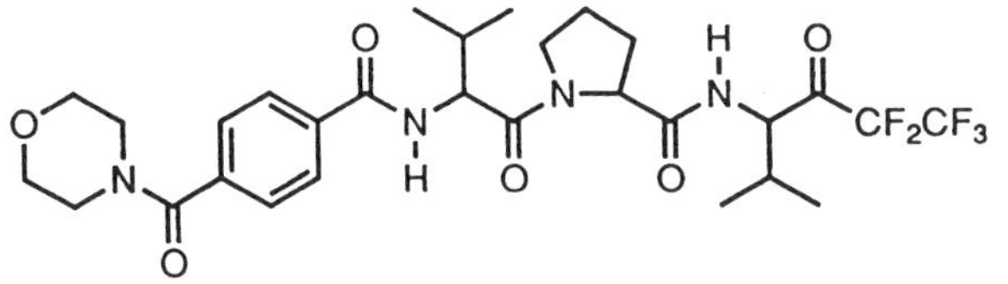


MDL 101,146
$K_I$ = 25 nM

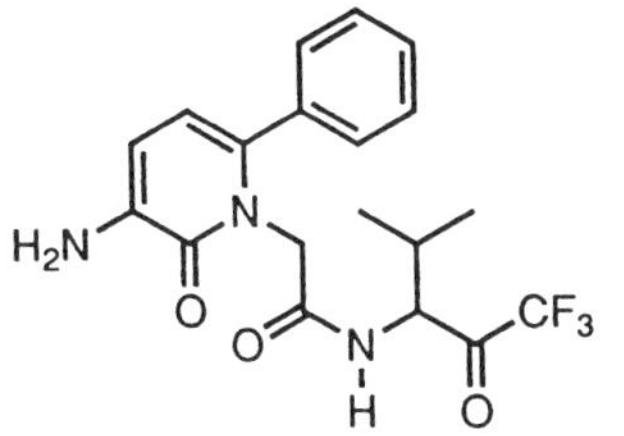


2-(3-amino-2-oxo-6-phenyl-1,2-dihydro-1-pyridyl)-N-(3,3,3-trifluoro-1-isopropyl-2-oxopropyl) acetamide
$K_I$ = 62 nM

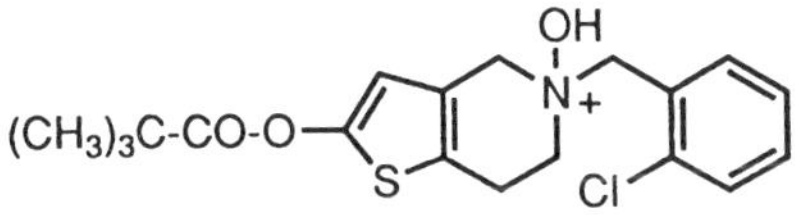


SR 26831
$IC_{50}$ = 80 nM

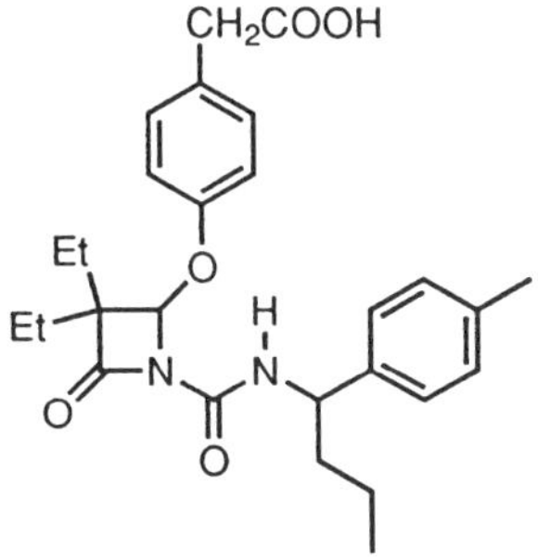


L-680,833
$k_{inact} / K_I = 622{,}000\ M^{-1}s^{-1}$

**Figure 3** Structures and inhibition constants of orally active inhibitors of human leukocyte elastase.

#### *Other Reversible Inhibitors*

Trifluoroacetyl peptides and trifluoroacetyldipeptide anilides inhibit HLE with wide range of $K_I$ values (37). The most potent inhibitors are $CF_3CO$-Lys-Ala-$NHC_6H_4$-4-R and $CF_3CO$-Lys-Leu-$NHC_6H_4$-4-R (R = isopropyl or cyclohexyl), which inhibit HLE with $K_I$ values in the submicromolar range. The crystal structure of the complexes of $CF_3CO$-AA-Ala-NH-$C_6H_4$-4-$CF_3$ (AA = Lys or Leu) with PPE have been determined (38,39). These two compounds show a reverse binding mode with PPE. The trifluoroacetyl group at N-terminus occupies the S1 binding pocket, and several hydrogen bonds are formed between the backbone of inhibitor and residues 214–216 of the enzyme. In the E–I complex of Leu-Ala derivative, the side chain of Leu makes hydrophobic contacts with Val-99 at the S2 subsite, and the Ala residue and trifluoromethylanilide do not have specific interactions with the active site of PPE.

A benzoylaminoacetic acid derivative ONO-5046 competitively inhibits HLE with a $K_I$ of 0.2 μM, but it does not inhibit other trypsin-like and chymotrypsin-like serine proteases at 100 μM (40). Other HLE inhibitors include anthraquinone derivatives (41), SC-39026 (a substituted alkyl benzoic acid derivative) (42), peptides with alkyl groups at the N- or C-terminus (43), *cis*-unsaturated fatty acids (44), elasnin (an alkyl substituted 2-hydroxy-4-pyrone) (45), and other 4-hydroxy-2-pyrone derivatives (46). The fact that oleic acid can inhibit HLE ($K_I = 9$ μM) (44) but not PPE suggests that HLE has an unusual hydrophobic binding site for fatty acid or other compounds containing hydrophobic chains.

## B. Irreversible Peptide Inhibitors

### *Peptide Chloromethyl Ketones*

These active site-directed irreversible inhibitors are the first class of selective inhibitors developed for HLE (47). The most effective chloromethyl ketone is MeO-Suc-Ala-Ala-Pro-Val-$CH_2Cl$, with $k_{obs}/[I]$ of 1560 $M^{-1}s^{-1}$. This compound does not inhibit human leukocyte cathepsin G, but it is an alkylating agent and reacts slowly with nucleophiles such as glutathione. Recently, a series of peptidyl chloromethyl ketones containing Tyr-Leu-Val sequence have been reported, and Boc-Ala-Tyr-Leu-Val-$CH_2Cl$ is the best inhibitor with a $k_{obs}/[I]$ value of 4950 $M^{-1}s^{-1}$ (48). In the crystal structures of HLE with MeO-Suc-Ala-Ala-Pro-Val-$CH_2Cl$ or MeO-Suc-Ala-Ala-Pro-Ala-$CH_2Cl$ (5,6), the P1 residue is located in the S1 pocket, one covalent bond is formed between the P1 carbonyl group and Oγ of Ser-195, and another bond is formed between the methylene group of the inhibitor and $N^{\varepsilon}$ of His-57 of HLE (Fig. 4). Both a hemiketal and an alkylated product have been detected by electrospray ionization mass spectrometry in the reaction mixture of PPE with MeO-Suc-Ala-Ala-Pro-Val-$CH_2Cl$ (49).

### *Peptide Phosphonates*

Peptidyl derivatives of diphenyl (α-aminoalkyl)phosphonates (Fig. 4) are specific and effective inhibitors of HLE (50,51). The tripeptide Boc-Val-Pro-$Val^P(OPh)_2$, which has the same sequence found in a potent trifluoromethyl ketone (23), is the best irreversible HLE phosphonate inhibitor, with $k_{obs}/[I]$ of 27,000 $M^{-6}1s^{-1}$. This phosphonate also inhibits PPE quite potently, but it does not inhibit chymotrysin or other chymases. The tetrapeptide MeO-Suc-Ala-Ala-Pro-$Val^P(OPh)_2$ inhibits both HLE and PPE effectively, with $k_{obs}/[I]$ values of 7100 $M^{-1}s^{-1}$;

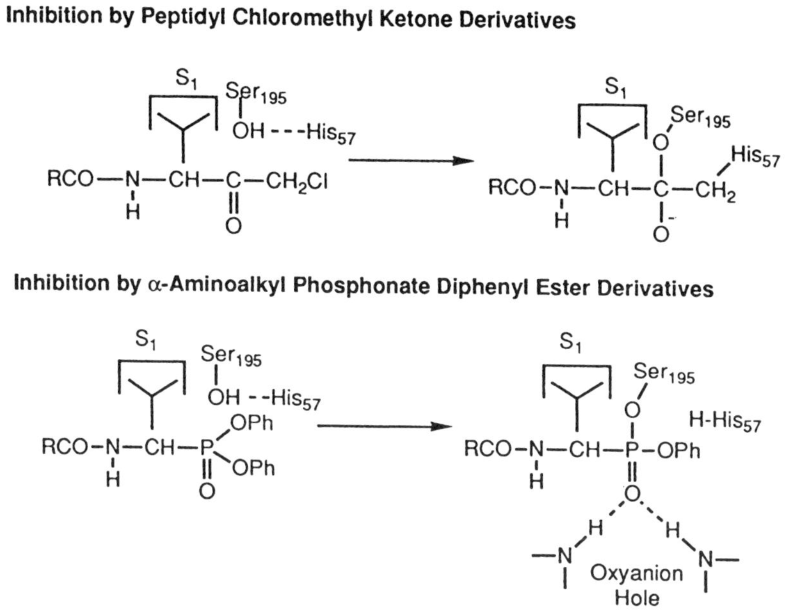


**Figure 4** Inhibition mechanism of elastase by peptide chloromethyl ketones and α-aminoalkylphosphonate diphenyl esters.

however, the corresponding Met derivative inhibits HLE poorly. Studies on inhibition of chymotrypsin by Suc-Val-Pro-$Phe^P(OPh)_2$ using $^{31}P$ NMR indicate that only one of the two diastereomers of the inhibitor is reacting with the enzyme. The enzyme–inhibitor complex has only one signal at 25.98 ppm in the $^{31}P$ NMR spectrum corresponding to the Ser-195 phosphonate ester. The mechanism of inhibition involves nucleophilic substitution by the hydroxyl group of Ser-195 at the phosphorus atom via a pentacovalent intermediate to give a product that resembles the tetrahedral intermediate formed during hydrolysis of peptide substrates (Fig. 4). The phosphonylated HLE is extremely stable and the half-time for reactivation is >48 hours; however, the second phenoxy group is lost at an unknown rate by an aging process.

### *Other Irreversible Inhibitors*

Azapeptides such as Ac-Ala-Ala-Anle-$OCH_2CF_3$ can react with HLE to form a stable acyl enzyme (carbazate derivative) that is more stable to hydrolysis than the normal acyl enzyme (ester) formed from a peptide substrate (52). In addition to acting as inhibitors, azapeptide *p*-nitrophenyl esters containing Aala, Anle, and Anva at the P1 position can be used as active titrants for HLE.

Low-molecular-weight peptidyl carbamates have been used as active-site-directed HLE inhibitors (53,54). In spite of their high inhibitory potency in vitro, their therapeutic usage has been limited due to short biological half-lives. Thus, macromolecular forms of peptidyl carbamate inhibitors of HLE have been designed for the prolongation of their half-lives in biological systems (55). These derivatives were synthesized by coupling of a low-molecular-weight peptidyl carbamate with a linear hydrophilic ploymer. The covalent linkage between the flexible linear polymer and the peptidyl carbamate inhibitor does not affect its in vitro inhibitory potency toward HLE. These macromolecular peptidyl carbamates inhibit HLE quite potently, and the $K_I$ values of 2–36 nM have been obtained after preincubation of enzyme and inhibitor.

Benzenesulfonyl fluorides with 2-fluoroacyl substituents are potent and specific inhibitors of HLE (56). The sulfonyl fluoride 2-($CF_3CF_2CONH$)-$C_4H_4SO_2F$ is the best inhibitor in the series, with $k_{obs}/[I]$ of 1700 $M^{-1}s^{-1}$, which is slightly better than the chloromethyl ketone MeO-Suc-Ala-Ala-Pro-Val-$CH_2Cl$. This compound is selective toward HLE since it inhibits cathepsin G and chymotrypsin quite slowly. Sulfonyl fluorides inhibit HLE by reacting with the active-site Ser-195 to form a sulfonyl derivative, and the fluoroacyl group interacts with the primary binding site S1 to increase the inhibition specificity.

Amino acid–derived azolides and sulfonate salts irreversibly inhibit HLE by forming various stable acyl enzymes (57,58). The inhibitory potency depends on the nature of amino acid esters, and compounds derived from methyl esters of Val, Nva, or Nle are the most potent. A series of 4-(acyloxy)benzophenones, (acyloxy)-4-pyrones (59), MR 889 (a cyclic thiolactone) (60,61), CE-0266 (a 4-(methylsulfinyl)phenyl butyrate derivative) (62), SR 26831 (an orally active compound) (Fig. 3) (63), N-(sulfonyloxy)phthalimides (64), and N-hydroxysuccimide derivatives (65,66) have also been reported as HLE inhibitors.

### C. Heterocyclic Inhibitors

Heterocyclic elastase inhibitors can act as simple acylating agents or mechanism-based inhibitors. Benzoxazinones (67–70), 3-alkoxy-4-chloroisocoumarins (71), isobenzofuranones (72), and saccharin derivatives (73–77) inhibit HLE by reaction of the active site Ser-195 with the carbonyl group of the heterocyclic ring. Some of these compounds show good selectivity toward HLE, and others are broad-spectrum inhibitors of serine proteases. Inhibition by many heterocyclic derivatives is achieved by a rapid acylation reaction combined with a slow deacylation rate. For example, 2-ethoxy-5-ethylbenzoxazinone, which contains an electron-withdrawing group at the 2 position and a small alkyl group at the 5 position, inhibits HLE with a $K_I$ of 42 pM. The stability of the acyl enzyme can be improved by introducing into the ring structure substituents that stabilize the acyl enzyme by steric or electronic effects. For example, 2-isopropylamino-5-

methylbenzoxazinone forms an acyl enzyme that deacylates with a half-time of 10.8 hours (69).

Mechanism-based inhibitors—also known as suicide inhibitors, $k_{cat}$ inhibitors, or enzyme-activated inhibitors—often contain a masked functional group that is unmasked upon reaction with the active-site residue of the enzyme. The initial step of the reaction usually involves formation of an acyl enzyme with Ser-195 and simultaneous unmasking of the reactive group, which can then react with another active-site residue to form an irreversibly inactivated enzyme. Mechanism-based inhibitors include cephalosporins, ynenol lactones, enol lactones, 3,4-dichloroisocoumarin, 3-alkoxy-7-amino-4-chloroisocoumarins, and halomethyldihydrocoumarins (78). Structures and inhibition constants of several mechanism-based inhibitors are shown in Fig. 5.

### *Cephalosporins*

Cephalosporins with various substituents (Fig. 4) are potent and time-dependent inhibitors of HLE (79–83). Various cephalosporin *t*-butyl esters containing small, α-oriented, electron-withdrawing groups at C-7 position, such as Cl or OMe, have the greatest activity. The oxidation state of the sulfur atom is very important with regard to the inhibitory potency. The sulfones exhibit considerably greater activity than the corresponding sulfides or β-sulfoxides, while the α-sulfoxides are inactive. Several representative compounds have also been tested against other serine proteases. Most of these β-lactams inhibit PPE and HLE very effectively, but their inhibition rates with chymotrypsin are slower. There is no significant activity against trypsin or cathepsin G, although some inhibitory activities have been observed against thrombin and plasmin. A variety of 7α-methoxycephalosporin ester and amide sulfones have also been tested against HLE, and the most potent $IC_{50}$ values are obtained with neutral, lipophilic derivatives, with the esters being more active than the corresponding amides. Several 3′-substituted cephalosporin *t*-butyl ester sulfones have also been tested, and the potency is determined by the electron-withdrawing ability and the size of the substituent. The crystal structure of the complex of PPE with 3-acetoxymethyl-7-α-chloro-3-cephem-4-carboxylate-1,1-dioxide *t*-butyl ester has been determined at 1.84 Å resolution (84). The inhibition mechanism shown in Fig. 6 is based on this structure and other biochemical evidence. It involves reaction of Ser-195 with the carbonyl group of the β-lactam ring to form a tetrahedral intermediate, which then collapses to form an acyl enzyme. Elimination of acetate leads to the formation of an exocyclic methylene at the 3′ position followed by elimination of HCl and formation of a double bond between C6 and C7. Deacylation by either aminolysis or hydrolysis can regenerate the free enzyme. Nucleophilic attack by His-57 on the exocyclic methylene prior to deacylation forms a stable inactive enzyme derivative. It is clear that the 7-α-chloro substituent of the unreacted inhibitor

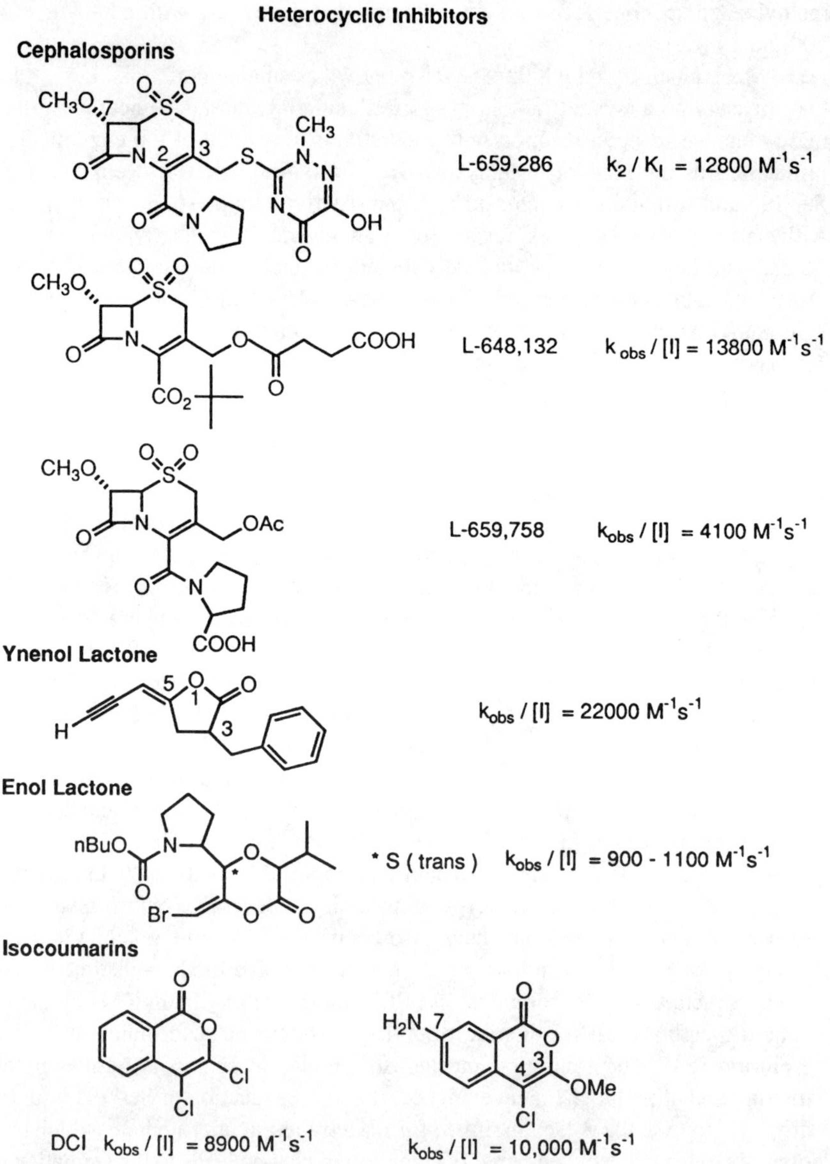


**Figure 5** Structures and inhibition constants of several heterocyclic mechansim-based inhibitors of human leukocyte elastase.

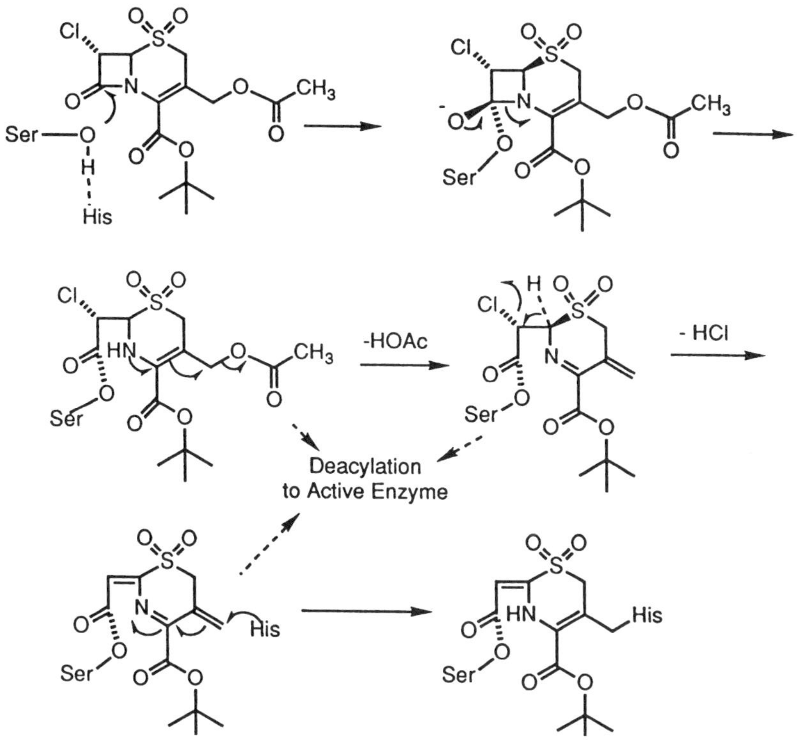


**Figure 6** Mechanism of inhibition of neutrophil elastase by cephalosporins. (Adapted from Ref. 84.)

originally fits into the S1 pocket, and this is consistent with the fact that elastase prefers β-lactam inhibitors with small 7-α-substituents.

A similar mechanism of inhibition of HLE by two cephalosporins, L-658,758 and L-659,286, has also been proposed (85). This mechanism of inhibition has been proved in the inhibition of PPE by two cephalosporins using electrospray ionization mass spectrometry (86). Several 7α-chloro and 7α-methoxy cephalosporin thioester sulfones with various C-3′ substituents have shown time-dependent inhibition toward HLE with $K_I$ ranging from micro- to nanomolar values and second-order rate constants reaching $10^6$ $M^{-1}s^{-1}$ (87).

### *Monocyclic β-Lactams*

Highly substituted monocyclic β-lactams have been investigated as irreversible inhibitors of HLE (88–92). The most potent inhibitor of HLE in the series is

L-680,833 (Fig. 3) (91), with $k_{inact}/K_I$ value of 622,000 $M^{-1}s^{-1}$. This compound also shows oral activity (91). The β-lactams with alkyl substituents, such as diethyl at C-3 position, are more potent toward HLE than PPE, which indicates that the C-3 substituent binds in the S1 site of the enzyme. Substituents on the C-4 position do not appear to interact strongly with HLE; however, they have profound effects on in vivo activity. The mechanism of inhibition involves the initial formation of a Michaelis complex, acylation of the catalytic serine residue, and loss of the leaving group at C-4 of the original β-lactam ring, followed by partitioning between regeneration of active enzyme and production of a stable enzyme–inhibitor complex (93). This E–I complex can be obtained by alkylation of the histidine, which has not been detected in the β-lactam-derived HLE–inhibitor complex using electrospray ionization mass spectrometry (94).

### Ynenol Lactones

Ynenol lactones that are both substituted α- to the lactone carbonyl and unsubstituted at the acetylene terminus are rapid inhibitors of HLE; they inhibit PPE and trypsin more slowly (95). Substitution at the acetylene terminus of these compounds reduced their ability to inhibit HLE. Ynenol lactones that are α-unsubstituted are alternative substrate inhibitors of HLE. The ynenol lactone 3-benzyl -5(E)-(prop-2-ynylidene)tetrahydro-2-furanone (Fig. 5) inhibited HLE quite potently. Rapid removal of the inhibitor during the course of inhibition produced a mixture of acyl enzyme and irreversibly inactivated enzyme, which partially recovered activity. Irreversibly inactivated enzyme could not be reactivated with hydroxylamine. All these results are consistent with a mechanism involving acylation of Ser-195 by the ynenol lactone, followed by isomerization of the acyl enzyme to give a tethered allenone that is attacked by a nucleophile such as His-57 to form an alkylated enzyme.

### Enol Lactones

Protio and halo enol lactones containing Pro-Val pseudo dipeptides have been tested against HLE and other serine proteases (96). The protio enol lactones are substrates of HLE, while the bromo enol lactone (Fig. 5) is an effective inhibitor of HLE and chymotrypsin. The pseudo dipeptidyl bromo enol lactone is more specific toward HLE than the monosubstituted halo enol lactones. Inactivation of HLE by this bromo enol lactone is partially recoverable upon treatment with the nucleophile hydrazine, which indicates that two species of inactivated enzyme are produced. The more stable species could involve the alkylation of His-57 by the inhibitor moiety in the acyl enzyme, and the less stable, hydrazine-reactivatable species could involve the alkylation of Asp-102 or the hydrolysis of the bromomethyl ketone group in the initially formed acyl enzyme to form a new, more stable acyl enzyme.

### *3,4-Dichloroisocoumarin and 3-Alkoxy-7-Amino-4-Chloroisocoumarins*

3,4-Dichloroisocoumarin (DCI) (Fig. 5) is a general serine protease inhibitor that contains a masked acid chloride group (97). Among various serine poteases, DCI inhibits HLE most effectively, with a $k_{obs}/[I]$ value of 8900 $M^{-1}s^{-1}$. The acyl enzyme derivative has been detected in the DCI-derived PPE–inhibitor complex using electrospray ionization mass spectrometry (49).

7-Amino-4-chloroisocoumarins with a small methoxy or ethoxy group at 3 position (Fig. 5) are potent inhibitors of HLE (71,98). They also inhibit PPE and other chymotrysin-like enzymes more slowly. The 3-alkoxy substituent of the isocoumarins probably interacts with the S1 subsite of the enzyme, since compounds with small alkoxy groups inhibit HLE and PPE most effectively while those with aromatic groups are potent inhibitors of chymotrypsin-like enzymes. Addition of a nucleophile, such as hydroxylamine to HLE inactivated by 3-alkoxy-7-amino-4-chloroisocoumarins, results in a slow and incomplete regain in enzyme activity, which indicates that several inactivated enzyme species are formed during the inactivation reaction. The mechanism of inhibition involves initial formation of an acyl enzyme with unmasking of the 4-aminobenzyl chloride functional group, which can then eliminate chloride to give a quinone imine methide intermediate. This intermediate can react either with an enzyme nucleophile such as His-57 to give an alkylated enzyme or with a solvent molecule to give a new acyl enzyme that can regenerate active enzyme upon deacylation. The crystal structures of three complexes of isocoumarins with PPE have been solved to atomic resolution (99–101). The structural analysis of PPE inhibited by 7-amino-4-chloro-3-methoxyisocoumarin at pH 5 in acetate buffer confirmed the acylation mechanism with the formation of an ester bond between the Ser-195 and the carbonyl group of the inhibitor and an acetate ion from the buffer displacing the chlorine to give a stable acyl enzyme. The resulting structure has the acetoxy group in the S1 pocket (99). In the crystal structure of PPE inhibited by 4-chloro-3-ethoxy-7-guanidinoisocoumarin, the ethoxy group is in the S1 pocket, and the chlorine atom has not been displaced but is near His-57. The 7-guanidino group formed three hydrogen bonds with Thr-41 (100). The structural study of PPE complexed with 7-amino-3-(2-bromoethoxy)-4-chloroisocoumarin provided the first structural evidence for irreversible binding of an isocoumarin inhibitor to PPE through both Ser-195 and His-57 in the active site (101).

## IV. In Vivo Studies and Therapeutic Utility

Pathological similarities between elastase-induced lung damage in experimental animals and human emphysema have been known for quite some time. Polymorphonuclear leukocytes (PMNs) are a major source of elastase during inflammation, and neutrophil elastase is capable of producing emphysematous damage when instilled into the lungs of animals. As a result, neutrophil elastase inhibitors have been evaluated extensively in various emphysema animal models as potential therapeutic agents for treatment of human diseases. The inhibitors include MeO-Suc-Ala-Ala-Pro-Val-$CH_2Cl$, substituted β-lactams (L-659,286, L-648,132, and L-658,758), peptide trifluoromethyl ketones (ICI 200,880, ICI 200,355, and BI-RA-260), peptide boronic acids (MeO-Suc-Ala-Ala-Pro-boro-Val-OH and its pinacol ester), peptide aldehydes (ICI 186,756 and Ro 31-3537), and furoyl saccharin. Several inhibitors including a N-protected peptidyl pentafluoroethyl ketone (MDL 101,146) (32), 3-amino-6-phenylpyridone and 3-amino-pyrimidone trifluoromethyl ketones (33,36), monocyclic β-lactams (e.g., L-680,833) (91), and SR 268321 (63) have shown oral activity.

Emphysema induced in hamsters by intratracheal instillation of PPE or HLE can be ameliorated by intratracheal instillation of MeO-Suc-Ala-Ala-Pro-Val-$CH_2Cl$ (AAPV-CMK) (102,103). One milligram of AAPV-CMK is given to hamsters 1 hour before instillation of 300 or 360 μg of HLE, or 1 or 4 hours after instilling 360 μg of HLE. The animals were studied for 8 weeks after the treatment. The AAPV-CMK given 4 hours after HLE did not ameliorate the emphysema. The AAPV-CMK given 1 hour before HLE ameliorated the emphysema, but not the bronchial secretory cell metaplasia. A molar ratio of instilled AAPV-CMK to HLE of 128 was required for 50% in vivo effectiveness in ameliorating emphysema. Clearance studies indicated that 6.9% of the instilled AAPV-CMK could still be lavaged from the lungs 1 hour after instillation. These bioassays demonstrated the in vivo effectiveness of this inhibitor.

Several cephalosporin inhibitors have been tested in an animal model of acute lung damage (104–106). The acute lung injury was measured as hemorrhage occurring within hours after intratracheal instillation of HLE. Hemorrhage occurred within minutes of elastase instillation, reached maximal values within 1 hour, remained constant for up to 5 hours, and correlated well with the amount of enzyme instilled. Thus, inhibition of hemorrhage is a good measure of the effectiveness of HLE inhibitors given by the intratracheal route. The compounds L-659,286, L-648,132 (Fig. 5), MeO-Suc-Ala-Ala-Pro-Val-$CH_2Cl$, and α1-PI, but not Tos-Lys-$CH_2Cl$, inhibited the hemorrhage caused by HLE. These specific HLE inhibitors have no effect on thermolysin-induced lung hemorrhage. The duration of the activity of these compounds in this model correlated with their persistence in lung lavage fluid as determined by HPLC analysis of the compound recovered by bronchoalveolar lavage. The inhibitors persisted for several hours in bronchoalveolar lavage fluid. The inhibitors L-659,286, MeO-Suc-Ala-Ala-Pro-Val-$CH_2Cl$, and α1-PI also suppressed further development of an ongoing hemorrhage when given 20 minutes after instillation of HLE. The cephalosporins L-659,286 and L-658,758 had $ED_{50}$ of 15 and 5 μg, respectively, for the inhibition of HLE-induced lung hemorrhage.

The ability of two cephalosporins, L-659,286 and L-658,758, to inhibit endogenous elastase, a therapeutic target at sites of inflammation, has also been tested. When elastase is released by exocytosis from stimulated PMNs, its local concentration far exceeded that of α1-PI for a short period of time. Under these transient conditions, some of the released elastase forms complexes with α1-PI, while some of the elastase hydrolyzes protein substrates in plasma, which results in the generation of several specific cleavage products. A highly specific and sensitive radioimmunoassay has been developed for one of these products, the Aα-(1-21) or N-terminal fragment of the Aα-chain of fibrinogen produced by HLE cleavage (107). This assay can be used to measure the activity of elastase when it is released from PMNs. The β-lactam L-658,758 (Fig. 5) inhibits the formation of Aα-(1-21) and α1-PI-PMN elastase complexes in a concentration-dependent manner, with $IC_{50}$ values of 14.5 and 38.3 μM, respectively. These inhibitors also inhibited Aα-(1-21) formation when isolated PMNs were stimulated to degranulate into a matrix of fibrinogen. The efficacy of L-658,758 in inhibiting Aα-(1-21) formation was also demonstrated after in vivo administration to a chimpanzee.

Two trifluoromethyl ketones, ICI 200,880 and ICI 200,355 (Fig. 1), are potent and specific inhibitors of HLE; these two compounds displayed long retention times when administered directly to the lungs of hamster but were rapidly eliminated after intravenous administration (27,108). Pretreatment of hamsters with either inhibitor before intratracheal admininstration of HLE produced a dose- and time-dependent inhibition of enzyme-induced increases in lung weight, total lavageable red cells, and total lavageable white cells. Aerosol administration of ICI 200,880 produced similar results. Subcutaneous administration of either 50 or 100 μmol/kg (twice a day) of ICI 200,880 for 14 or 28 days prevented the time-dependent increase in alveolar diameter produced by a single intratracheal dose of PPE when the inhibitor was initially administered 24 hours after the enzyme. Treatment of hamsters with the same protocol and doses of ICI 200,880 for 8 weeks prevented the destructive lesion induced by a single intratracheal dose of HLE. The trifluoromethyl ketone ICI 200,880 is currently being evaluated in humans.

The trifluoromethyl ketone BI-RA-260 (Fig. 1) has also been tested in hamsters in an elastase-induced pulmonary hemorrhage model (30). Intratracheal administration of this inhibitor, 5 minutes prior to the administration of HLE, effectively inhibited the hemorrhage, with an $ED_{50}$ of 4.8 μg. BI-RA-260 (20 μg) administered 24, 48, and 72 hours before the HLE challenge significantly reduced the hemorrhage. In a 21-day chronic model of emphysema in hamsters, the administration of 200 μg of HLE causes emphysema in the lungs, which can be quantitated histologically utilizing image analysis. The inhibitor BI-RA-260, when administered at 20 μg and 5 minutes prior to the HLE challenge, significantly inhibited pulmonary lesions associated with septal destruction and increased alveolar spaces.

The peptidyl aldehyde ICI 186,756 (Fig. 1) is a competitive and specific inhibitor of HLE, and effectively inhibits the hydrolysis of elastin by HLE (14). Pretreatment of hamsters with this inhibitor before intratracheal admininstration of HLE inhibits enzyme-induced increases in lung weight, total lavageable red cells, and total lavageable white cells measured 24 hours after HLE administration. However, similar lung effects produced by intratracheal admininstration of PPE were not inhibited by ICI 186,756. Treatment of hamsters with 43 μmol/kg (s.q.) of this inhibitor for 14 or 28 days modulated the increases in alveolar diameter produced by both PPE and HLE, respectively. Another peptide aldehyde, Ro 31-3537, has also been studied in a model of emphysema in the hamster induced by multiple sequential intratracheal doses of HLE (109). Concomitant intratracheal administration of 200 μg of inhibitor with the enzyme significantly reduced lung damage, as measured by quasistatic lung compliance and by histological assessment of the emphysema.

The peptidyl boronic acid MeO-Suc-Ala-Ala-Pro-boro-Val-OH is able to prevent emphysema induced by intratracheally administered PPE in hamsters when the inhibitor is given intratracheally or intraperitoneally (110). MeO-Suc-Ala-Ala-Pro-boro-Val-pinacol (Boroval) can diminish the effect of emphysema induced by PPE, and it also provides a degree of protection against PPE-induced increases in lung volume and mean linear intercept when administered intratracheally at 200 mg/kg either 15 minutes before, simultaneously with, or 15 minutes after instilling elastase (111). However, with HLE-induced emphysema in hamsters, pretreatment with as much as a 170-fold molar excess of Boroval, given intratracheally 1 hour before 0.3 mg HLE, did not prevent emphysema (112). Furoyl saccharin has also been shown to protect against the emphysema lesions induced by PPE in rabbits and hamsters (113).

Oral administration of MDL 101,146 (Fig. 3) to hamsters at 10, 25, and 50 mg/kg before an intratracheal instillation of HLE inhibited pulmonary hemorrhage, with an $ED_{50}$ of 15 mg/kg (30). The duration of this compound (50 mg/kg p.o.) for the inhibition of HLE-induced hemorrhage was between 2 and 4 hours. This compound also showed inhibition of HLE-induced hemorrhage by a single bolus i.v. injection or intratracheal administration. Several 3-amino-6-phenylpyridone trifluoromethyl ketones (Fig. 3) have shown oral inhibition toward HLE-induced hemorrhage at 2.5 mg/kg (36). One 3-amino-pyrimidone trifluoromethyl ketone derivative exhibited an oral $ED_{50}$ of 7.5 mg/kg, and had activity for more than 4 hours following oral dosing (33). The oral bioavailability of this pyrimidone derivative is 62–88% in rat, hamster, and dog. The i.v. or p.o. administration of SR 26831 in the rat prevented acute lung injury induced by intratracheal instillation of HLE in a dose-dependent manner (61). One monocyclic β-lactam, L-680,833 (Fig. 3), showed inhibitory activity in stimulated whole blood; it inhibited Aα-(1-21) fibrinopeptide production and HLE-α1-proteinase–inhibitor complex formation, with an $IC_{50}$ of 9 μM (91). The bioavailability of this compound has been shown by the inhibition of tissue damage induced in hamster lungs by intratracheal instillation of HLE and also by the inhibition of elastase activities released from human PMNs after their transfer into the pleural cavity of mice.

## V. Summary

A wide variety of low-molecular-weight synthetic inhibitors, including reversible and irreversible peptide inhibitors, and heterocyclic compounds have been shown to inhibit HLE very potently in vitro. However, to be therapeutically useful for treatment of human diseases, synthetic inhibitors must have a high degree of selectivity, stability, and minimal side reactions or toxic effects. Peptide chloromethyl ketones were the first class of compounds to be tested in animal models of emphysema and found to be effective, but the renal toxicity observed in these experiments prevented the further clinical use of chloromethyl ketones.

Reversible peptide inhibitors are often claimed to have greater therapeutic potential since they are less likely to react with other proteins of nucleophils in vivo. Peptide aldehydes are effective against emphysema in animal models; however, due to their instability in vivo, they are unlikely to be candidates for clinical use. Peptide boronic acids are able to prevent PPE-induced emphysema in hamsters, but further animal studies indicated that these compounds were rapidly cleared in animals and are ineffective against HLE-induced emphysema. Peptide trifluoromethyl ketones such as ICI 200,880 and ICI 200,355 proved to be effective in animal models of emphysema and have long retention times when administered to the lung. They are being evaluated in humans.

Another type of compound that looks quite promising is the mechanism-based inhibitor, including cephalosporins. These β-lactam derivatives inhibit hemorrhage in HLE-induced lung injury and have persisted for several hours in bronchoalveolar lavage fluids. Cephalosporins also inhibit elastase released from stimulated PMNs at sites of inflammation. Furoyl saccharin is effective in two acute animal models of emphysema; however, due to its hydrolytic instability, this compound is not likely to be therapeutically useful. Other potent mechanism-based inhibitors of HLE need to be further evaluated for stability, toxic effects, and in vivo effectiveness before their potential for future clinical use will be known.

Orally active elastase inhibitors, including 3-amino-6-pyridone trifluoromethyl ketones and monocyclic β-lactams, are quite effective in in vivo testing and have long retention times after oral administration. Thus, these peptide trifluoromethyl ketones and β-lactams appear to have the greatest potential for use as therapeutic agents for the treatment of human emphysema. It is clear that the use of synthetic elastase inhibitors in future clinical studies in humans will provide new insights into the role of HLE in various human diseases.

## Abbreviations

Aala, aza-alanine; Abu, aminobutanoic acid; Ac, acetyl; $AdSO_2$, 1-admantane-sulfonyl; Anle, aza-norleucine; Anva, aza-norvaline; APPA, 4-amidinophenyl pyruvic acid; Box, 2-benzoxazole; Boc, *t*-butyloxycarbonyl; CMK, chloromethyl ketone; HLE, human leukocyte elastase; MeO-Suc, methoxysuccinyl; PMN, polymorphonuclear leukocyte; p.o., per oral administration; PPE, porcine pancreatic elastase; s.q., subcutaneous administration; Z, benzyloxycarbonyl.

## References


1. Janoff A. Elastases and emphysema: Current assessment of the protease-antiprotease hypothesis. Am Rev Respir Dis 1985; 132:417–434.
2. Schecter I, Berger A. On the size of the active site in protease. 1. Papain. Biochem Biophys Res Commun 1967; 27:157–162.
3. Bode W, Wei A-Z, Huber R, Meyer E, Travis J, Neumann S. X-ray crystal structure of the complex of human leukocyte elastase (PMN elastase) and the third domain of the turkey ovomucoid inhibitor. EMBO J 1986; 5:2453–2458.
4. Bode W, Meyer E, Powers JC. Human leukocyte and porcine pancreatic elastase: X-ray crystal structures, mechanism, substrate specificity, and mechanism-based inhibitors. Biochemistry 1989; 28:1951–1963.
5. Wei A-Z, Mayr I, Bode W. The refined 2.3 Å crystal structure of human leukocyte elastase in a complex with a valine chloromethyl ketone inhibitor. FEBS Lett 1988; 234:367–373.
6. Navia MA, McKeever BM, Springer JP. Lin T-Y, Williams HR, Fluder EM, Dorn CP, Hoogsteen K. Structure of human neutrophil elastase in complex with a peptide chloromethyl ketone inhibitor at 1.84-Å resolution. Proc Natl Acad Sci USA 1989; 86:7–11.
7. Powers JC, Harper JW. Inhibitors of serine proteinases. In: Barrett AJ, Salvensen G, eds. Proteinase Inhibitors. Amsterdam: Elsevier, 1986:55–152.
8. Powers JC. Synthetic elastase inhibitors: Prospects for use in the treatment of emphysema. Am Rev Respir Dis 1983; 127:S54–S58.
9. Trainer A. Synthetic inhibitors of human neutrophil elastase. Trends Phamacol Sci 1987; 8:303–307.
10. Groutas WC. Inhibitors of leukocyte elastase and leukocyte cathepsin G. Agents for the treatment of emphysema and related ailments. Med Res Rev 1987; 7:227–241.
11. Edwards PD, Berstein PR. Synthetic inhibitors of elastase. Med Res Rev 1994; 14: 127–194.
12. Williams JW, Morrison JF. The kinetics of reversible tight-binding inhibition. Methods Enzymol 1979; 63:437–467.
13. Hassal CH, Johnson WH, Kennedy AJ, Roberts NA. A new class of inhibitors of human leukocyte elastase. FEBS Lett 1985; 183:201–205.
14. Williams JC, Stein RL, Strimpler AM, Reaves B, Krell RD. Biochemical and pharmacological characterization of ICI 186,756, a novel, potent, and selective inhibitor of human neutrophil elastase. Exp Lung Res 1991; 17:25–74.

15. Kettner CA, Shenvi AB. Inhibition of the serine proteases leukocyte elastase, pancreatic elastase, cathepsin G, and chymotrypsin by peptide boronic acids. J Biol Chem 1984; 259:15106–15114.
16. Takahashi LH, Radhakrishnan R, Rosenfield RE, Meyer EF. Crystallographic analysis of the inhibition of porcine pancreatic elastase by a peptidyl boronic acid: structure of a reaction intermediate. Biochemistry 1989; 28:7610–7617.
17. Zhong S, Jordan F, Kettner C, Polgar L. Observation of tightly bound $^{11}B$ nuclear magnetic resonance signals on serine proteases. Direct solution evidence for tetrahedral geometry around the boron in putative transition-state analogues. J Am Chem Soc 1991; 113:9429–9435.
18. Hori H, Yasutake A, Minematsu Y, Powers JC. Inhibition of human leukocyte elastase, porcine pancreatic elastase and cathepsin G by peptide ketones. In: Deber CM, Hruby VJ, Kopple KD, eds. Peptides: Structure and Function. Proceedings of the Ninth American Peptide Symposium. Pierce Chemical, 1985: 819–822.
19. Peet NP, Burkhart JP, Angelastro MR, Giroux EL, Mehdi S, Bey P, Kolb M, Neises B, Schirlin D. Synthesis of peptidyl fluoromethyl ketones and peptidyl α-keto esters as inhibitors of porcine pancreatic elastase, human neutrophil elastase, and rat and human neutrophil cathepsin G. J Med Chem 1990; 33:394–407.
20. Mehdi S, Angelastro MR, Burkhart JP, Koehl JR, Peet NP, Bey P. The inhibition of human neutrophil elastase and cathepsin G by peptidyl 1,2-dicarbonyl derivatives. Biochem Biophys Res Commun 1990; 166:595–600.
21. Walter J, Bode W. The x-ray crystal structure analysis of the refined complex formed by bovine trypsin and *p*-amidinophenyl pyruvate at 1.4 Å resolution. Hoppe-Seyler's Z Physiol Chem 1983; 364:949–959.
22. Edwards PD, Meyer EF, Vijayalakshmi J, Tuthill PA, Andisik DA, Gomes B, Strimpler A. Design, synthesis, and kinetic evaluation of a unique class of elastase inhibitors, and peptidyl α-ketobenxazoles, and the x-ray crystal structure of the covalent complex between porcine pancreatic elastase and Ac-Ala-Pro-Val-2-Benzoxazole. J Am Chem Soc 1992; 114:1854–1863.
23. Stein RL, Strimpler AM, Edwards PD, Lewis JJ, Mauger RC, Schwartz JA, Stein MM, Trainor DA, Wildonger RA, Zottola MA. Mechanism of slow-binding inhibition of human leukocyte elastase by trifluoromethyl ketones. Biochemistry 1987; 26:2682–2689.
24. Dunlap RP, Stone PJ, Abeles RH. Reversible, slow, tight-binding inhibition of human leukocyte elastase. Biochem Biophys Res Commun 1987; 145:509–513.
25. Govardhan CP, Abeles RH. Structure-activity studies of fluoroketone inhibitors of α-lytic protease and human leukocyte elastase. Arch Biochem Biophys 1990; 280: 137–146.
26. Bergeson SH, Edwards PD, Schwartz JA, Shaw A, Stein MM, Trainer DA, Wildoager RA, Wolania DJ. Peptide Derivatives. US patent 4,910,190, 1990.
27. Williams JC, Falcone RC, Knee C, Stein RL, Strimpler AM, Reaves B, Giles RE, Krell RD. Biologic characterization of ICI 200,880 and ICI 200,355, novel inhibitors of human neutrophil elastase. Am Rev Respir Dis 1991; 144:875–883.
28. Liang TC, Abeles RH. Complex of α-chymotrypsin and N-acetyl-L-leucyl-L-phenylalanyl trifluoromethyl ketone: structural studies with NMR spectroscopy. Biochemistry 1987; 26:7603–7608.

29. Takahashi LH, Radhakrishnan R, Rosenfield RE, Meyer EF, Trainor DA. Crystal structure of the covalent complex formed by a peptidyl α,α-difluoro-β-keto amide with porcine pancreatic elastase at 1.78-Å resolution. J Am Chem Soc 1989; 111: 3368–3374.
30. Skiles JW, Fuchs V, Miao C, Soreck R, Grozinger KG, Mauldin SC, Vitous J, Mui PW, Jacober S, Chow G, Matteo M, Skoog M, Weldon SM, Possanza G, Keirns J, Letts G, Rosenthal AS. Inhibition of human leukocyte elastase (HLE) by N-substituted peptidyl trifluoromethyl ketones. J Med Chem 1992; 35:641–662.
31. Skiles JW, Miao C, Sorcek R, Jacober S, Mui PW, Chow G, Weldon SM, Possanza G, Skoog M, Keirns J, Letts G, Rosenthal AS. Inhibition of human leukocyte elastase by N-substituted peptides contining α,α-difluorostatone residues at P1. J Med Chem 1992; 35:4795–4808.
32. Durham SL, Hare CM, Angelastro MR, Burkhart JP, Koehl JR, Marquart AL, Mehdi S, Peet NP, Janusz MJ. Pharmacology of N-[4-(4-morpholinylcarbonyl)benzoyl]-L-valyl-N-[3,3,4,4,4-pentafluoro-1-(1-methylethyl)-2-oxobutyl-L-prolinamide (MDL 101,146): a potent orally active inhibitor of human neutrophil elastase. J Pharm Exp Therap 1994; 270:185–191.
33. Brown FJ, Andisik DW, Bernstein PR, Bryant CB, Ceccarelli C, Damewood JR Jr, Edwards PD, Earley RA, Feeney S, Green RC, Gomes B, Kosmider BJ, Krell RD, Shaw A, Steelman GB, Thomas RM, Vacek EP, Veale CA, Tuthill PA, Warner P, Williams JC, Wolanin DJ, Woolson SA. Design of orally active, non-peptidic inhibitors of human leukocyte elastase. J Med Chem 1994; 37:1259–1261.
34. Warner P, Green RC, Gomes B, Strimpler AM. Non-peptidic inhibitors of human leukocyte elastase. 1. The design and synthesis of pyridone-containing inhibitors. J Med Chem 1994; 37:3090–3099.
35. Damewood JR Jr, Edwards PD, Feeney S, Gomes B, Steelman GB, Tuthill PA, Williams JC, Warner P, Woolson SA, Wolanin DJ, Veale CA. Nonpeptidic inhibitors of human leukocyte elastase. 2. Design, synthesis and in vitro activity of a series of 3-amino-6-arylpyridin-2-one trifluoromethyl ketones. J Med Chem 1994; 37:3303–3312.
36. Bernstein PR, Andisik DW, Bradley PK, Bryant CB, Ceccarelli C, Damewood JR Jr, Earley RA, Edwards PD, Feeney S, Gomes B, Kosmider BJ, Steelman GB, Thomas RM, Vacek EP, Veale CA, Tuthill PA, Williams JC, Wolanin DJ, Woolson SA. Nonpeptidic inhibitors of human leukocyte elastase. 3. Design, synthesis, X-ray crystallographic analysis, and structure-activity relationship for a series of orally active 3-amino-6-phenyl-1-pyridin-2-one trifluoromethyl ketones. J Med Chem 1994; 37:3313–3326.
37. Renaud A, Lestienne P, Hughes DL, Bieth JG, Dimicoli JL. Mapping the S′ subsites of porcine pancreactic and human leukocyte elastases. J Biol Chem 1983; 258:8312–8316.
38. Hughes DL, Sieker LC, Bieth J, Dimicoli JL. Crystallographic study of the binding of a trifluoroacetyl dipeptide anilide inhibitor with elastase. J Mol Biol 1982; 162:645–658.
39. de la Sierra IL, Papamichael E, Sakarellos C, Dimicoli JK, Prangé T. Interaction of the peptide $CF_3$-Leu-Ala-NH-$C_6H_4$-$CF_3$ (TFLA) with porcine pancreatic elastase: X-ray studies at 1.8 Å. J Mol Recog 1990; 3:36–44.

40. Kawabata K, Suzuki M, Sugitani M, Imaki K, Toda S, Miyamoto T. ONO-5046, a novel inhibitor of human neutrophil elastase. Biochem Biophys Res Commun 1991; 177:814–820.
41. Zembower DE, Kam CM, Powers JC, Zalkow LH. Novel anthraquinone inhibitors of human leukocyte elastase and cathepsin G. J Med Chem 1992; 35:1597–1605.
42. Nakao A, Partis RA, Jung GP, Mueller RA. SC-39026, a specific human neutrophil elastase inhibitor. Biochem Biophys Res Commun 1991; 147:666–674.
43. Lentini A, Farchione F, Ternai B, Kreua-Ongarjukool N, Tovivich P. Synthetic inhibitors of human leukocyte elastase. Part 3. Peptides with alkyl groups at N- or C-terminus: Non-toxic competitive inhibitors of human leukocyte elastase. Biol Chem Hoppe-Seyer 1987; 368:369–378.
44. Ashe BM, Zimmerman M. Specific inhibition of human granulocyte elastase by *cis*-unsaturated fatty acids and activation by the corresponding alcohols. Biochem Biophys Res Commun 1977; 75:194–199.
45. Omura S, Nakagawa A, Ohno H. Structure of elasnin, a novel elastase inhibitor. J Am Chem Soc 1979; 101:4386–4388.
46. Cook L, Ternai B. Similar binding sites for unsaturated fatty acids and alkyl 2-pyrone inhibitors of human sputum elastase. Biol Chem Hoppe-Seyler 1988; 369: 627–631.
47. Powers JC, Gupton BF, Harley AD, Nishino N, Whitley RJ. Specificity of porcine pancreatic elastase, human leukocyte elastase and cathepsin G: Inhibition with peptide chloromethyl ketones. Biochim Biophys Acta 1977; 485:156–166.
48. Tsuda Y, Okada Y, Nagamatsu Y, Okamoto U. Synthesis of peptide chloromethyl ketones and examination of their inhibitory effects on human spleen fibrinolytic proteinase (SFP) and human leukocyte elastase (LE). Chem Pharm Bull 1987; 35: 3576–3584.
49. Aplin RT, Robinson CV, Schofield CJ, Westwood NJ. Studies on the inhibition of porcine pancreatic elastase using electrospray mass spectrometry. J Chem Soc Commun 1992; 1650–1652.
50. Oleksyszyn J, Powers JC. Irreversible inhibition of serine proteases by peptide derivatives of (α-aminoalkyl)phosphonate diphenyl esters. Biochemistry 1991; 30: 485–493.
51. Oleksyszyn J, Powers JC. Amino acid and peptide phosphonate derivatives as specific inhibitors of serine peptidases. Methods Enzymol 1994; 244:423–441.
52. Powers JC Boone R, Carroll DL, Gupton F, Kam CM, Nishino N, Sakamoto M, Tuhy PM. Reaction of azapeptides with human leukocyte elastase and porcine pancreatic elastase: New inhibitors and active site titrants. J Biol Chem 1984; 259:4288–4294.
53. Digenis GA, Agha BJ, Tsuji K, Kato M, Shinogi M. Peptidyl carbamates incorporating amino acid isosteres as novel elastase inhibitors. J Med Chem 1986; 29:1468–1476.
54. Kato M, Agha BJ, Abdul-Raheem A, Tsuji K, Banks WR, Digenis GA. Peptidyl carbamates as novel elastase inhibitors: stucture activity relationship studies. J Enzyme Inhib 1993; 7:105–130.
55. Rypacek F, Banks WR, Noskova D, Digenis GA. Synthetic macromolecular inhibitors of human leukocyte elastase. 1. Synthesis of peptidyl carbamates bound to

water-soluable polymers: poly-α,β-[N-(2-hydroxyethyl)-D,L-aspartamide] and poly-α-[$N^5$-(2-hydroxyethyl)-L-glutamine]. J Med Chem 1994; 37:1850–1856.
56. Yoshimura T, Barker LN, Powers JC. Specificity and reactivity of human leukocyte elastase, porcine pancreatic elastase, human granulocyte cathepsin G, and bovine pancreatic chymotrypsin with arylsulfonyl fluorides: Discovery of a new series of potent and specific irreversible elastase inhibitors. J Biol Chem 1982; 257:5077–5084.
57. Groutas WC, Abrams WR, Theodorakis MC, Kasper AM, Rude SA, Badger RC, Ocain TD, Miller KE, Moi MK, Brubaker MJ, Davis KS, Zandler ME. Amino acid derived latent isocyanates: irreversible inactivation of porcine pancreatic elastase and human leukocyte elastase. J Med Chem 1985; 28:204–209.
58. Groutas WC, Brubaker MJ, Zandler ME, Stanga MA, Huang TL, Castrisos JC, Crowley JP. Sulfonate salts of amino acids: novel inhibitors of the serine proteinases. Biochem Biophys Res Commun 1985; 128:90–93.
59. Miyano M, Deason JR, Nakao A, Stealey MA, Villamil CI, Sohn DD, Mueller RA. (Acyloxy)benzophenones and (acyloxy)-4-pyrones. A new class of inhibitors of human neutrophil elastase. J Med Chem 1988; 31:1052–1061.
60. Luisetti M, Piccioni PD, Donnini M, Peona V, Pozzi E, Grassi C. Studies of MR 889, a new synthetic proteinase inhibitor. Biochem Biophys Res Commun 1989; 165: 568–573.
61. Baici A, Pelloso R, Hörler D. The kinetic mechanism of inhibition of human leukocyte elastase by MR889, a new cyclic thiolic compound. Biochem Pharmocol 1990; 39:919–924.
62. Cunningham RT, Mangold SE, Spruce LW, Ying QL, Simon SR, Wieczorek M, Ross S, Cheronis JC, Kirschenheuter GP. Synthesis and evaluation of CE-0266: A new human neutrophil elastase inhibitor. Bioorg Chem 1992; 20:345–355.
63. Herbert HM, Frehel D, Rosso MP, Seban E, Castet C, Pepin O, Maffrand JP, Le Fur G. Biochemical and pharmacological activities of SR 26831, a potent and selective elastase inhibitor. J Pharm Exp Therap 1992; 260:809–816.
64. Neumann U, Gütschow M. N-(Sulfonyloxy)phthalimide and analogues are potent inactivators of serine proteases. J Biol Chem 1994; 269:21561–21567.
65. Groutas WC, Brubaker MJ, Stanga MA, Castrisos JC, Crowley JP, Schatz EJ. Inhibition of human leukocyte elastase by derivatives of N-hydroxysuccinimide: A structure-activity-relationship study. J Med Chem 1989; 32:1607–1611.
66. Groutas WC, Venkataraman R, Brubaker, MJ, Epp JB, Chong LS, Stanga MA, McClenahan JJ, Tagusagawa F. 3-(Alkylthio)-N-hydroxysuccinimide derivatives: potent inhibitors of human leukocyte elastase. Biochim Biophys Acta 1993; 1164: 283–288.
67. Teshima T, Griffin JC, Powers JC. A new class of heterocyclic serine inhibitors: Inhibition of human leukocyte elastase, porcine pancreatic elastase, cathepsin G, and bovine chymotrypsin $A_\alpha$ with substituted benzoxazinones, quinazolines, and anthranilates. J Biol Chem 1982; 257:5085–5091.
68. Stein RL, Strimpler AM, Viscarello BR, Wildoger RA, Mauger RC, Trainor DA. Mechanism for slow-binding inhibitors of human leukocyte elastase by valine-derived benzoxazinones. Biochemistry 1987; 26:4126–4130.

69. Kranze A, Spencer RE, Tam TF, Liak TJ, Copp LJ, Thomas EM, Rafferty SP. Design and synthesis of 4H-3,1-benzoxazin-4-ones as potent alternate substrate inhibitors of human leukocyte elastase. J Med Chem 1990; 33:464–479.
70. Uejima Y, Kokubo M, Oshida J, Kawabata H, Kato Y, Fujii K. 5-Methyl-4H-3,1-benzoxazin-4-one derivatives: Specific inhibitors of human leukocyte elastase. J Pharm Exp Therap 1993; 265:516–523.
71. Harper JW, Powers JC. Reaction of serine proteases with substituted 3-alkoxy-4-chloroisocoumarins and 3-alkoxy-7-amino-4-chloroisocoumarins: New reactive mechanism based inhibitors. Biochemistry 1985; 24:7200–7213.
72. Hemmi K, Harper JW, Powers JC. Inhibition of human leukocyte elastase, cathepsin G, chymotrypsin $A_{\alpha}$, and porcine pancreatic elastase with substituted isobenzofuranones and benzopyrandiones. Biochemistry 1985; 24:1841–1848.
73. Zimmerman M, Morman H, Mulvey D, Jones H, Frankshun R, Ashe BM. Inhibition of elastase and other serine proteases by heterocyclic acylating agents. J Biol Chem 1980; 255:9848–9851.
74. Ashe BM, Clark RL, Jones H, Zimmerman M. Selective inhibiton of human leukocyte elastase and bovine α-chymotrypsin by novel heterocycles. J Biol Chem 1981; 256:11603–11606.
75. Kerneur C, Hornebeck W, Robert L, Moczar E. Inhibition of human leukocyte elastase by fatty acyl-benzisothiasolinone, 1,1-dioxide conjugates (fatty acyl saccharins). Biochem Pharm 1993; 45:1889–1895.
76. Subramanyam C, Bell MR, Carabateas P, Court JJ, Dority JA Jr, Ferguson E, Gordon R, Hlasta DJ, Kumar V, Saindane M. 2,6-Disubstituted aryl carboxylic acids, leaving groups "par excellence" for benzisothiazolone inhibitors of human leukocyte elastase. J Med Chem 1994; 37:2623–2626.
77. Groutas WC, Kuang R, Venkataraman R. Substituted 3-oxo-1,2,5-thiadiazolidine 1,1-dioxides: a new class of potential mechanism-based inhibitors of human leukocyte elastase and cathepsin G. Biochem Biophys Res Comm 1994; 198:341–349.
78. Vilain AC, Okochi V, Vergely I, Reboud-Ravaux M, Mazaleyrat JP, Wakselman M. Acyloxybenzyl halides, inhibitors of elastases. Biochim Biophys Acta 1991; 1076:401–405.
79. Doherty JB, Ashe BM, Argenbright LW, Barker PL, Bonny RJ, Chandler GO, Dahlgren ME, Dorn GP, Finke PE, Firestone RA, Fletcher D, Hagmann WK, Mumford R, O'Grady L, Maycock AL, Pisano JM, Shah SK, Thompson KR, Zimmerman M. Cephalosporin antibiotics can be modified to inhibit human leukocyte elastase. Nature 1986; 322:192–194.
80. Doherty JB, Ashe BM, Barker PL, Blacklock TJ, Butcher JW, Chandler GO, Dahlgren ME, Davies P, Dorn GP, Finke PE, Firestone RA, Fletcher D, Hagmann WK, Halgren T, Knight WB, Mumford R, Maycock AL, Navia MA, O'Grady L, Pisano JM, Shah SK, Thompson KR, Weston H, Zimmerman M. Inhibition of human leukocyte elastase. 1. Inhibition by C-7-substituted cephalosporin *tert*-butyl esters. J Med Chem 1990; 33:2513–2521.
81. Finke PE, Ashe BM, Knight WB, Maycock AL, Navia MA, Shah SK, Thompson KR, Underwood DJ, Weston H, Zimmerman M, Doherty JB. Inhibition of human leukocyte elastase. 2. Inhibition by substituted cephalosporin esters and amides. J Med Chem 1990; 33:2522–2528.

82. Shah SK, Brause KA, Chandler GO, Finke PE, Ashe BM, Weston H, Knight WB, Maycock AL, Doherty JB. Inhibition of human leukocyte elastase. 3. Synthesis and activity of 3′-substituted cephalosporins. J Med Chem 1990; 33:2529–2535.
83. Finke PE, Shah SK, Ashe BM, Ball RG, Blacklock TJ, Bonney RJ, Brause KA, Chandler GO, Cotton MN, Davies P, Dellea PS, Dorn CP Jr, Fletcher DS, O'Grady LA, Hagmann WK, Hand KM, Knight WB, Maycock AL, Mumford RA, Osinga DG, Sohar P, Thompson KR, Weston H, Doherty JB. Inhibition of human leukocyte elastase. 4. Selection of a substituted cephalosporin (L-658,758) as a topical aerosol. J Med Chem 1992; 35:3731–3744.
84. Navia MA, Springer JP, Lin TY, Williams HR, Firestone RA, Pisano JM, Doherty JB, Finke PE, Hoogsteen K. Crystallographic study of a β-lactam inhibitor complex with elastase at 1.84 Å resolution. Nature 1987; 327:79–82.
85. Knight WB, Maycock AL, Green BG, Ashe BM, Gale P, Weston H, Finke PE, Hagmann WK, Shah SK, Doherty JB. Mechanism of inhibition of human leukocyte elastase by two cephalosporin derivatives. Biochemistry 1992; 31:4980–4986.
86. Aplin RT, Robinson CV, Schofield CJ, Westwood NJ. An investigation into the mechanism of elastase inhibition by cephalosporins using electrospray ionization mass spectrometry. Tetrahedron 1993; 47:10903–10912.
87. Alpegiani M, Baici A, Bissolino P, Carminati P, Cassinelli G, Del Nero S, Franceschi G, Orezzi P, Perrone E, Rizzo V, Sacchi N. Synthesis and evaluation of new elastase inhibitors. I. 1,1-Dioxocephem-4-thiolesters. Eur J Med Chem 1992; 27:875–890.
88. Knight WB, Green BG, Chabin RM, Gale P, Maycock AL, Weston H, Kuo DW, Westler WM, Dorn CP, Finke PE, Hagmann WK, Hale JJ, Liesch J, MacCross M, Navia MA, Shah SK, Underwood D, Doherty JB. Specificity, stability, and potency of monocyclic β-lactam inhibitors of human leukocyte elastase. Biochemistry 1992; 31:8160–8170.
89. Shah SK, Dorn CP Jr, Finke PE, Hale JJ, Hagmann WK, Brause KA, Chandler GO, Kissinger AL, Ashe BM, Weston H, Knight WB, Maycock AL, Delles PS, Fletcher DS, Hand KM, Mumford RA, Underwood D, Doherty JB. Orally active β-lactam inhibitors of human leukocyte elastase-1: Activity of 3,3-diethyl-2-azetidinones. J Med Chem 1992, 35:3745–3754.
90. Hagmann WK, Kissinger AL, Shah SK, Finke PE, Dorn CP Jr, Brause KA, Ashe BM, Weston H, Maycock AL, Knight WB, Dellea PS, Fletcher DS, Hand KM, Osinga D, Davies P, Doherty JB. Orally active β-lactam inhibitors of human leukocyte elastase-2: Effect of C-4 substitution. J Med Chem 1993; 36:771–777.
91. Doherty JB, Shah SK, Finke PE, Dorn CP Jr, Hagmann WK, Hale JJ, Kissinger AL, Thompson KR, Brause KA, Chandler GO, Knight WB, Maycock AL, Ashe BM, Weston H, Gale P, Mumford RA, Andersen OF, Williams HR, Nolan TE, Frankenfield DL, Underwood D, Vyas KP, Kari PH, Dahlgren ME, Mao J, Fletcher DS, Dellea PS, Hand KM, Osinga D, Peterson LB, Williams DT, Metzger JM, Bonney RJ, Humes JL, Pacholok SP, Hanlon WA, Opas E, Stolk J, Davies P. Chemical, biochemical, pharmacokinetic, and biological properties of L-680,833: A potent, orally active monocyclic β-lactam inhibitor of human polymorphonuclear leukocyte elastase. Proc Natl Acad Sci USA 1993; 90:8727–8731.
92. Wakselman M, Joyeau R, Kobaiter R, Boggetto N, Vergely I, Maillard J, Okochi V,

Montagne JJ, Reboud-Ravaux M. Functionalized N-aryl azetidinones as novel mechanism-based inhibitors of neutrophil elastase. FEBS Lett 1991; 282:377–381.
93. Chabin R, Green BG, Gale P, Maycock AL, Weston H, Dorn CP, Finke PE, Hagmann WK, Hale JJ, MacCross M, Shah SK, Underwood D, Doherty JB, Knight WB. Mechanism of inhibition of human leukocyte elastase by monocyclic β-lactams. Biochemistry 1993; 32:8970–8980.
94. Knight WB, Swiderek KM, Sakuma T, Calaycay J, Shively JE, Lee TD, Covey TR, Shushan B, Green BG, Chabin R, Shah S, Mumford R, Dickinson TA, Griffin PR. Electrospray ionization mass spectrometry as a mechanistic tool: mass of human leukocyte elastase and a β-lactam-derived E-I complex. Biochemistry 1993; 32: 2031–2035.
95. Copp LJ, Krantz A, Spencer RW. Kinetics and mechanism of human leukocyte elastase inactivation by ynenol lactones. Biochemistry 1987; 26:169–178.
96. Reed PE, Katzenellenbogen JA. Proline-valine pseudo peptide enol lactones: Effective and selective inhibitors of chymotrypsin and human leukocyte elastase. J Biol Chem 1991; 266:13–21.
97. Harper JW, Hemmi K, Powers JC. Reaction of serine proteases with substituted isocoumarins: discovery of 3,4-dichloroisocoumarin, a new general mechanism based serine protease inhibitor. Biochemistry 1985; 24:1831–1841.
98. Powers JC, Kam CM. Isocoumarin inhibitors of serine peptidases. Methods Enzymol 1994; 244:442–457.
99. Meyer EF, Presta LG, Radhakrishnan R. Stereospecific reaction of 3-methoxy-4-chloro-7-aminoisocoumarin with crystalline porcine pancreatic elastase. J Am Chem Soc 1985; 107:4091–4093.
100. Powers JC, Oleksyszyn J, Narasimhan SL, Kam CM, Radhakrishnan R, Meyer EF. Reaction of porcine pancreatic elastase with 7-substituted-3-alkoxy-4-chloroisocoumarins: design of potent inhibitors using the crystal structure of the complex formed with 4-chloro-3-ethoxy-7-guanidinoisocoumarin. Biochemistry 1990; 29: 3108–3118.
101. Vijayalakshmi J, Meyer EF, Kam CM, Powers JC. Structural study of porcine pancreatic elastase complexed with 7-amino-3-(2-bromoethoxy)-4-chloroisocoumarin as nonreactivatable doubly covalent enzyme-inhibitor complex. Biochemistry 1991; 30:2175–2183.
102. Stone PJ, Lucey EC, Calore JD, Snider GL, Franzblau C, Costillo MJ, Powers JC. The moderation of elastase-induced emphysema in the hamster by intratracheal pretreatment or post-treatment with succinyl-alanyl-prolyl-valine-chloromethyl ketone. Am Rev Respir Dis 1981; 124:56–59.
103. Lucey EC, Stone PJ, Powers JC, Snider GL. Amelioration of human leukocyte elastase-induced emphysema in hamster by pretreatment with oligopeptide chloromethyl ketone. Eur Respir J 1989; 2:421–427.
104. Bonny RJ, Ashe B, Maycock A, Dellea P, Hand K, Osinga D, Fletcher D, Mumford R, Davies P, Frankenfield D, Nolan T, Schaeffer L, Hagmann W, Finke P, Shah S, Dorn C, Doherty J. Pharmacological profile of the substituted beta-lactam L-659,286: a member of a new class of human PMN elastase inhibitors. J Cell Biochem 1989; 39:47–53.

105. Fletcher DS, Osinga DG, Hand KM, Dellea PS, Ashe BM, Mumford RA, Davies P, Hagmann W, Finke PE, Doherty JB, Bonny RJ. A comparison of α1-proteinase inhibitor methoxysuccinyl-Ala-Ala-Pro-Val-chloromethylketone and specific β-lactam inhibitors in an acute model of human polymorphonuclear leukocyte elastase-induced lung hemorrhage in the hamster. Am Rev Respir Dis 1990; 141: 672–677.
106. Davies P, Ashe BM, Bonny RJ, Dorn C, Finke P, Fletcher D, Hanlon WA, Humes JL, Maycock A, Mumford R, Navia MA, Opas EE, Pacholok S, Shah S, Zimmerman M, Doherty JB. The discovery and biologic properties of cephalosporin-based inhibitors of PMN elastase. Ann NY Acad Sci 1991; 624:219–229.
107. Mumford RA, Williams H, Mao J, Dahlgren ME, Frankenfield D, Nolan T, Schaffer L, Doherty JB, Fletcher D, Hand K, Bonny R, Humes JL, Pacholok S, Hanlon W, Davies P. Direct assay of Aα(1-21), a PMN elastase-specific cleavage product of fibrinogen, in the chimpanzee. Ann NY Acad Sci 1991; 624:167–178.
108. Williams JC, Stein RL, Giles RE, Krell RD. Biochemistry and pharmacology of ICI200,880, a synthetic peptide inhibitor of human neutrophil elastase. Ann NY Acad Sci 1991; 624:230–243.
109. Kennedy AJ, Cline A, Ney UM, Johnson WH, Roberts NA. The effect of a peptide aldehyde reversible inhibitor of elastase on a human leukocyte elastase-induced model of emphysema in the hamster. Eur J Respir Dis 1987; 71:472–478.
110. Soskel NT, Watanabe S, Hardie R, Shenvi AB, Punt JA, Kettner C. A new peptide boronic acid inhibitor of elastase-induced lung injury in hamsters. Am Rev Respir Dis 1986; 133:639–642.
111. Soskel NT, Watanabe S, Hardie R, Shenvi AB, Punt JA, Kettner C. Effects of dosage and timing of administration of a peptide boronic acid inhibitor on lung mechanics and morphometrics in elastase-induced emphysema in hamsters. Am Rev Respir Dis 1986; 133:635–638.
112. Stone PJ, Lucey EC, Snider GL. Induction and exacerbation of emphysema in hamsters with human neutrophil elastase inactivated reversibly by a peptide boronic acid. Am Rev Respir Dis 1990; 141:47–52.
113. Lungarella G, Gardie C, Fonzi L, Comparini L, Share NN, Zimmerman M, Martorana PA. Effect of novel synthetic protease inhibitor furoyl saccharin on elastase-induced emphysema in rabbits and hamsters. Exp Lung Res 1986; 11:35–47.

# 24

## α1AT Deficiency and Liver Transplantation

**DAVID H. VAN THIEL**

Baptist Medical Center of Oklahoma
Oklahoma City, Oklahoma

**THOMAS E. STARZL**

University of Pittsburgh Medical Center
Pittsburgh, Pennsylvania

### I. Introduction

Alpha 1–antitrypsin ($\alpha_1$AT) is a 52 kDa alpha 1–glycoprotein that is produced by hepatocytes and secreted into the blood, where it acts as a circulating serine protease inhibitor (1–4). It is a prototypical "suicide" protease inhibitor that combines with its complementary serine protease—be it polymorphonuclear leukocyte serine protease or pancreatic elastase—resulting in its own elimination from the plasma.

α1AT deficiency is a heritable autosomal recessive metabolic disease that results in the synthesis and secretion of a defective alpha 1–glycoprotein without enzymatic activity Z form that occurs as a consequence of a single amino acid substitution (Gly 342 to Lys 342) (1). It occurs as a result of a single nucleotide substitution in the DNA encoding for the normal M form of the serine protease inhibitor α1AT.

As noted in earlier chapters, many different alleles for the $\alpha_1$AT gene exist. The frequency of various $\alpha_1$AT protease inhibitor (PI) phenotypes in almost a thousand whites in Minnesota is shown in Table 1. The most common phenotype is M1, having a frequency of 0.724 (1). The mutant phenotype responsible for $\alpha_1$AT deficiency, PiZ, has an estimated frequency of 0.014 (1–5). Thus, the

**Table 1** Distribution of PI Phenotypes and Allele Frequencies in Whites Living in Minnesota

| Phenotypes | No. observed | Allele frequencies |
|---|---|---|
| M1 | 478 | PI*M1 = 0.724 |
| M1M2 | 177 | PI*M2 = 0.137 |
| M1M3 | 121 | PI*M3 = 0.095 |
| M1S | 28 | PI*S = 0.023 |
| M1Z | 18 | PI*Z = 0.014 |
| M1F | 4 | PI*F = 0.003 |
| M1I | 5 | PI*I = 0.003 |
| M1P | 2 | PI*P = *0.001* |
| M2 | 19 | Total = 1.000 |
| M2M3 | 24 | |
| M2S | 4 | |
| M2Z | 4 | |
| M3 | 9 | |
| M3Z | 3 | |
| M3S | 5 | |
| S | 2 | |
| SF | 1 | |
| | Total = 904 | |

frequency of homozygous $\alpha_1$AT PiZZ individuals can be calculated to be about 1/5000 individuals. The normal range for $\alpha_1$AT levels in serum is 0.85 to 2.13 mg/ml. Individuals who are PiZZ have very low, but not zero, levels of the protein in their serum, with levels typically being below 0.3 mg/ml.

Individuals who are heterozygotes for the Z allele have reduced levels that range from levels half of those of the lower limit of normal to nearly normal levels (Fig. 1) (1,6–16). In contrast, heterozygotes with alleles other than Z often have increased levels of $\alpha_1$AT in their serum, as shown in Figure 1 (6–16).

## II. $\alpha$1AT Deficiency and Liver Disease

Individuals with $\alpha_1$AT deficiency are uniquely susceptible to the development of two disease processes (1–3): panacinar early-onset emphysema and hepatocellular liver disease that presents as either neonatal hepatitis (17–23) in infants or severe protein synthetic liver failure in adults (24–37). The latter presumably occurs as a result of an intrahepatic accumulation of abnormal $\alpha_1$AT protein within hepatocytes (38,39).

In a review of the cause of death of adults with $\alpha_1$AT, 69% were reported to

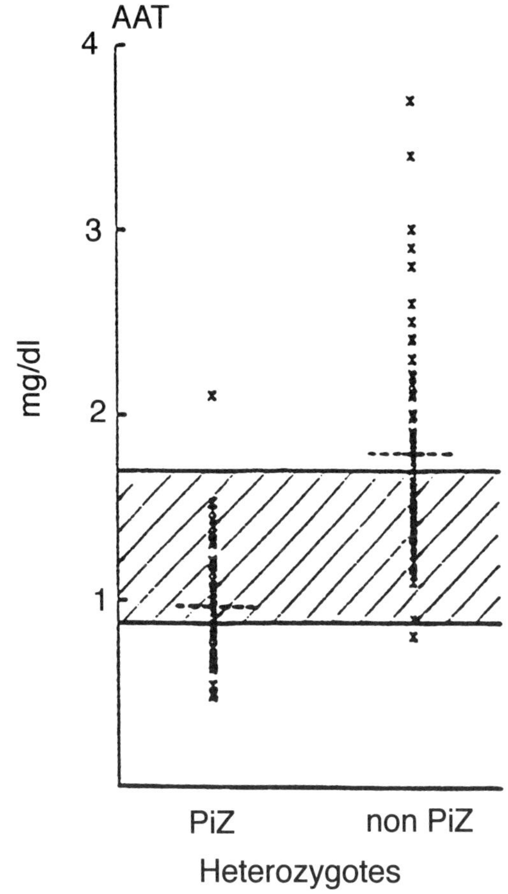


**Figure 1** Serum α1AT levels in heterozygotes with and without a Z allele.

have died as a direct result of either respiratory failure associated with emphysema or a complication of their pulmonary disease (25). A much smaller fraction, 13%, died as result of either hepatic failure or bleeding esophageal varices (Fig. 2) (27,29–32,34,35). As impressive as these figures are, they underestimate the problem of liver disease as a cause of death in individuals with $\alpha_1$AT deficiency, as the study from which these data were obtained examined the case of death of only adults with PiZZ $\alpha_1$AT deficiency and, as a result, failed to include deaths as a result of $\alpha_1$AT deficiency occurring in children (17–23). In the latter cases, essentially all the deaths are a result of liver disease or one of its complications, such as portal hypertension. In our own experience, the number of cases with

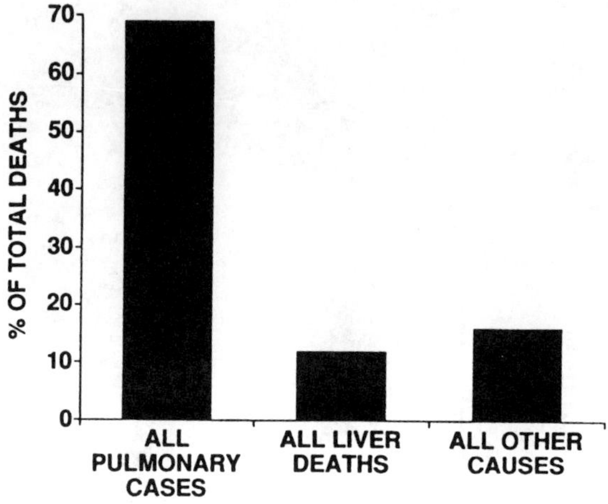


**Figure 2** Cause of death in adults with α1AT deficiency.

$\alpha_1$AT liver disease presenting for liver transplantation in infants or children exceeds the number of cases of adults who present with liver disease due to $\alpha_1$AT deficiency. If the deaths that occur in both children and adults with $\alpha_1$AT deficiency were determined, it would appear that liver disease accounts for 59% of the total deaths whereas pulmonary disease accounts for 23%. Even these figures underestimate the role of $\alpha_1$AT as a cause of lethal liver disease because an increased prevalence of "cryptogenic" cirrhosis associated with $\alpha_1$AT heterozygotes for the PiZ allele (particularly MZ) has been reported and the deaths of these individuals would not be included in these totals (7–15,40–42).

Neonatal hepatitis is a common clinical presentation of individuals with $\alpha_1$AT deficiency during infancy (17–23,37). Almost 30% of infants with neonatal hepatitis ultimately can be shown to be homozygous for the Z allele. Nearly 6% of the cases of neonatal hepatitis will be heterozygotes (MZ) for the Z allele. Thus, the prevalence of neonatal hepatitis in $\alpha_1$AT Z heterozygotes is twice that seen in individuals who have a "normal" MM phenotype. As noted above, adults with cryptogenic cirrhosis have a statistically increased incidence of heterozygosity for the Z allele ($p < 0.001$), which is almost ten-fold greater than the rate of cryptogenic cirrhosis in large, clinical liver-disease populations (Fig. 3) (7–16,40–42). Interestingly, the rates of autoimmune, viral, and alcoholic liver disease in $\alpha_1$AT heterozygotes for the Z allele appear to be reduced by about 50%. Only the reduction in the prevalence of alcoholic liver disease, however, achieved a level of statistical significance ($p < 0.01$).

More recently, the relationship between $\alpha_1$AT deficiency and liver disease has been shown to be more complex than simply a deficiency of a normal

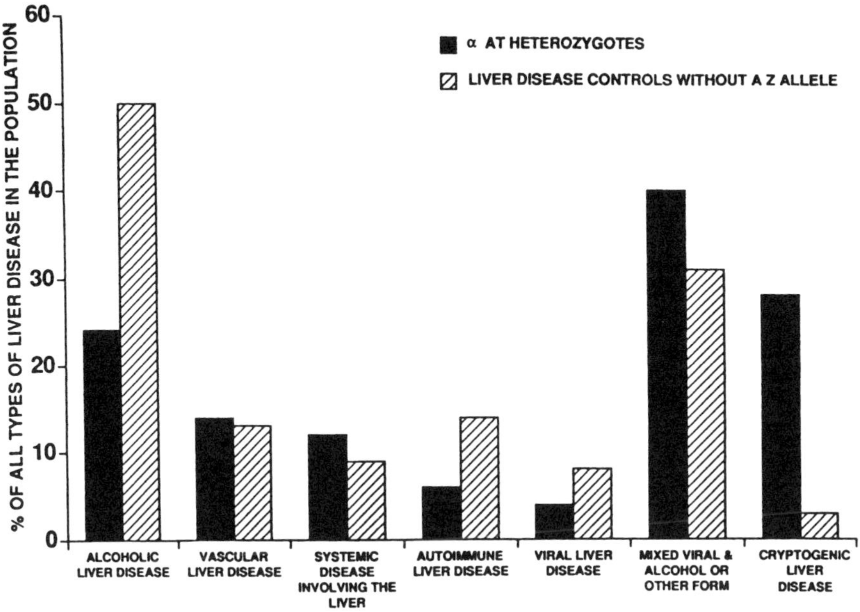


**Figure 3** Frequency of Z allele in patients with cryptogenic cirrhosis seen as adults.

circulating secretory serine protease; it may also involve immunological or at least genetic factors, as the rate of $\alpha_1$AT deficiency with liver disease is almost threefold higher ($\chi^2 = 7.124$; $p < 0.01$) in individuals who are HLA Dr3–positive (43,44). In contrast, HLA Dr4 appears to be protective, with a halving of the rate of liver disease in individuals who are homozygous for the Z allele ($\chi^2 = 4.010$; $p < 0.05$). The observation that HLA Dr3 occurs at an increased frequency in patients with $\alpha_1$AT deficiency and liver disease, however, could not be confirmed in our own series of orthotopic liver-transplant (OLTx) patients (45). Nonetheless, RFIP studies have noted that the association with HLA Dr3 and $\alpha_1$AT-deficiency liver disease is associated with the Dw24 and Dw25 subtypes (both $p < 0.05$) and that both Dr3 Dw24 and Dr3 Dw25 occur two and four times more frequently in individuals with $\alpha_1$AT deficiency and liver disease than in controls (42,43).

The role of other genetic or environmental factors in the pathogenesis of the liver disease associated with $\alpha_1$AT deficiency and the Z allele is either less clear or totally unknown (46). It should be noted, however, that a role for environmental factors may exist, as is the situation with smoking and the association of $\alpha_1$AT deficiency and panacinar emphysema (1,2,24,46,47). Individuals who smoke and are homozygous for the Z allele develop clinically evident emphysema a full decade or more earlier than do homozygotes who do not smoke (1–3).

The clinical presentation of children with $\alpha_1$AT deficiency is rather consistent, with greater than 75% presenting with neonatal hepatitis (jaundice) and smaller numbers presenting with either asymptomatic hepatosplenomegaly or hematemesis (Fig. 4) (17–23). In the vast majority of cases with neonatal hepatitis, the jaundice resolves within 8 months. A minority (<20%) die in the first year of life, usually in the seventh or eighth month of life. Most, however, do not die but live to develop liver disease that requires transplantation as either an older child or an adult. Table 2 shows the differential diagnosis of $\alpha_1$AT disease in children segmented into those who present initially with evidence for liver disease as infants (<1 year of age) and those who are more than 1 year old at the time of initial presentation. In most cases, after the initial period of neonatal hepatitis characterized by cholestasis, the disease progresses as does any other hepatocellular disease, with the development of portal hypertension and protein synthetic defects that characterize the disease process. Six clinical findings are used to identify children with $\alpha_1$AT deficiency who have a poor prognosis: the presence of hepatomegaly, a palpably hard liver, failure to thrive, clubbing of fingers, and two or more overt signs of portal hypertension (ascites and varices). Typically, the disease in children follows a characteristic histopathological progression from

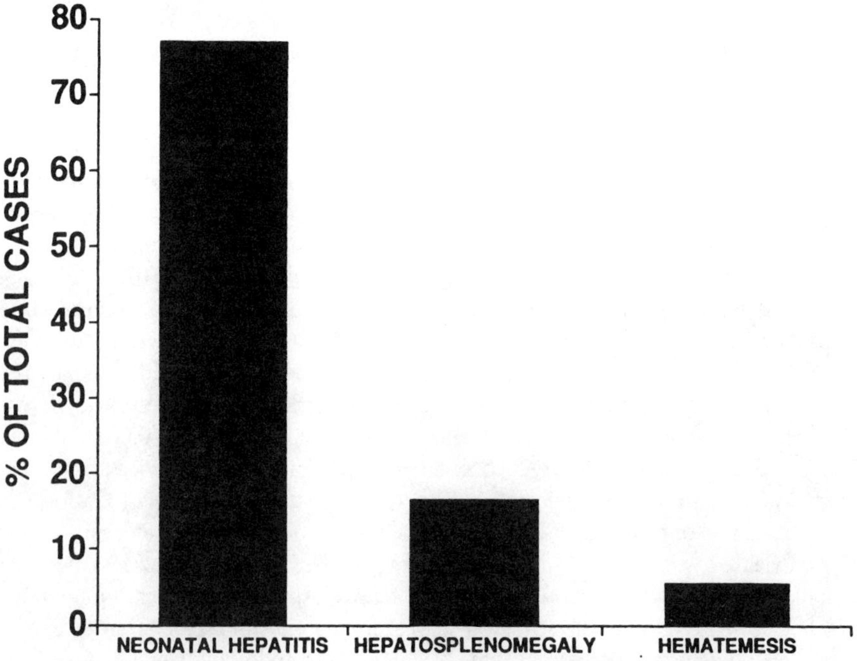


**Figure 4** Frequency of various types of clincal presentations of children with $\alpha$1AT deficiency.

**Table 2** Differential Diagnosis of α1AT-Deficiency Liver Disease

| Neonates to 1 year | >1 year |
|---|---|
| Neonatal hepatitis | Cystic fibrosis |
| TORCH[a] | Autoimmune chronic active hepatitis |
| Blood-group incompatibility | Wilson's disease |
| Cystic fibrosis | Microcytic liver disease |
| Galactosemia | Congenital hepatic fibrosis |
| Tyrosinemia | Chronic viral hepatitis |

[a]TORCH = toxoplasmosis, rubella, cytomegalovirus hepatitis.

the newborn period through 2 years of age, when cirrhosis is usually present (Table 3). Signs and symptoms of portal hypertension typically occur after age 2 and lead to a need for transplantation or to death by age 8 ± 0.3 years (range 8 months to 13 years) (Fig. 4).

The situation is quite similar in adults, with most cases either giving a history of neonatal jaundice or silently developing cirrhosis that presents clinically when a complication of the cirrhosis becomes evident, typically, a problem related to portal hypertension such as ascites, variceal bleeding, or hepatic encephalopathy (24–37).

## III. Liver Transplantation

Table 4 shows the frequency of the dominant clinical features of patients with $\alpha_1$AT deficiency at a time point immediately prior to OLTx. Table 5 shows the age distribution of cases with $\alpha_1$AT deficiency who have received a liver transplant in Pittsburgh. Table 6 shows the percentage of the total cases on an annual basis who were transplanted in Pittsburgh for $\alpha_1$AT deficiency. As is evident from Table 5, two peaks in age at time of OLTx occur: the first at ages 2–11 years and the second between 18 and 59 years. Table 6 shows that the fraction of total transplant cases

**Table 3** Hepatic Histology in Children with α1AT Deficiency Liver Disease: Effect of Age

| | |
|---|---|
| Giant cell hepatitis | 3 months or less |
| Hepatitis | 3 months to 3 years |
| Portal fibrosis | 4 months to 18 years |
| Cirrhosis | 6 months to 18 months |

**Table 4** Dominant Clinical Features in Patients with $\alpha 1$AT Deficiency Immediately Before Liver Transplantation

| Clinical features | % |
|---|---|
| Ascites | 80 |
| Variceal hemorrhage | 59 |
| Jaundice | 38 |
| Encephalopathy | 10 |

with $\alpha_1$AT deficiency has remained rather stable through the years, ranging from 4 to 9%, with minor variations above this figure.

The rate of graft and patient survival following liver transplantation for all cases with $\alpha_1$AT deficiency is 68% and 76%, respectively, through 5 years (Figure 5A). The rate of graft and patient survival for children and adults with $\alpha_1$AT deficiency through 5 years is shown in Figure 5B. Little difference in graft survival is evident, but patient survival through 5 years is clearly better for children (81%) than it is for adults (71%). The vast majority of cases (81.3%) require only one graft; 13.5% require a second graft and 5.2% require a third graft.

As for the technical details of the transplant operation, because most cases with $\alpha_1$AT deficiency are neither very young (<1 year of age) nor very old (>65 years of age), little or no surgical difficulty is experienced as a result of the required vascular of biliary-tract reconstructions. The major problem during the operative procedure is a result of the portal hypertension and coagulopathy that characterize the disease. In adults, this problem is resolved in large measure as a result of the use of the portal systemic bypass developed by Denmark et al. (49) and used initially by Shaw et al. (50). In children, the bypass is frequently not used

**Table 5** Age Distribution of $\alpha 1$AT-Deficient Patients at Time of Liver Transplantation

| | *n* | % |
|---|---|---|
| Infant (under 2 years) | 5 | 5.2 |
| Child (2–11) | 40 | 41.7 |
| Adolescent (12–17) | 4 | 4.2 |
| Adult (18–59) | 39 | 40.6 |
| Senior (over 60) | 8 | 8.3 |

**Table 6** Number of Cases Transplanted for $\alpha$1AT Deficiency and the Years in Which the Transplant Procedure was Performed

| | *n* | % |
|---|---|---|
| 1981 | 6 | 6.3 |
| 1982 | 4 | 4.2 |
| 1983 | 7 | 7.3 |
| 1984 | 9 | 9.4 |
| 1985 | 9 | 9.4 |
| 1986 | 15 | 15.6 |
| 1987 | 8 | 8.3 |
| 1988 | 12 | 12.5 |
| 1989 | 8 | 8.3 |
| 1990 | 13 | 13.5 |
| 1991 | 5 | 5.2 |
| Total | 96 | 100.0% |

and bleeding can at times be a difficult management problem during the initial parts of the transplant operation.

Following transplantation, the $\alpha_1$AT phenotype of the serine protease present in blood becomes that of the organ donor and the serum level returns to the normal range (51–53). As a result, not only is liver function returned to normal with OLTx but also the hepatic disease is cured (51–53). Moreover, because of the normal serum levels, most likely either the pulmonary disease is stabilized or its rate of progression is markedly slowed. This does not occur with portal caval shunting, the only other surgical procedure shown to have benefit in children with this disease (54,55). A major question that remains to be resolved is whether the act of liver replacement also cures or at least halts the progression of the pulmonary disease that occurs as a consequence of $\alpha_1$AT deficiency. Studies to examine the serine antiprotease activity, $\alpha_1$AT levels, and phenotype in alveolar lavage specimens in long-term survivors of OLTx for $\alpha_1$AT deficiency are currently in progress in Pittsburgh. Similarly, studies characterizing the presence or absence—and, if present, the severity—of the pulmonary disease in liver recipients following successful OLTx for $\alpha_1$AT are currently in progress.

With the recent demonstration that donor lymphodendritic cell seeding from liver allografts occurs following successful OLTx (56,57), it has become understandable why liver allograft recipients transplanted for metabolic diseases (both

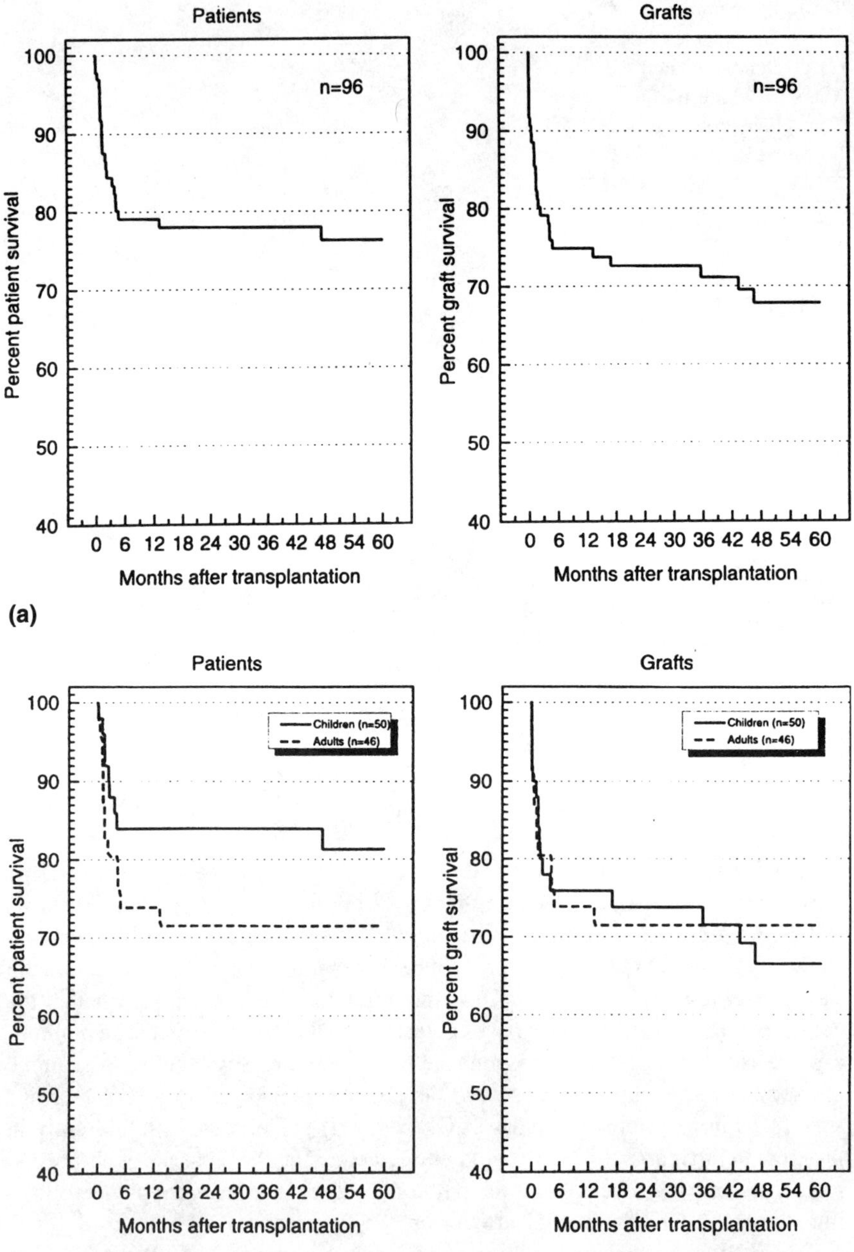


(b)

**Figure 5** Graft and patient survival of (a) all individuals transplanted for α1AT deficiency at the University of Pittsburgh and (b) for the same cases divided into children and adults.

hepatically based and nonhepatically based) such as type 4 glycogen storage disease (57), type II hyperlipoproteinemia (58), Wilson's disease (59), Wolman's disease (60), Nieman-Pick disease (61), Gaucher's disease (unpublished observations), and seablue histiocyte syndrome (unpublished observations) have experienced benefits well beyond what was anticipated from liver transplantation. Because the lungs are natural repositories of dendritic cells, it is to be expected that donor-specific α1AT-positive dendritic cells would be found in the bronchi and alveolar walls of liver allograft recipients who were α1AT-deficient prior to OLTx. The presence of these cells locally in the lungs following OLTx as well as the fact that normal levels of $\alpha_1$AT are achieved in the serum of patients transplanted for $\alpha_1$AT deficiency would be expected to either slow or, more likely, halt the progression of any $\alpha_1$AT deficiency-dependent pulmonary disease following successful OLTx.

## IV. Conclusion

Based on these recent observations (56,57), the role that whole-organ transplantation plays in the management of metabolic disease in general may need to be reevaluated. It may well be that all such procedures, regardless of the organ being transplanted, result in a gain of metabolic function determined by the content of lymphodendritic cells that migrate from the donor organ throughout the body of the recipient (56,57). The concept that a kidney, spleen, liver, or other organ could bring a systemic supply of a missing lyzozomal enzyme has been suggested before (62–64) but was abandoned because of the lack of a rationale and the inability to demonstrate benefit.

Even if the abnormality of $\alpha_1$AT deficiency in the lungs were not cured as a result of liver transplantation, patient survival and quality of life would be greatly enhanced. It appears more likely, however, that because the level of $\alpha_1$AT is either normal or greatly enhanced as a result of OLTx, the lung disease is likely to be stabilized or at least its rate of progression markedly reduced following successful OLTx. One might anticipate further that, since the liver disease is cured, the risk for the development of a hepatocellular carcinoma would decline dramatically (8,65–71). Because individuals with $\alpha_1$AT deficiency are not at increased risk for a biliary cancer prior to liver transplantation, following transplantation the risk for this condition should not be altered (28).

## References

1. Perlmutter DH. The cellular basis for liver injury in $\alpha_1$-antitrypsin deficiency. Hepatology 1991; 13:172–185.
2. Banda MJ, Rice AG, Griffin GL, Senior RM. The inhibitory complex of human

$\alpha_1$-proteinase inhibitor and human leukocyte elastase is a neutrophil chemoattractant. J Exp Med 1988; 167:1608–1615.
3. Janoff A. Elastases and emphysema: Current assessment of the protease-antiprotease hypothesis. Am Rev Respir Dis 1985; 132:417–433.
4. Banda MJ, Rice AG, Griffin GL, Senior RM. The inhibitory complex of human $\alpha_1$-proteinase inhibitor and human leukocyte elastase is a neutrophil chemoattractant. J Exp Med 1988; 167:1608–1615.
5. Cook PJL. The genetics of $\alpha_1$-antitrypsin: A family study in England and Scotland. Ann Hum Genet Lond 1975; 38:275–287.
6. Hodges JR, Millward-Sadler GH, Barbatis C, Wright R. Heterozygous MZ alpha$_1$-antitrypsin deficiency in adults with chronic active hepatitis and cryptogenic cirrhosis. N Engl J Med 1981; 304:557–560.
7. Eriksson S, Moestrup T, Hägerstrand I. Liver, lung and malignant disease in heterozygous (Pi MZ) $\alpha_1$-antitrypsin deficiency. Acta Med Scand 1975; 198:243–247.
8. Lieberman J, Silton RM, Agliozzo CM, McMahon J. Hepatocellular carcinoma and intermediate $\alpha_1$-antitrypsin deficiency (MZ phenotype). Am J Clin Pathol 1975; 64: 304–310.
9. Sparos L, Tountas Y, Chapuis-Cellier C, Theodoropoulos G, Trichopoulos D. Alpha$_1$-antitrypsin levels and pheotypes and hepatitis B serology in liver cancer. Br J Cancer 1984; 49:567–570.
10. Eriksson S, Lindmark B, Olsson S. Lack of association between hemochromatosis and $\alpha_1$-antitrypsin deficiency. Acta Med Scand 1986; 219:291–294.
11. Eriksson S, Carlson J, Velez R. Risk of cirrhosis and primary liver cancer in alpha$_1$-antitrypsin deficiency. N Engl J Med 1986; 314:736–739.
12. Fargion S, Klasen EC, Lalatta F, Sangalli G, Tommasini M, Fiorelli G. $\alpha_1$-antitrypsin in patients with hepatocellular carcinoma and chronic active hepatitis. Clin Genet 1981; 19:134–139.
13. Crowley JJ, Sharp HL, Freier E, Ishak KG, Schow P. Fatal liver dissease associated with $\alpha_1$-antitrypsin deficiency PiM$_1$/PiM$_{duarte}$. Gastroenterology 1987; 93:242–244.
14. Kueppers F, Dickson ER, Summerskill WH. Alpha$_1$-antitrypsin phenotypes in chronic active liver disease and primary biliary cirrhosis. Mayo Clin Proc 1976; 51:286–288.
15. Vecchio FM, Fabiano A, Orsini G, Ragusa D, Massi G. Alpha-1-antitrypsin MZ phenotype and cryptogenic chronic liver disease in adults. Digestion 1983; 27: 100–104.
16. Sharp HL, Bridges RA, Krivit W, Freier EF. Cirrhosis associated with alpha-1-antitrypsin deficiency: A previously unrecognized inherited disorder. J Lab Clin Med 1969; 6:934–939.
17. Sveger T. Liver disease in alpha$_1$-antitrypsin deficiency detected by screening of 200,000 infants. N Engl J Med 1976; 294:1316–1321.
18. Moroz SP, Cutz E, Cox DW, Sass-Kortsak A. Liver disease associated with alpha$_1$-antitrypsin deficiency in childhood. J Pediatr 1976; 88:19–25.
19. Sveger T. The natural history of liver disease in $\alpha_1$- antitrypsin deficient children. Acta Pediatr Scand 1988; 77:847–851.
20. Psacharopoulos HT, Mowat AP, Cook PJL, Carlile PA, Portmann B, Rodeck CH. Outcome of liver disease associated with $\alpha_1$ antitrypsin deficiency (PiZ). Arch Dis Childhood 1983; 58:882–887.

21. Ghishan FK, Greene HL. Liver disease in children with PiZZ $\alpha_1$-antitrypsin deficiency. Hepatology 1988; 8:307–310.
22. Alper CA, Johnson AM. Alpha$_1$-antitrypsin deficiency and disease. Pediatrics 1970; 46:837–840.
23. Cottrall K, Cook PJL, Mowat AP. Neonatal hepatitis syndrome and alpha-1-antitrypsin deficiency: An epidemiological study in south-east England. Postgrad Med J 1974; 50:376–380.
24. Berg NO, Eriksson S. Liver disease in adults with alpha$_1$-antitrypsin deficiency. N Engl J Med 1972; 287:1264–1267.
25. Larsson C. Natural history and life expectancy in severe alpha$_1$-antitrypsin deficiency, PiZ. Acta Med Scand 1978; 204:345–351.
26. Cox DW, Smyth S. Risk for liver disease in adults with alpha$_1$-antitrypsin deficiency. Amer J Med 1983; 74:221–227.
27. Triger DR, Millward-Sakler GH, Czaykowski AA, Trowell J, Wright R. Alpha-1-antitrypsin deficiency and liver disease in adults. Quart J Med, New Series 1976; 178: 351–372.
28. Rabinovitz M, Gavaler JS, Kelly RH, Prieto M, Van Thiel DH. Lack of increase in heterozygous $\alpha_1$-antitrypsin deficiency phenotypes among patients with hepatocellular and bile duct carcinoma. Hepatology 1992; 15:407–410.
29. Carlson J, Eriksson S. Chronic cryptogenic liver disease and malignant hepatoma in intermediate alpha$_1$-antitrypsin deficiency identified by a PiZ-specific monoclonal antibody. Scand J Gastroenterol 1985; 20:835–842.
30. Eriksson S, Hägerstrand I. Cirrhosis and malignant hepatoma in $\alpha_1$-antitrypsin deficiency. Acta Med Scand 1974; 195:451–458.
31. Eriksson S. $\alpha_1$-antitrypsin deficiency and liver cirrhosis in adults. Acta Med Scand 1987; 221:461–467.
32. Eriksson SG. Liver disease in $\alpha_1$-antitrypsin deficiency. Scand J Gastroenterol 1985; 20:907–911.
33. Rawlings W, Moss J, Cooper HS, Hamilton SR. Hepatocellular carcinoma and partial deficiency of alpha-1 antitrypsin (MZ). Ann Intern Med 1974; 81:771–773.
34. Rakela J, Goldschmiedt M, Ludwig J. Late manifestation of chronic liver disease in adults with alpha-1-antitrypsin deficiency. Dig Dis Sci 1987; 32:1358–1362.
35. Gherardi GJ. Alpha-1-antitrypsin deficiency and its effect on the liver. Hum Pathol 1971; 2:173–175.
36. Larsson C, Eriksson S. Liver function in asymptomatic adult individuals with severe $\alpha_1$-antitrypsin deficiency (Pi Z). Scand J Gastroenterol 1977; 12:543–546.
37. Sharp HL. The current status of alpha-1-antitrypsin, a protease inhibitor in gastrointestinal disease. Gastroenterology 1976; 70:611–621.
38. Carlson JA, Rogers BB, Sifers RN, Finegold MJ, Clift SM, DeMayo FJ, Bullock DW, Woo SLC. Accumulation of PiZ$\alpha_1$-antitrypsin causes liver damage in transgenic mice. J Clin Invest 1989; 83:1183–1189.
39. Dycaico MJ, Grant SGN, Felts K, Nichols WS, Geller SA, Hager JH, Pollard AJ, Kohler SW, Short HP, Jirik FR, Hanahan D, Sorge JA. Neonatal hepatitis induced by $\alpha_1$-antitrypsin: A transgenic mouse model. Science 1988; 24:1409–1412.
40. Craig JR, Dunn AE, Peters RL. Cirrhosis associated with partial deficiency of alpha-1-antitrypsin: A clinical and autopsy study. Hum Pathol 1975; 6:113–120.

41. Bell H, Schrumpf E, Fagerhol MK. Heterozygous MZ alpha-1-antitrypsin deficiency in adults with chronic liver disease. Scan J Gastroenterol 1990; 25:788–792.
42. Reid CL, Wiener GJ, Cox DW, Richter JE, Geisinger KR. Diffuse hepatocellular dysplasia and carcinoma associated with the Mmalton variant of $\alpha_1$-antitrypsin. Gastroenterology 1987; 93:181–187.
43. Doherty DG, Donaldson PT, Whitehouse DB, Mieli-Vergani G, Duthie A, Hopkinson DA, Mowat AP. HLA phenotypes and gene polymorphisms in juvenile liver disease associated with α-1-antitrypsin deficiency. Hepatology 1990; 12:218–223.
44. Nemeth A, Möller E. HLA in juvenile liver disease with alpha-one-antitrypsin deficiency. Acta Pediatr Scand 1987; 76:603–607.
45. Casavilla A, Gordon R, Van Thiel DH, Starzl TE. Lack of an association between HLA antigens DR3 and alpha-1-antitrypsin deficiency in liver transplant recipients. Submitted.
46. Rabinovitz M, Gavaler JS, Kelly RH, Van Thiel DH. The association between heterozygous $\alpha_1$-antitrypsin deficiency and genetic hemochromatosis. Hepatology 1993; 18:703–708.
47. Wewers MD, Gadek JE, Keogh BA, Fells GA, Crystal RG. Evaluation of danazol therapy for patients with PiZZ alpha-1-antitrypsin deficiency. Am Rev Respir Dis 1986; 134:476–480.
48. Eriksson S. The effect of tamoxifen in intermediate $alpha_1$-antitrypsin deficiency associated with the phenotype PiSZ. Ann Clin Res 1983; 15:95–98.
49. Denmark SW, Shaw BW Jr, Starzl TE, et al. Veno-venous bypass without systemic anticoagulation in canine and human liver transplantation. Surg Forum 1983; 34:380–382.
50. Shaw BW Jr, Martin DJ, Marquez JM, et al. Advantages of venous bypass during orthotopic transplantation of the liver. Semin Liver Dis 1985; 5:344–348.
51. Hood JM, Koep LJ, Peters RL, Schróter, Weil R, Redeker AG, Starzl TE. Liver transplantation for advanced liver disease with alpha-1-antitrypsin deficiency. N Engl J Med 1990; 302:272–275.
52. Esquivel CO, Marino IR, Fioravanti V, Van Thiel DH. Liver transplantation for metabolic disease of the liver. Gastroenterology 1988; 17:167–175.
53. Gartner JC, Zitelli BJ, Malatack JJ, Shaw BW, Iwatsuki S, Starzl TE. Orthotopic liver transplantation in children: Two-year experience with 47 patients. Pediatrics 1984; 74:140–145.
54. Starzl TE. Portacaval shunt in three children with alpha-1-antitrypsin deficiency and cirrhosis: 9 to 12⅓ years later. Hepatology 1990; 11:152–154.
55. Starzl TE, Porter KA, Francavilla A, Iwatsuki S. Reversal of hepatic alpha-1-antitrypsin deposition after portal caval shunt. Lancet 1983; ii:424–426.
56. Starzl TE, Demetris AJ, Murase N, Ildstad S, Ricordi C. Cell migration, chimerism, and graft acceptance. Lancet 1992; 390:617–618.
57. Starzl TE, Demetris AJ, Trucco M, Ricordi C, Isdstad S, Murase N, Kendall RS. Chimerism after liver transplantation in patients with type IV glycogen storage disease. N Engl J Med 1993; 328:745–749.
58. Starzl TE, Bilheimer DW, Bahnson HT, Shaw BW Jr, Hardesty RL, Griffith BP, Iwatsuki S, Zitelli BJ, Gartner JC Jr, Malatack JJ, Urbach AH. Heart-liver transplantation in a patient with familial hypercholesterolaemia. Lancet 1984; i:1382–1383.

59. Bellary SV, Van Thiel DH. Wilson's disease: A diagnosis made in two individuals greater than 40 years of age. J Hepatol. In press.
60. Ferry GD, Whisennand HH, Finegold MJ, Alpert E, Globmicki A. Liver transplantation for cholesteryl ester storage disease. J Ped Gastroenterol Nutr 1991; 12:376–378.
61. Daloze P, Delvin EE, GLorieux JH, et al. Replacement therapy for inherited enzyme deficiency: Liver replacement in Niemann-Pick disease Type A. Am J Med Genet 1977; 1:229–239.
62. Parkman R. The application of bone marrow transplantation to the treatment of genetic diseases. Science 1986; 232:1373–1378.
63. Groth C, Collste H, Dreborg S, Hakansson G, Lundgren G, Svennerholm L. Attempts at enzyme replacement in Gaucher disease by renal transplantation. Acta Paediatr Scand 1979; 68:475–479.
64. Desnick RJ, Simjmons RL, Allen KY, Woods JE, Anderson CF, Najarian JS, Krivit W. Correction of enzymatic deficiencies by renal transplantation: Fabry's disease. Surgery 1972; 72:203–211.
65. Piggott M, Wagaine-Twabwe D, Ramcharan JE, Taylor D. Alpha$_1$-antitrypsin deficiency and liver disease. Br Med J 1981; 283:1262–1263.
66. Chio L, Oon C. Changes in serum alpha$_1$-antitrypsin, alpha$_1$ACII glycoprotein and beta$_2$ glycoprotein I in patients with malignant hepatocellular carcinoma. Cancer 1979; 43:596–604.
67. Vergalla J, Jones EA, Kew MC. Alpha-1-antitrypsin deficiency and hepatocellualr carcinoma. S Afr Med J 1983; 64:950–951.
68. Zwi S, Hurwitz SS, Cohen C, Prinsloo I, Kagan E. Alpha$_1$-antitrypsin deficiency—An association with hepatic malignancy. S Afr Med J 1975; 59:1887–1890.
69. Rubel LR, Ishak KG, Benjamin SB, Knuff TE. $\alpha_1$-antitrypsin deficiency and hepatocellular carcinoma. Arch Pathol Lab Med 1982; 106:678–681.
70. Lindmark B, Millward-Sadler H, Callea F, Eriksson S. Hepatocyte inlcusions of $\alpha_1$-antichymotrypsin in a patient with partial deficiency of $\alpha_1$-antichymotrypsin and chronic liver disease. Histopathology 1990; 16:221–225.
71. Schleissner LA, Cohen AH. Alpha$_1$-antitrypsin deficiency and hepatic carcinoma. Am Rev Resp Disease 1975; 3:863–868.

# 25

# Lung Transplantation for α1AT-Deficiency Emphysema

**ELBERT P. TRULOCK and JOEL D. COOPER**

Washington University School of Medicine
and Barnes Hospital
St. Louis, Missouri

## I. Introduction

Between 1963 and 1973, 36 patients underwent lung transplantation in medical centers throughout the world (1–3). Chronic obstructive pulmonary disease (COPD) was the primary indication for transplantation in nine of these patients, and was a coexistent condition in five or six others. In at least four of these recipients, antitrypsin-deficiency emphysema was the cause of the COPD. Only one recipient with COPD lived longer than 1 month, and there were no long-term survivors among these recipients. Respiratory failure, pneumonia, rejection, and airway complications were the main causes of death, but the moribund condition of some recipients before the operation undoubtedly contributed to the disappointing results.

In this initial series, single-lung transplantation in recipients with obstructive lung disease was complicated by hyperinflation of the native lung with compression of the allograft, and serial ventilation-perfusion lung scans showed increasing perfusion but decreasing ventilation to the allograft in some cases (4). Because of this experience, the notion evolved that a single-lung allograft in parallel with an emphysematous lung was an inherently unworkable combination, and in 1970 Bates (5) speculated about the need for bilateral simultaneous lung transplantation to balance ventilation and perfusion.

For the next decade, there was a hiatus in human lung transplantation, but, with the introduction of cyclosporine to the immunosuppressive regimen, the current era of successful heart–lung and lung transplantation began in the early 1980s (6). Beginning in 1983, the Toronto Lung Transplant Group successfully performed single-lung transplantation in patients with pulmonary fibrosis (7–9). The low static compliance and the high vascular resistance of the remaining fibrotic lung preferentially directed both ventilation and perfusion to the transplanted lung. Posttransplantation lung function was good, and no untoward interaction between the two lungs was encountered.

The earlier problems with single-lung allografts in patients with severe obstructive lung disease continued to influence transplantation strategy, however. Although experiments with single-lung transplantation in canines with papain-induced emphysema had shown that significant ventilation-perfusion mismatching would not occur unless a complication developed in the allograft, only one human single-lung transplant for emphysema had been very successful (10,11). Hence, Patterson et al. (12) adhered to the conventional wisdom and in 1986 devised the en bloc double-lung operation for patients with obstructive lung disease. The early results, including three recipients with antitrypsin-deficiency emphysema, were excellent (12,13).

The double-lung operation was patterned after heart–lung transplantation. With the recipient on cardiopulmonary bypass, the native lungs were extracted and the donor lungs were implanted en bloc through a median sternotomy (12). When the indications for this operation were extended, the cardiac and hemorrhagic complications associated with cardiopulmonary bypass significantly increased the morbidity and mortality of the procedure. To overcome these difficulties, the bilateral sequential technique was developed in 1989 (14). This modification, which subsequently became the standard operation for bilateral transplantation, simplified the surgical approach, eliminated the need for cardiopulmonary bypass in the majority of recipients, and reduced perioperative mortality (15).

While double-lung transplantation was initially considered the appropriate procedure for patients with severe obstructive lung disease, in 1988 Mal et al. (16) successfully performed single-lung transplants in two patients with COPD, one of whom had antitrypsin deficiency emphysema, and other reports soon appeared (17). Over the ensuing years, single-lung transplantation for COPD became the most frequently performed lung-transplant operation (15,18), and several centers have now reported series with excellent results (19–24).

With the evolution and success of both single and bilateral procedures, transplantation has become an option for many patients with advanced emphysema caused by antitrypsin deficiency. Functional results and medium-term survival rates have been good, but chronic allograft rejection—i.e., bronchiolitis obliterans syndrome—has emerged as a major problem for these as well as other recipients. This chapter surveys the status of lung transplantation for antitrypsin-deficiency emphysema, with some comparisons to COPD, and discusses the controversy about antitrypsin-replacement therapy afterward.

## II. Current Activity

Data on lung transplantation have been maintained by two international registries, the Registry of the International Society for Heart and Lung Transplantation (ISHLT) and the St. Louis International Lung Transplant Registry (15,18). Both have shown an exponential rise in activity since the late 1980s (Fig. 1), and COPD and antitrypsin-deficiency emphysema have been among the usual indications (Table 1).

The operations for antitrypsin-deficiency emphysema and COPD are compared in Figure 2. Single-lung transplantation has been the more popular operation in each group, but bilateral lung transplantation has been performed more often for antitrypsin-deficiency emphysema than for COPD (29% vs. 17%, respectively). Perhaps this choice has been influenced by the lower age of the recipients with antitrypsin-deficiency emphysema or by lingering concerns about single-lung transplantation for severe emphysema.

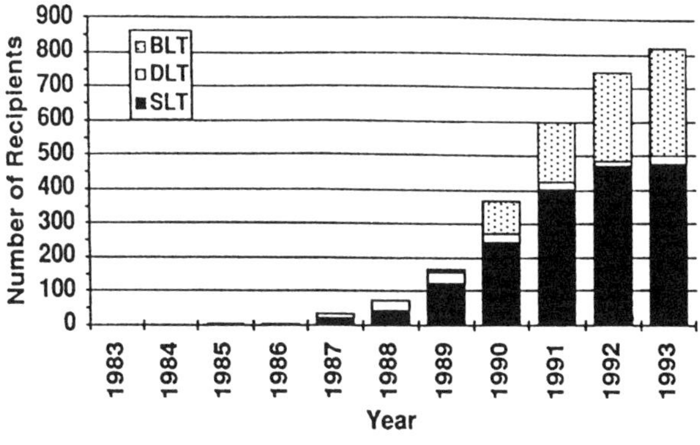


**Figure 1** Annual lung-transplant activity, by type of operation, from the St. Louis International Lung Transplant Registry (September 1994 update). SLT, single-lung transplantation; DLT, double-lung transplantation; BLT, bilateral sequential lung transplantation.

**Table 1** Indications for Lung Transplantation

| Diagnosis | *n* | % |
|---|---|---|
| COPD | 911 | 29 |
| Antitrypsin-deficiency emphysema | 411 | 13 |
| Idiopathic pulmonary fibrosis | 523 | 16.5 |
| Cystic fibrosis | 466 | 15 |
| Primary pulmonary hypertension | 262 | 8 |
| Eisenmenger's syndrome | 81 | 2.5 |
| Retransplantation | 87 | 3 |
| Bronchiectasis | 82 | 2.5 |
| Lymphangiomyomatosis | 49 | 1.5 |
| Sarcoidosis | 46 | 1.5 |
| Others | 242 | 7.5 |

*Source*: From Ref. 18.

## III. Recipient Selection

Patients with a variety of end-stage lung diseases have undergone transplantation. The distribution of indications for transplantation primarily reflects the prevalence and the natural history of the various lung diseases, but it is also influenced by selection criteria for transplantation and other biases. The typical diagnoses have been COPD, antitrypsin-deficiency emphysema, cystic fibrosis, idiopathic pul-

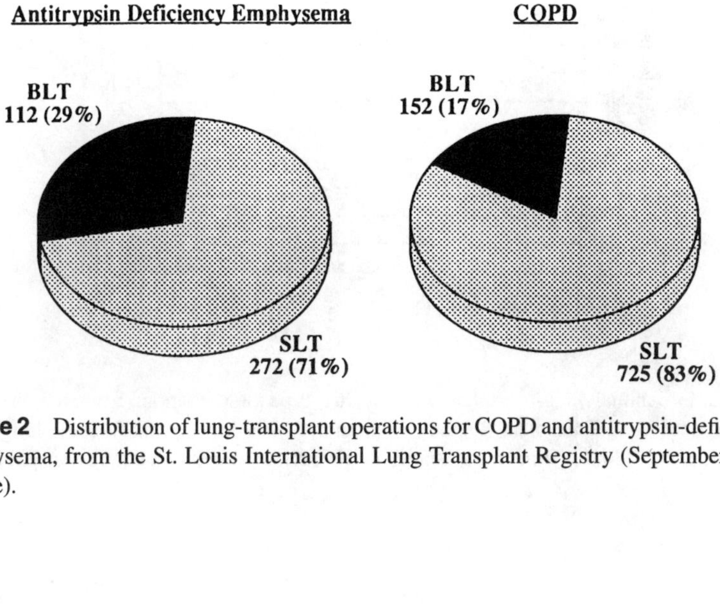


**Figure 2** Distribution of lung-transplant operations for COPD and antitrypsin-deficiency emphysema, from the St. Louis International Lung Transplant Registry (September 1994 update).

monary fibrosis, and primary pulmonary hypertension (Table 1). Less experience has accrued with most other diseases, and transplantation for some of them remains debatable.

Alpha 1–antitrypsin (α1AT) deficiency is associated with premature development of panlobular emphysema and accelerated loss of lung function, especially in cigarette smokers (25,26). Estimates of longevity in patients with antitrypsin-deficiency emphysema have predicted a lifespan shorter than that in the normal population (26). Because most patients with antitrypsin-deficiency emphysema are relatively young and otherwise healthy, they are usually good candidates for lung transplantation. Thus, while antitrypsin-deficiency emphysema is the cause of only a small portion of all COPD, it has been a frequent indication for lung transplantation.

Most lung-transplant programs screen referrals and select candidates according to a predetermined protocol (27–29). Specific recipient-selection criteria vary somewhat among centers and depend on the program's experience and emphasis, but the general principles are similar. Some representative guidelines are outlined in Table 2, and the major contraindications are listed in Table 3. However, many issues—such as age, ventilator dependence, high-dose corticosteroid therapy, previous cardiothoracic surgery, and other medical conditions—must be assessed in the context of the individual case.

Typical age restrictions have been 50–55 years for bilateral lung transplantation and 60–65 years for single-lung transplantation. In the St. Louis International Registry, only 5% of the recipients have been more than 60 years of age, and in 1993 only 2% of the recipients in the United States were older than 65 years (18,30). In an analysis from the transplant center in Toronto, age greater than 50 years was not associated with excess morbidity or mortality, but only a few recipients were older than 60 years (31). In the two international registries and in the Scientific Registry of Transplant Recipients in the United States, the tendency has been toward poorer results in patients older than 60–65 years than in younger adults (15,18,30).

Ventilator dependence has traditionally been regarded as a strong relative, if

**Table 2** Recipient Selection: General Criteria

| |
|---|
| Clinically and physiologically severe disease |
| Medical therapy ineffective or unavailable |
| Limited life expectancy, usually <2 years |
| Ambulatory with rehabilitation potential |
| Acceptable nutritional status, usually 80–120% of ideal body weight |
| Satisfactory psychosocial profile and support system |
| No contraindications |

**Table 3** Recipient Selection: Contraindications

| |
|---|
| Acutely ill or unstable clinical status |
| Uncontrolled or untreatable pulmonary or extrapulmonary infection |
| Uncured neoplasm |
| Significant disease or dysfunction of other vital organs, especially the heart, liver, kidney, and central nervous system |
| Active cigarette smoking |
| Drug or alcohol dependency |
| Unresolvable psychosocial problems or noncompliance with medical management |

not absolute, contraindication to lung transplantation. Indeed, registry data have confirmed that patients who are ventilator-dependent at the time of transplantation have a higher mortality rate after transplantation. In the United States, recipients classified as being "on life support" had survival rates of 61% at 1 month and 37% at 1 year versus 86% and 61%, respectively, in recipients categorized as "in intensive care" (30). Preoperative ventilation (single-lung recipients) and intensive care (bilateral/double-lung recipients) were identified as statistically significant risk factors for postoperative mortality in a multivariate analysis of the ISHLT data (15). Patients who have developed respiratory failure while waiting have had successful operations (32–34), but evaluation of patients with ventilator-dependent respiratory failure cannot be recommended because of the donor shortage and the poor results.

Many advanced lung diseases are treated with corticosteroids, and cytotoxic drugs are used for some of the interstitial diseases. Neither of these therapies is an obstacle to transplantation. In the first few years of lung transplantation, perioperative corticosteroid treatment was avoided because of the historical experience with bronchial dehiscence and the experimental evidence that it diminished bronchial breaking strength (35). However, with current surgical techniques, pretransplantation corticosteroid therapy has not increased the incidence of airway complications, and maintenance prednisone treatment in doses up to 0.2–0.3 mg/kg/day before transplantation is permissible if needed to manage the underlying disease (36,37).

Prior cardiothoracic surgery, pleurodesis, or pleurectomy can increase the technical difficulty of extracting the native lung and thereby the operative risk of lung transplantation. The potential problems created by these procedures are highly variable. Simple pneumothorax that was treated by closed-tube thoracostomy (with or without pleurodesis), open-lung biopsy, or uncomplicated lobectomy is not usually an impediment to transplantation later. More complex cases must be decided individually, but a previous thoracic procedure alone rarely precludes lung transplantation.

A scheme for evaluating candidates is shown in Table 4. The tests focus on quantifying the severity of the lung disease, screening for associated cardiac disease, and assessing the performance status of the patient. Many candidates are at risk for coronary artery disease because of their age and/or other risk factors, including past cigarette smoking. The usefulness of noninvasive provocative tests is usually limited by poor exercise tolerance coupled with a submaximal heart rate, but routine coronary angiography has had a relatively low yield (12%) in asymptomatic candidates whose only risk factor was cigarette smoking (38). However, while angiography cannot be justified by its positivity rate, the value of a negative preoperative study in operative and postoperative decision-making should not be underestimated.

**Table 4** Scheme for Evaluating Potential Recipients

| |
|---|
| Comprehensive medical examination appropriate for age and sex |
| Chest radiograph, electrocardiogram, and routine blood tests |
| Additional studies to assess the status of any nonpulmonary medical conditions |
| Other laboratory tests |
| ABO blood type |
| HLA typing and panel reactive antibodies (PRA) |
| Serological tests for hepatitis A, B and C; HIV; EBV; and CMV |
| Pulmonary studies |
| Standard PFTs and ABG |
| Quantitative ventilation-perfusion scintigraphy |
| Sputum culture[a] |
| Computed tomography[a] |
| Cardiopulmonary exercise test[a] |
| Cardiovascular studies |
| Radionuclide ventriculography or transthoracic echocardiography (with saline contrast[a]) |
| Right-heart catheterization |
| Transesophageal echocardiography[a] |
| Left-heart catheterization with coronary angiography[a] |
| Rehabilitation and physical therapy assessment |
| Six-minute walk test |
| Psychosocial evaluation |
| Nutritional assessment |

[a]As clinically indicated in selected patients.

## IV. Timing of Transplantation

When should transplantation be undertaken? This question cannot be answered precisely. Recent clinical events, trends in physiological parameters, overall functional status, and quality of life must be integrated into the decision. Enhancing quality of life is an important motivation for many patients who are referred for transplantation; however, prognosis should be the main determinant in timing the procedure. Actuarial survival after transplantation is shown in Figure 3, and these results must be weighed against the prognosis of the underlying disease without transplantation. Transplantation would be appropriate when other therapeutic options have been exhausted and when life expectancy would be improved by intervention.

Both the number of patients awaiting transplantation and the average waiting time before transplantation have been increasing. For example, in the United States the median waiting time to transplantation for lung recipients listed in 1992 was 410 days. Donor lungs must be matched for blood type and body size, within tolerance. Thereafter, according to current U.S. policy, they are distributed to

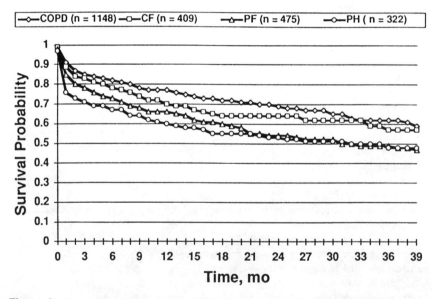

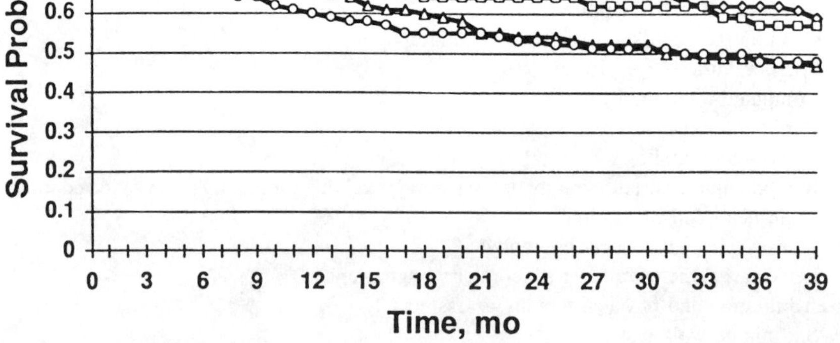


**Figure 3** Actuarial survival after lung transplantation, by diagnosis, from the St. Louis International Lung Transplant Registry (April 1994 update). COPD, chronic obstructive pulmonary disease (including antitrypsin-deficiency emphysema); CF, cystic fibrosis; PF, pulmonary fibrosis; PH, pulmonary hypertension (primary or Eisenmenger's syndrome).

recipients in order of their time on the waiting list. There is no priority for severity of illness or clinical status. Hence, an inevitable delay must be incorporated into the referral, evaluation, listing, and transplantation strategy.

COPD has been the fifth leading cause of death in the United States since the late 1970s, but antitrypsin deficiency has been estimated to be the cause of only about 2% of all cases of emphysema. In epidemiological studies of patients with COPD, age and baseline postbronchodilator $FEV_1$ have been identified as the most reliable prognostic indices (39), but other relevant factors include nutritional status and pulmonary hypertension. Nonhypoxemic patients less than 60 years of age with a postbronchodilator $FEV_1$ less than 30% of the predicted normal value had a 2-year actuarial survival rate above 70% and a 3-year survival rate of approximately 60% in both the Intermittent Positive Pressure Breathing Trial and the Nocturnal Oxygen Therapy Trial (39). These rates are comparable to the outcome after lung transplantation (Fig. 3).

The survival rate of patients with antitrypsin deficiency has been substantially less than that in the overall population in several studies. In a cohort of patients with symptomatic antitrypsin-deficiency emphysema followed at the National Institutes of Health, the probabilities of survival to 50 and 60 years of age were 52% and 16%, respectively. These are in sharp contrast to survival rates of 92% and 85%, respectively, at the same ages for the overall U.S. population (26). Unlike COPD, prognostic indices relating lung function to outcome have not been clearly delineated for antitrypsin-deficiency emphysema, probably because of the relatively small number of patients in most studies. However, extrapolation from the data for COPD is not unreasonable.

On the basis of this analysis and clinical experience, criteria have been derived for timing the initial referral of patients with COPD or antitrypsin deficiency for lung transplantation (Table 5). By comparison with the physiological profile of actual recipients (Table 6), transplantation will be premature for some patients who fulfill these criteria. Nonetheless, the goal is to anticipate the inherent delay and to avoid missing the window of opportunity.

**Table 5** Criteria for Timing the Referral

| |
|---|
| Postbronchodilator $FEV_1$ $<30\%$ of predicted normal |
| Chronic hypercapnia |
| Moderate to severe secondary pulmonary hypertension |
| Clinical course |
| Rapidly declining lung function |
| Recurrent life-threatening exacerbations |

**Table 6** Lung Function Before and After Transplantation in Recipients with COPD or Antitrypsin-Deficiency Emphysema (AT Def.)

| | Single-lung transplantation | | | | Bilateral lung transplantation | | | |
|---|---|---|---|---|---|---|---|---|
| | COPD | | AT Def. | | COPD | | AT Def. | |
| Time | *n* | $FEV_1$, L (%) | *n* | $FEV_1$, L (%) | *n* | $FEV_1$, L (%) | *n* | $FEV_1$, L (%) |
| Pretransplant | 38 | 0.48 ± 0.13 (18 ± 4) | 8 | 0.56 ± 0.14 (19 ± 5) | 24 | 0.49 ± 0.13 (16 ± 5) | 27 | 0.60 ± 0.14 (17 ± 5) |
| Posttransplant | | | | | | | | |
| 3 mo | 33 | 1.52 ± 0.52 (56 ± 140) | 7 | 1.52 ± 0.19 (53 ± 12) | 21 | 2.69 ± 0.85 (83 ± 15) | 23 | 3.07 ± 0.92 (97 ± 36) |
| 6 mo | 34 | 1.59 ± 0.46 (58 ± 12) | 6 | 1.63 ± 0.39 (56 ± 8) | 21 | 2.92 ± 0.74 (91 ± 12) | 25 | 3.33 ± 0.78 (94 ± 17) |
| 1 yr | 31 | 1.48 ± 0.37 (55 ± 11) | 6 | 1.52 ± 0.40 (52 ± 6) | 15 | 2.85 ± 0.66 (93 ± 14) | 20 | 3.37 ± 1.10 (95 ± 26) |
| 2 yr | 25 | 1.37 ± 0.35 (49 ± 14) | 5 | 1.33 ± 0.32 (45 ± 10) | 8 | 2.85 ± 0.79 (93 ± 15) | 14 | 2.92 ± 0.83 (87 ± 28) |
| 3 yr | 13 | 1.22 ± 0.37 (49 ± 20) | 3 | 1.12 ± 0.14 (45 ± 8) | 4 | 2.01 ± 0.35 (75 ± 24) | 9 | 2.55 ± 0.81 (76 ± 33) |

Data are presented as mean ± SD. Values in parentheses are percent of predicted normal.

## V. Choice of Procedure

Both single- and bilateral lung transplantation have been performed for COPD and antitrypsin-deficiency emphysema (13,16,17,19–24,40). Standard pulmonary-function-test results have, not surprisingly, been better after bilateral lung transplantation, but the difference in exercise capacity has been less dramatic (40–42). There was no significant difference in actuarial survival at 1, 2, and 3 years after transplantation between single- and bilateral lung recipients with COPD, including antitrypsin-deficiency emphysema, in the St. Louis International Lung Transplant Registry (18). However, single-lung transplant recipients with "emphysema" had somewhat better survival during the first year than bilateral recipients in the ISHLT Registry (15).

Single-lung transplantation is a simpler, shorter operation, and it has a lower perioperative complication rate than bilateral transplantation (21). Obviously, utilization of single-lung transplantation could potentially extend the limited supply of donor organs to more recipients. Thus, it offers distinct advantages for older or higher-risk patients, patients with a previous thoracic procedure in one hemithorax, and patients with a significant asymmetry in the distribution of bullae or in the functional contribution between the two lungs. When there has been no significant disparity between the two native lungs, graft position—right versus left—has not significantly affected posttransplantation lung function (43).

Single-lung transplantation has two shortcomings, however. As originally described, a single-lung allograft in parallel with an emphysematous lung has a propensity to hyperinflation of the native lung and ventilation-perfusion imbalance between the native lung and the allograft if complications develop in the allograft that decrease its compliance or increase its airway resistance (4,11). While such situations still arise, they are usually manageable and resolve when the primary problem in the allograft has been adequately treated. Perhaps what is more important, single-lung transplantation provides less reserve lung function as a buffer for any future decrements related to infection or rejection. With less margin, recipients who develop chronic rejection may become symptomatic and functionally impaired with relatively little loss of function.

Bilateral lung transplantation restores lung function into the normal range, but it is a longer operation with a higher perioperative complication rate (21). It may be preferable for younger recipients, patients with extensive bullae in both lungs, and patients with a bronchitic or bronchiectatic component to their emphysema. Additionally, it offers greater latitude for donor–recipient size-matching than single-lung transplantation.

In the end, the "best" transplant procedure is usually the one that can be done when the patient needs it. If the patient is a candidate for either operation, single- and bilateral lung transplantations are complementary because they widen the size spectrum of the donor lung(s) that can be used for the recipient.

In the last few years, interest in surgical therapy for emphysema—without giant bullae or compressed lung—has been rejuvenated. Currently, the operations range from laser ablation of bullous areas through a thoracoscopic approach to selective surgical resection of severely emphysematous regions through a median sternotomy or staged sequential lateral thoracotomies. Thus far, most candidates for these operations have had COPD unrelated to antitrypsin deficiency, and the majority have had lung function above the range for transplantation or have had some contraindication to transplantation. Therefore, the role of these operations in the management of patients with antitrypsin-deficiency emphysema is still uncertain, and no specific recommendations can be made at this time.

## VI. Results

The outcome of lung transplantation can be gauged by actuarial survival, lung function and exercise performance, and quality of life. Quality of life has not been extensively studied, and this section focuses on survival statistics and physiological results.

Actuarial survival has been better for recipients with COPD or antitrypsin-deficiency emphysema than for recipients with other diagnoses (Fig. 3). The differences in survival appear relatively early and probably reflect the greater complexity of transplantation for the other diseases.

The Registry of the International Society for Heart and Lung Transplantation has reported somewhat better actuarial survival for recipients with COPD than for those with antitrypsin-deficiency emphysema (15), but there has been little difference between these two groups in the St. Louis International Lung Transplant Registry (Fig. 4). In the recipients with antitrypsin-deficiency emphysema, bilateral lung transplantation currently appears to offer a slight advantage in medium-term survival rates (Fig. 5).

Our center has experience with more than 100 recipients with COPD or antitrypsin-deficiency emphysema, and no differences in outcome have been discerned between these two groups. Actuarial survival at Barnes Hospital through 1994 is illustrated in Figure 6. During the first 5 years after transplantation, there has been no consistent difference in the survival rates between recipients with COPD and those with antitrypsin-deficiency emphysema. Furthermore, the incidence of acute rejection, cytomegalovirus pneumonia, and chronic rejection has been comparable in the two groups.

A physiological profile of recipients with COPD or antitrypsin-deficiency emphysema is presented in Table 6. Before transplantation, spirometry showed severe airflow limitation in all patients, with the mean values of $FEV_1$ ranging from 16% to 19% of the predicted norm; no significant differences were detected among the subgroups. After transplantation, lung function improved significantly

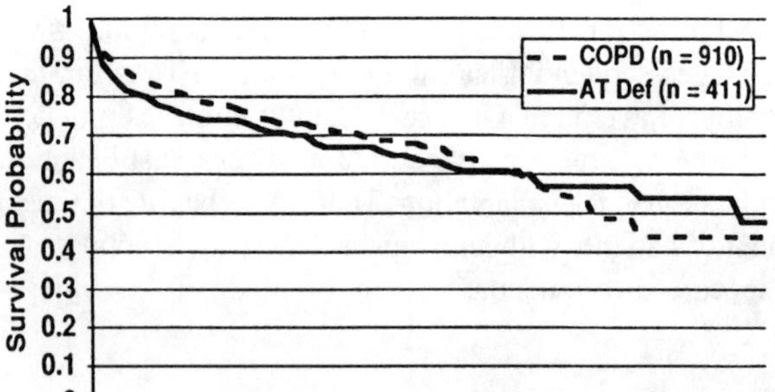


**Figure 4** Actuarial survival after lung transplantation for COPD and antitrypsin-deficiency emphysema (AT Def), from the St. Louis International Lung Transplant Registry (August 1994).

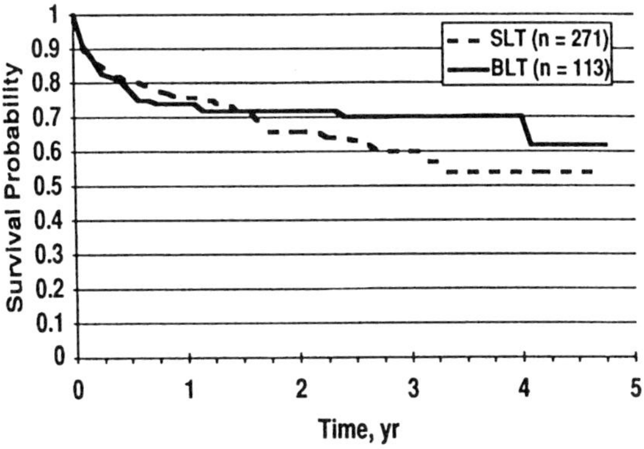


**Figure 5** Actuarial survival for single- versus bilateral lung transplantation for antitrypsin-deficiency emphysema, from the St. Louis International Lung Transplant Registry (August 1994).

in each subgroup. Regardless of the diagnosis, the $FEV_1$ of the bilateral transplant recipients was, not unexpectedly, higher than that of the single-lung recipients. However, for each operation there was no significant difference at any time between the recipients with COPD and those with antitrypsin-deficiency emphysema. There was a gradual downward trend in lung function at 2 to 3 years after transplantation. This was caused by the development of chronic rejection in some of the recipients. If recipients with this complication were excluded, lung function remained stable over time.

Other comparisons of performance have included cardiopulmonary exercise

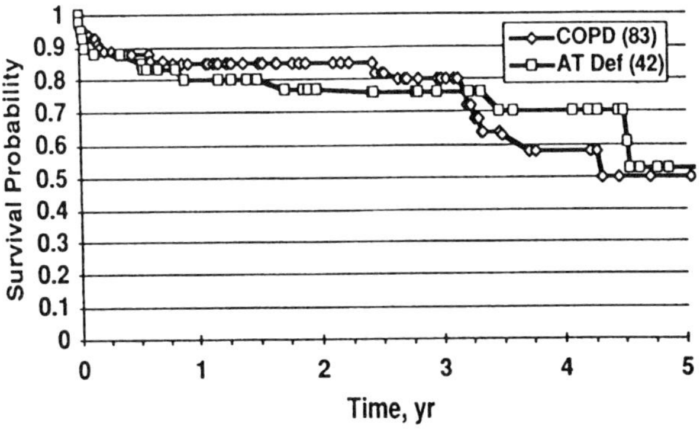


**Figure 6** Actuarial survival for recipients with COPD and antitrypsin-deficiency emphysema (AT Def) at Barnes Hospital, 1988–1994.

testing and 6-minute walking distance. These tests have shown a longer 6-minute walking distance and a higher maximum oxygen uptake in bilateral recipients, but no difference between recipients with COPD and those with antitrypsin-deficiency emphysema.

In summary, lung function and exercise tolerance are improved significantly by either single- or bilateral lung transplantation in patients with antitrypsin-deficiency emphysema. In results from our center, no substantial differences in lung function or medium-term outcome have been apparent between recipients with antitrypsin-deficiency emphysema and those with COPD.

## VII. Antitrypsin-Replacement Therapy After Transplantation

The safety and biochemical efficacy of α1AT-replacement therapy have been demonstrated (44,45). The impact of replacement therapy on the subsequent clinical or physiological course remains uncertain, but guidelines for selecting and treating patients with antitrypsin-deficiency emphysema have been promulgated (46). While a modest number of patients with antitrypsin deficiency have undergone transplantation, there is no widely accepted policy or practice regarding replacement therapy afterward.

Persuasive arguments can be offered for and against augmentation therapy for recipients with antitrypsin deficiency. Lower-respiratory-tract defenses are breached at many levels after lung transplantation, and rejection and infection are the two most common complications. In this setting the consequences of inflammatory insults could be amplified, and replacement therapy after transplantation would be a logical extension of the proteinase–antiproteinase hypothesis. However, α1AT-replacement therapy is inconvenient and expensive, and its importance in this situation is unknown. Moreover, emphysema develops very slowly in nonsmoking, antitrypsin-deficient patients, and recurrent emphysema caused by antitrypsin deficiency is unlikely to be a limiting factor in the life expectancy of a lung-transplant recipient.

The proteinase–antiproteinase balance in the bronchoalveolar lavage (BAL) fluid of antitrypsin-deficient lung- and heart–lung-transplant recipients and nondeficient, control recipients has been investigated during periods of clinical stability and during lower-respiratory-tract illnesses in only one study (47). During periods of clinical stability, neither the antitrypsin-deficient recipients nor the controls had detectable free elastase activity in their BAL fluid. During respiratory illnesses, which included acute lung injury and pneumonia in both groups and one episode of rejection in the antitrypsin-deficient group, three of seven antitrypsin-deficient recipients and one of four controls had measurable free elastase activity. On the basis of these results, King and her colleagues (47) concluded that α1AT supplementation "during respiratory tract inflammation may be indicated to inhibit elastase-mediated injury to the transplanted lung."

In our opinion, such an approach cannot be endorsed yet. The proteinase–antiproteinase balance is occasionally overwhelmed in nondeficient patients, and supplementation of antitrypsin-deficient recipients may not be effective during some insults. Furthermore, many of these episodes are relatively short-lived when other definitive therapy is administered.

The subset of recipients with chronic allograft rejection merits special mention, however. This complication has afflicted approximately 35% of recipients at most centers regardless of their underlying disease, and the response to treatment with augmented immunosuppression has been disappointing. It is characterized by chronic lower-respiratory-tract inflammation (bronchiolitis) and ultimately fibrosis (bronchiolitis obliterans), and the BAL cell profile in these recipients is characterized by an increased proportion of neutrophils. The proteinase–antiproteinase balance has not been studied in this situation, but α1AT supplementation might be rational for antitrypsin-deficient lung-transplant recipients with chronic rejection.

## VIII. Summary

Lung transplantation is an option for appropriately selected patients with end-stage emphysema caused by antitrypsin deficiency. The functional results have been excellent after single- or bilateral lung transplantation, and the medium-term survival results have been encouraging. However, the role of antitrypsin-replacement therapy after lung transplantation remains uncertain, and further study is needed.

## References

1. Wildevuur CRH, Benfield JR. A review of 23 human lung transplantations by 20 surgeons. Ann Thorac Surg 1970; 9:489–515.
2. Veith FJ, Koerner SK. Problems in the management of human lung transplant patients. Vasc Surg 1974; 8:273–282.
3. Veith FJ, Koerner SK. The present status of lung transplantation. Arch Surg 1974; 109:734–740.
4. Stevens PM, Johnson PC, Bell RL, Beall AC, Jenkins DE. Regional ventilation and perfusion after lung transplantation in patients with emphysema. N Engl J Med 1970; 282:245–249.
5. Bates DV. The other lung. N Engl J Med 1970; 282:277–279.
6. Veith FJ, Kamholz SL, Mollenkopf FP, Montefusco CM. Lung transplantation 1983. Transplantation 1983; 35:271–278.
7. Toronto Lung Transplant Group. Unilateral lung transplantation for pulmonary fibrosis. N Engl J Med 1986; 314:1140–1145.

8. Toronto Lung Transplant Group. Experience with single-lung transplantation for pulmonary fibrosis. JAMA 1988; 259:2258–2262.
9. Grossman RF, Frost A, Zamel N, Patterson GA, Cooper JD, Myron PR, et al. Results of single-lung transplantation for bilateral pulmonary fibrosis. N Engl J Med 1990; 322:727–733.
10. Veith FJ, Koerner SK, Attai LA, Bardfeld P, Boley SJ, Bloomberg A, et al. Single-lung transplantation in emphysema. Lancet 1972; i:1138–1139.
11. Veith FJ, Koerner SK, Siegelman SS, Torres M, Bardfeld PA, Attai LA, et al. Single lung transplantation in experimental and human emphysema. Ann Surg 1973; 178: 463–476.
12. Patterson GA, Cooper JD, Goldman B, Weisel RD, Pearson FG, Waters PF, et al. Technique of successful clinical double-lung transplantation. Ann Thorac Surg 1988; 45:626–633.
13. Cooper JD, Patterson GA, Grossman R, Maurer J, Toronto Lung Transplant Group. Double-lung transplant for advanced chronic obstructive lung disease. Am Rev Respir Dis 1989; 139:303–307.
14. Pasque MK, Cooper JD, Kaiser LR, Haydock DA, Triantafillou A, Trulock EP. Improved technique for bilateral lung transplantation: rationale and initial clinical experience. Ann Thorac Surg 1990; 49:785–791.
15. Hosenpud JD, Novick RJ, Breen TJ, Daily OP. The registry of the International Society for Heart and Lung Transplantation: eleventh official report—1994. J Heart Lung Transplant 1994; 13:561–570.
16. Mal H, Andreassian B, Pamela F, Duchatelle J-P, Rondeau E, Dubois F, et al. Unilateral lung transplantation in end-stage pulmonary emphysema. Am Rev Respir Dis 1989; 140:797–802.
17. Trulock EP, Egan TM, Kouchoukos NT, Kaiser LR, Pasque MK, Ettinger N, et al. Single lung transplantation for severe chronic obstructive pulmonary disease. Chest 1989; 96:738–742.
18. Report of the St. Louis International Lung Transplant Registry. September 1994.
19. Kaiser LR, Cooper JD, Trulock EP, Pasque MK, Triantafillou A, Haydock D, et al. The evolution of single lung transplantation for emphysema. J Thorac Cardiovasc Surg 1991; 102:333–341.
20. Marinelli WA, Hertz MI, Shumway SJ, Fox JMK, Henke CA, Harmon KR, et al. Single lung transplantation for severe emphysema. J Heart Lung Transplant 1992; 11:577–583.
21. Low DE, Trulock EP, Kaiser LR, Pasque MK, Dresler C, Ettinger N, et al. Morbidity, mortality, and early results of single versus bilateral lung transplantation for emphysema. J Thorac Cardiovasc Surg 1992; 103:1119–1126.
22. Mal H, Sleiman C, Jebrak G, Messian O, Dubois F, Darne C, et al. Functional results of single-lung transplantation for chronic obstructive lung disease. Am J Respir Crit Care Med 1994; 149:1476–1481.
23. Levine SM, Anzueto A, Peters JI, Cronin T, Sako EY, Jenkinson SG, et al. Medium term functional results of single-lung transplantation for endstage obstructive lung disease. Am J Respir Crit Care Med 1994; 150:398–402.
24. Brunsting LA, Lupinetti FM, Cascade PN, Becker FS, Daly BD, Martinez FJ, et al.

Pulmonary function in single lung transplantation for chronic obstructive pulmonary disease. J Thorac Cardiovasc Surg 1994; 107:1337–1345.
25. Pierce JA. Antitrypsin and emphysema: perspective and prospects. JAMA 1988; 259: 2890–2895.
26. Brantly ML, Paul LD, Miller BH, Falk RT, Wu M, Crystal RG. Clinical features and history of the destructive lung disease associated with alpha-1-antitrypsin deficiency of adults with pulmonary symptoms. Am Rev Respir Dis 1988; 138:327–336.
27. Marshall SE, Kramer MR, Lewiston NJ, Starnes VA, Theodore J. Selection and evaluation of recipients for heart-lung and lung transplantation. Chest 1990; 98:1488–1494.
28. Morrison DL, Maurer JR, Grossman RF. Preoperative assessment for lung transplantation. Clin Chest Med 1990; 11:207–215.
29. Trulock EP. Recipient selection. Chest Surg Clin NA 1993; 3:1–18.
30. 1994 Annual Report of the U. S. Scientific Registry for Transplant Recipients and the Organ Procurement and Transplantation Network—Transplant Data: 1988–1993. UNOS, Richmond, VA, and the Division of Organ Transplantation, Bureau of Health Resources Development, Health Resources and Services Administration, U.S. Department of Health and Human Services, Bethesda, MD.
31. Snell GI, De Hoyos A, Winton T, Maurer JR. Lung transplantation in patients over the age of 50. Transplantation 1993; 55:562–566.
32. Low DE, Trulock EP, Kaiser LR, Pasque MK, Ettinger NA, Dresler C, et al. Lung transplantation of ventilator-dependent patients. Chest 1992; 101:8–11.
33. Massard G, Shennib H, Metras D, Camboulives J, Viard L, Mulder DS, et al. Double-lung transplantation in mechanically ventilated patients with cystic fibrosis. Ann Thorac Surg 1993; 55:1087–1092.
34. Flume PA, Egan TM, Westerman JH, Paradowski LJ, Yankaskas JR, Detterbeck FC, et al. Lung transplantation for mechanically ventilated patients. J Heart Lung Transplant 1994; 13:15–21.
35. Lima O, Cooper JD, Peters WJ, Ayabe H, Townsend E, Luk SC, et al. Effects of methylprednisolone and azathioprine on bronchial healing following lung autotransplantation. J Thorac Cardiovasc Surg 1981; 82:211–215.
36. Calhoon JH, Grover FL, Gibbons WJ, Bryan CL, Levine SM, Bailey SR, et al. Single lung transplantation: alternative indications and technique. J Thorac Cardiovasc Surg 1991; 101:816–825.
37. Schäfers H-J, Wagner TOF, Demertzis S, Hamm M, Wahlers T, Cremer J, et al. Preoperative corticosteroids: a contraindication to lung transplantation? Chest 1992; 102:1522–1525.
38. Liebowitz DW, Caputo AL, Shapiro GC, Schulman LL, McGregor CC, Di Tullio MR, et al. Coronary angiography in smokers undergoing evaluation for lung transplantation: Is routine use justified? J Heart Lung Transplant 1994; 13:701–703.
39. Anthonisen NR. Prognosis in chronic obstructive pulmonary disease: results from multicenter trials. Am Rev Respir Dis 1989; 140(suppl):S95–S99.
40. Patterson GA, Maurer JR, Williams TJ, Cardoso PG, Scavuzzo M, Todd TR, et al. Comparison of outcomes of double and single lung transplantation for obstructive lung disease. J Thorac Cardiovasc Surg 1991; 101:623–632.

41. Levy RD, Ernst P, Levine SM, Shennib H, Anzueto A, Bryan CL, et al. Exercise performance after lung transplantation. J Heart Lung Transplant 1993; 12:27–33.
42. Howard DA, Iademarco E, Trulock EP. The role of cardiopulmonary exercise testing in lung and heart-lung transplantation. Clin Chest Med 1994; 15:405–420.
43. Levine SM, Anzueto AR, Gibbons WJ, Calhoon JH, Jenkinson SG, Trinkle JK, et al. Graft position and pulmonary function after single lung transplantation for obstructive lung disease. Chest 1993; 103:444–448.
44. Wewers MD, Casolaro MA, Sellers SE, Swayze SC, McPhaul KM, Wittes JT, et al. Replacement therapy for alpha 1-antitrypsin deficiency associated with emphysema. N Engl J Med 1987; 316:1055–1062.
45. Hubbard A, Sellers S, Czerski D, Stephens L, Crystal RG. Biochemical efficacy and safety of monthly augmentation therapy for alpha-1-antitrypsin deficiency. JAMA 1988; 260:1259–1264.
46. Buist AS, Burrows B, Cohen A, Crystal RG, Fallat RJ, Gadek JE, et al. Guidelines for the approach to the patient with severe hereditary alpha-1-antitrypsin deficiency. Am Rev Respir Dis 1989; 140:1494–1497.
47. King MB, Campbell EJ, Gray BH, Hertz MI. The proteinase-antiproteinase balance in alpha-1-proteinase inhibitor-deficient lung transplant recipients. Am J Respir Crit Care Med 1994; 149:966–971.

# AUTHOR INDEX

*Italic numbers give the page on which the complete reference is listed.*

## A

## C

## D

## F

## G

## I



## J

## L

## O

## P

## Q



## R

## S

# T

## U



## V

# SUBJECT INDEX

## B



## C

## D



## E

## N



## O



## P

## R



## S